Medical Therapy of Acute Stroke

Neurological Disease and Therapy

Series Editor
William C. Koller
Department of Neurology
University of Kansas Medical Center
Kansas City, Kansas

Volume 1 Handbook of Parkinson's Disease
Edited by William C. Koller

Volume 2 Medical Therapy of Acute Stroke
Edited by Mark Fisher

Medical Therapy of Acute Stroke

edited by

MARK FISHER

University of Southern California
School of Medicine
Los Angeles, California

MARCEL DEKKER, INC. New York and Basel

Library of Congress Cataloging-in-Publication Data

Medical therapy of acute stroke.

(Neurological disease and therapy ; v. 2)
Includes index.
1. Cerebrovascular disease--Treatment. I. Fisher, Mark. II. Series. [DNLM: 1. Acute Disease. 2. Cerebrovascular Disorders--therapy. WL 355 M489]
RC388.5.M44 1989 616.8'1 88-33507
ISBN 0-8247-7870-7 (alk. paper)

This book is printed on acid-free paper.

MARCEL DEKKER, INC.
270 Madison Avenue, New York, New York 10016

Current printing (last digit):
10 9 8 7 6 5 4 3 2 1

PRINTED IN THE UNITED STATES OF AMERICA

Series Introduction

Neurology has been called the last frontier of medical science. Indeed, our knowledge of the functioning of the nervous system in health and disease has increased at a rapid rate. In the past, neurologists were mainly concerned with the diagnosis of disease. Currently, however, therapeutics is a major aspect of the practice of neurology, with established and investigational therapeutics for all the major neurological diseases. Our knowledge of the pathophysiology of disease states and modes of possible therapeutic intervention now makes it possible to devote a series of books to individual neurological disorders.

The first book of this series was concerned with the diagnosis and treatment of Parkinson's disease. Acute cerebrovascular disease is the subject of this volume. Dr. Fisher and his colleagues bring us up to date on promising developments in medical treatment of acute stroke. This book is essential reading for clinicians in neurological specialties.

William C. Koller, M.D., Ph.D.

Foreword

Stroke is the generic term that we use for clinical syndromes, the pathological substrates for which are cerebral infarction, intracerebral hemorrhage, or subarachnoid hemorrhage. In the early part of this century, the common clinical term for stroke was apoplexy, from the Greek term meaning "to strike down." Apoplexy was the usual term used on death certificates for stroke of any type but undoubtedly was used for many other conditions that caused sudden, unexpected death. In 1900, for example, the stroke mortality rate reported in the United States was three times that reported in 1976. Thus, mortality statistics for stroke have not given us accurate chronological trends and have provided no reliable data on types of stroke.

The introduction of computerized tomography has enabled us to distinguish reliably among the different types of stroke. This major step in technology has allowed us to initiate therapy for acute stroke on a more rational and systematic basis.

Most of the attention to medical therapy has been directed to cerebral infarction, which may result from a number of different primary pathological processes, including arteriolar disease related to hypertension, atherothrombotic disease in the cervical or cerebral arteries, and cardiogenic emboli. It is frequently difficult, and sometimes impossible, to determine the intravascular pathological substrate for cerebral infarction. Sometimes none of these pathological conditions is apparent. In other patients, all of these conditions may be present as potential explanations. It is the clinician's challenge to diagnose and correct conditions that put the patient at an increased risk of stroke.

Although many modalities for medical therapy are discussed throughout this volume, the primary clinical management for acute stroke is still supportive care to prevent such problems as pneumonia, pulmonary emboli, and cardiac complications. We are now approaching the time when rapid aggressive treatment of patients with acute cerebral infarction may result in better preservation of brain tissue and thus less neurological impairment. Mark Fisher and his collaborators have provided a clear presentation of the state of our knowledge of the process of cerebral ischemia and have presented a critical assessment of the various medical treatments that have been proposed, some of which have been well tested. Recent development of agents that lyse intra-arterial thrombi and other agents that promise neuronal protection provide hope that the future will bring opportunities to modify the effects of acute brain ischemia.

Jack P. Whisnant, M.D.
Chairman, Department of Health Sciences Research
Roy E. and Merle Meyer Professor of Neuroscience
Mayo Clinic and Mayo Medical School
Rochester, Minnesota

Preface

This book is representative of a new trend in cerebral vascular disease. Stroke patients, particularly those with ischemic stroke, have often been something less than first-class citizens in the hospital. Indeed, in what other illness are patients so frequently labeled "victims"? In what other disease of acute onset has therapeutic nihilism been so widespread? Perhaps the "victimization" of stroke patients, has, for some, provided something of an intellectual justification for a passive therapeutic approach.

Happily, this attitude is changing, and changing quickly. The great advances in treatment of myocardial infarction have undoubtedly contributed to a different orientation by physicians toward stroke patients; many treatment modalities described in this book originated with cardiologists. Among neurologists, the recent advances in neuroimaging have led to an increasing emphasis on therapy of neurological illnesses; no other neurological disorder has more possibilities for a variety of interventions than does stroke.

This book has been designed to be both a sourcebook of information on stroke therapy as well as a guidebook for stroke treatment. The first two chapters provide some clinical and basic science background on stroke. Chapters 3 through 12 review various stroke treatment strategies. The final three chapters provide specific recommendations for current therapy.

I would like to take this opportunity to name certain individuals who particularly influenced the development of this editor: W. O. Farber, Josephine Moore, Ram Singh, John Marshall, W. W. Tourtellotte, Adam Wechsler, Mark Goldberg, and Leslie Weiner. I wish to offer many, many thanks to my colleagues who wrote chapters, making this book possible. And to the reader, I extend this invitation to consider therapies in acute stroke.

Mark Fisher

Contents

Contributors

Harold P. Adams, Jr., M.D. University of Iowa, Iowa City, Iowa

Thomas Brott, M.D. University of Cincinnati College of Medicine, Cincinnati, Ohio

Bruce M. Coull, M.D. The Oregon Health Sciences University School of Medicine, Portland, Oregon

J. Donald Easton, M.D. Brown University–Rhode Island Hospital, Providence, Rhode Island

*Robert J. Fallis, M.D.** Brigham and Women's Hospital, Harvard Medical School, Boston, Massachusetts

Mark Fisher, M.D. University of Southern California School of Medicine, Los Angeles, California

Robert B. Francis, Jr., M.D. University of Southern California School of Medicine and Coagulation Laboratory, University of Southern California Medical Center, Los Angeles, California

Steven L. Giannotta, M.D. University of Southern California School of Medicine, Los Angeles, California

G. B. Hieshima, M.D. University of California, San Francisco, California

R. T. Higashida, M.D. University of California, San Francisco, California

Edward L. Hogan, M.D. Medical University of South Carolina, Charleston, South Carolina

Chung Y. Hsu, M.D., Ph.D. Medical University of South Carolina, Charleston, South Carolina

E. Paul MacCarthy, M.D. University of Cincinnati College of Medicine, Cincinnati, Ohio

John Marshall, M.D. The National Hospital, London, England

**Present affiliation*: Neuroimmunology Branch, National Institutes of Health, Bethesda, Maryland

Herbert J. Meiselman, Sc.D. University of Southern California School of Medicine, Los Angeles, California

L. Mela-Riker, M.D. The Oregon Health Sciences University School of Medicine, Portland, Oregon

John H. Neal, M.D. University of Southern California School of Medicine, Los Angeles, California

William Pearce, Ph.D. Loma Linda University School of Medicine, Loma Linda, California

Richard A. Shubin, M.D. University of Southern California School of Medicine, Los Angeles, California

Y. Tan, M.D. Shanghai Medical University, Shanghai, China

F. Y. Tsai, M.D. University of Missouri School of Medicine, Kansas City, Missouri

Frank M. Yatsu, M.D. University of Texas Medical School at Houston, Houston, Texas

Medical Therapy of Acute Stroke

1

Clinical Aspects of Stroke

John Marshall
The National Hospital, London, England

I. INTRODUCTION

Ischemia exists when the blood supply is insufficient to meet the metabolic needs of a tissue. The metabolic needs of the brain are high; despite contributing only about 2% to body weight, it takes about 20% of cardiac output. A fall in the blood supply can therefore have disastrous effects on cerebral function.

Our understanding of cerebral ischemia has greatly advanced in recent years. Previously it was considered very much as an "all-or-none" phenomenon. The teaching, much influenced by dramatic events such as a cardiac arrest during surgery, was that deprivation of oxygen for a period of 3 minutes resulted in the death of neurons. Experimental work has modified this picture by introducing the concept of ischemic thresholds (1). These are levels of cerebral blood flow (CBF) below which first the electrical activity of neurons and then the energy-providing mechanisms fail. These changes can, however, be reversed. The final stage is marked by efflux of potassium from the cells, at which point irreversible damage is done. These concepts will be considered in detail in Chapter 2. Their importance for the physician is that they provide both a stimulus and a basis for intervention because all is not lost at the first manifestation of ischemia.

II. CLINICAL CLASSIFICATION

Before the introduction of the concept of ischemic thresholds, physicians were already revising their ideas about cerebral ischemia and stroke. Traditionally, strokes were divided into hemorrhage, thrombosis, and embolism, which were pathological categories applied to clinical situations. All were thought to produce irreversible and usually devastating changes in the brain. Clincal observation directed increasing attention to what were variously known as minor strokes, or little strokes, and finally as transient ischemic attacks (TIAs). These are focal neurological deficits of abrupt onset and short duration with a marked tendency to recur in patients with cerebrovascular disease. Their clinical significance rests on the fact that TIAs frequently give warning of impending major stroke. Their scientific significance lies in their being a clinical counterpart of the ischemic models used in experimental work.

Ischemia, whether experimental or as encountered in the clinical situation, is reversible. If allowed to continue for too long, it leads to infarction. The time scale is therefore important, and for this reason ischemic strokes have come to be classified in temporal terms. Deficits that last less than 24 hours are labeled TIAs, though in practice TIAs are of much shorter duration, a matter of minutes or an hour or two. Deficits of more than 24 hours but less than 3 weeks are referred to as reversible ischemic neurological deficits (RINDs), while anything over 3 weeks is called a completed stroke.

The site of the ischemia is not without importance, for the natural history of events occurring in the carotid territory is markedly different from those in the vertebrobasilar territory (2). To be complete, classification of a cerebrovascular event requires three modes: the site of the lesion, i.e., carotid versus vertebrobasilar; the duration, i.e., TIA, RIND, or completed stroke; and finally its pathology, i.e., hemorrhage, thrombus, or embolism. It is only on this basis that therapy can proceed rationally. Unfortunately, in the clinical situation, it is not possible to allocate every event to a precise category, but every effort should be made to do so.

III. EPIDEMIOLOGY

A. Risk Factors

Because cerebrovascular disease ranks third as a cause of death in Western developed countries and is a major cause of disability in survivors, much attention has been devoted to its epidemiology (3). Strokes occur in about 150 per 100,000 population per annum, and about 70 of these result in death (4). The most important, though unavoidable, risk factor is age, with the incidence of stroke rising steeply from the age of 60 years.

Foremost among the avoidable risk factors is undoubtedly hypertension. Risk of stroke increases progressively with level of pressure above the normal for the person's age and sex, and persists when the hypertension relates to systolic pressure alone.

Cardiac disease is also an important risk factor. The main offender in this respect is ischemic heart disease, whether manifested clinically as angina, myocardial infarction, or congestive failure or whether detectable only by changes in the electrocardiogram. Evidence of left ventricular hypertrophy in the ECG increases the risk of stroke by a factor of 10 (5).

Extracranial vascular disease, in particular carotid atheroma, increases the risk of stroke. Other peripheral vascular disease is less significant though also relevant.

The presence of diabetes mellitus also increases the risk of stroke. The role of cholesterol and lipids is less clear and the source of much controversy. There does appear to be a relationship, particularly between excess lipids in earlier life and later stroke, though precisely which of the lipid fractions is responsible is unclear.

A high hemoglobin level is related to vascular incidents of all kinds, including stroke (6). This applies to a PCV of 0.50 upwards, which might not be considered clinically to merit the term polycythemia.

Smoking produces a threefold increase in the risk of stroke (7). The role of the contraceptive pill remains controversial.

B. Changes in Pattern

The most significant fact to emerge from epidemiological studies is the decline in the incidence of stroke. This has been in progress certainly since 1940 and possibly longer. It applies to both intracerebral hemorrhage and infarction but not to subarachnoid hemorrhage. The main reason for the decline is the control of hypertension. This is disputed, because the decline in stroke began before efficient hypotensive therapy became widely available. This fact does not, however, disprove the relevance of blood pressure control, as better socioeconomic conditions with reduced incidence of renal disease may well have caused a decline in the prevalence of hypertension prior to the introduction of hypotensives. Hypertension is a risk factor for both cerebral hemorrhage and infarction, the incidence of both being reduced by control of blood pressure.

C. Therapeutic Conclusions

The main therapeutic conclusions to be drawn from the epidemiological data are that blood pressure should be controlled, cardiac disease monitored and treated wherever possible, diabetes detected early and treated, the hemoglobin level checked and reduced when raised, and smoking avoided.

IV. CEREBRAL HEMORRHAGE

A. Mechanism

The most devastating manifestation of cerebrovascular disease is cerebral hemorrhage, coming as it does without warning. The cause in the vast majority of cases is high blood pressure. Other causes such as cryptic arteriovenous malformations and blood dyscrasias are responsible for only a small minority of cases. The relationship to hypertension, which is increasingly being detected early and controlled, is the reason the incidence of cerebral hemorrhage has steadily declined, to a greater extent than cerebral infarction.

Hypertension leads to the formation of microaneurysms, particularly on the short penetrating striate arteries of the brain (8). Rupture of a single microaneurysm may lead to only a microscopic hemorrhage, giving rise ultimately to a lacune. There is evidence that simultaneous rupture of a number of microaneurysms may be the mechansm of a massive cerebral hemorrhage. The alternative is rupture of a nonaneurysmal artery in which the pathological changes of fibrinoid necrosis associated with hypertension are present.

B. Clinical Presentation

The presentation traditionally associated with cerebral hemorrhage is one of very sudden onset, with headache, vomiting, and rapid loss of consciousness.

The loss of consciousness is deep, and the hemiplegia is manifest even in the unconscious state by the blowing in and out of the affected cheek with respiration and by the way in which the affected limbs fall when lifted. Respiration is usually compromised.

This remains the picture of massive cerebral hemorrhage. The prognosis is grave, with death following in 24-48 hours in 80% of cases (9). What is new is the realization that not all cerebral hemorrhages are massive and not all present as described or carry a bad prognosis. This realization has come about through the introduction of the computerized tomograph (CT) scan. This has shown that cases that on clinical grounds would have been diagnosed as an infarct are in fact caused by small intracerebral hemorrhage (Fig. 1). It was already known from autopsy data that the ability to distinguish at the bedside between hemorrhage and infarction was poor (10), but the serious possibility of error was not fully appreciated until the advent of the CT scan.

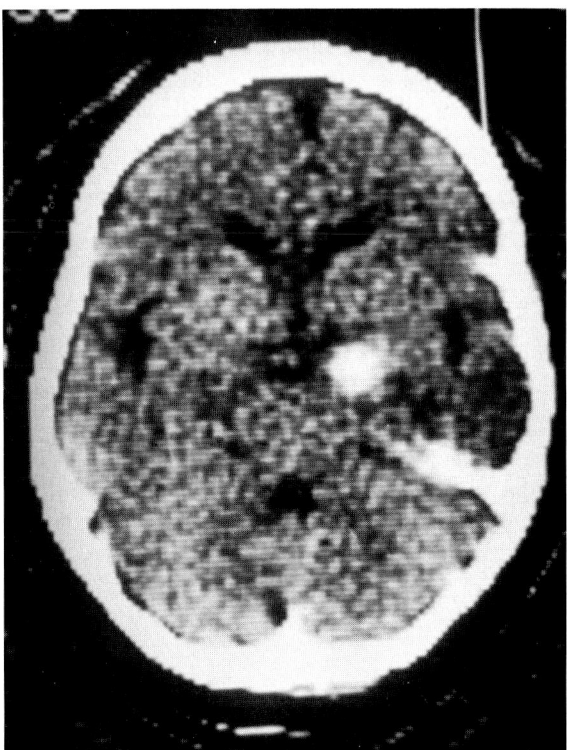

Figure 1 CT scan showing small, deep, intracerebral hemorrhage.

A cerebral hemorrhage may therefore present without loss of consciousness, though usually there is headache and early vomiting, and the residual hemiplegia or other focal neurological deficit can be mild. Distinction between hemorrhage and infarction is, of course, crucial if therapy such as anticoagulation, which could have an adverse effect in the case of an incorrect diagnosis, is to be given. Treatment of stroke, other than general measures, cannot safely be undertaken without a CT scan.

Prognosis for the small lacunar type of hemorrhage is surprisingly good. Even when the initial neurological deficit is profound, there is often rapid improvement within a matter of days, leaving only minor disability or even no disability at all.

V. TRANSIENT ISCHEMIC ATTACKS

A. Mechanism

The study of TIAs has been important not only for the management of patients but also for understanding the mechanisms of ischemia. TIAs were originally attributed to vasospasm. This was an understandable error, as it was difficult to conceive of any mechanism other than spasm that could suddenly produce focal ischemia and just as suddenly restore blood supply. Spasm of cerebral arteries does occur in migraine, hypertensive encephalopathy, subarachnoid hemorrhage, and during surgical manipulation; it is not the cause of the commonly encountered TIA.

The first mechanism of TIAs to be correctly recognized was the hemodynamic crisis (11). This envisaged that in the presence of focal narrowing of an artery any general fall in blood flow from whatever cause would first produce ischemia beyond the site of the narrowing. This undoubtedly occurs, for example, in hypertensive patients whose hypotensive drugs are poorly controlled or in some episodes of cardiac dysrhythima. It is not the explanation for the great majority of TIAs.

These have been shown to be caused by emboli often of the fibrin-platelet type (12). These impact in a vessel, briefly interrupting the blood supply. They then disintegrate so that blood flow is restored before irreversible damage is done, thus producing a TIA. Prolonged impaction with irreversible damage produces not a TIA but a RIND or a completed stroke. The best clinical evidence for this is ophthalmoscopic observation of the retina during an attack of amaurosis fugax, in which the arrest of a white body in retinal artery and its subsequent dispersal can be seen (13).

Disintegration of an embolus depends on many factors. The constitution of the embolus itself is important; fibrin-platelet emboli readily disintegrate, whereas an organized thrombus is more stable. The degree of activation of the fibrinolytic mechanisms, perfusion pressure, and velocity of blood flow are also important.

One of the objections to the embolic hypothesis for TIAs is their tendency to recur in the same site. It was argued that emboli would be scattered and would not consistently find their way to the same site. Laminar flow in arteries does cause a high percentage of emboli arising from a lesion on an arterial wall to follow the same course through the vascular tree. Only a small number go elsewhere, a fact that can be recognized clinically. A careful history from a patient experiencing many TIAs often reveals that while most follow a stereotyped pattern, other patterns will occasionally occur.

B. Source of Emboli

Recognition of the frequency with which emboli are responsible for TIAs led to increased interest in their source. The traditional source of emboli was the heart. However, emboli from this source are more often well-organized thrombi, which, in the form of emboli, produce infarction rather than transient ischemia. Attention was directed to the great vessels, especially the internal carotid artery, as a more likely source. Clinical, radiological, surgical, and pathological observations showed that atheromatous plaques in the arteries are often overlaid by thrombi, which give rise to emboli and produce TIAs. The plaques are commonly stenosing, but it is the production of emboli rather than interference with blood flow that causes TIAs.

Though emboli from the heart usually lead to infarction, TIAs can also occur. In a large study of patients with rheumatic endocarditis and valvular disease, a condition traditionally associated with embolic cerebral infarction, some 13% of patients were experiencing TIAs (14).

C. Clinical Presentation

When considering the clinical manifestations of transient ischemia it is important to distinguish between the carotid and vertebrobasilar territory. In the former, the classical manifestation is amaurosis fugax, abrupt loss of vision in one eye lasting 2 or 3 minutes and recovering rapidly. Depending upon where the embolus lodges, the visual loss may involve the entire field or the upper or lower half. It is often described by patients as like a shutter coming down.

Another presentation of carotid TIAs is heaviness or weakness of an upper or lower limb or both. Combination of amaurosis fugax on one side with weakness of the limbs on the opposite side is virtually pathognomonic of a TIA resulting from emboli from an internal carotid stenosis. Unilateral sensory symptoms rather than weakness may also occur. When the dominant cerebral hemisphere is involved, transient dysphasia may be the form taken by the TIAs.

ing on management in both the acute and chronic stages. The second reason is that emboli tend to disintegrate, restoring blood flow to ischemic or infarcted tissue. This has relevance to management in the acute stage. For example, early anticoagulation to prevent further emboli may cause hemorrhage when the initial embolus disintegrates and blood flow is restored to infarcted tissue. These problems will be dealt with in the chapters on therapy.

B. Clinical Presentation

A cerebral infarct presenting as a stroke may or may not have been preceded by a TIA. Opinions differ on how frequently warning episodes occur; much depends on the thoroughness with which enquiry is made; probably about two-thirds of strokes are preceded by some warning.

Immediate loss of consciousness, if it occurs at all, is usually brief and is more likely to occur with embolism than with thrombosis. The focal neurological deficit (hemiplegia, hemianopia, dysphasia) usually develops gradually over many minutes or hours. Headache at the onset is uncommon and immediate vomiting rare. In some instances the neurological deficit may evolve over many hours, and when the time exceeds 6 hours the term stroke in evolution or progressive stroke is usually applied. This situation is to be contrasted with instances of large infarcts, which subsequently provoke the formation of massive edema. Here, after an initial period of stabilization, which may last 12-24 hours, the patient begins to deteriorate, with increasing neurological deficit and depression of the level of consciousness.

C. Prognosis

Prognosis for completed stroke due to infarction using clinical criteria alone is difficult in the early stage. The same degree of initial neurological deficit can be caused by a large cortical infarct or by a small lacunar infarct in the internal capsule. Recovery from the latter is, however, likely to add to the large number of patients with persisting and severely disabling hemiplegia. CT scan can help in this regard, but even this is of limited value in the first 24 hours because the changes produced by even quite large infarcts may not be sufficiently manifest at this stage.

Apart from the prognosis for the neurological deficit, the overall outlook is important. Two-thirds of patients who have had a stroke die later from a myocardial infarct or other cardiac event rather than from a second stroke. The patient's blood pressure and cardiac and general vascular status and the presence or absence of a persisting source of emboli are more important prognostic factors than the severity and type of the cerebrovascular accident and neurological deficit.

VII. DIFFUSE CEREBRAL ISCHEMIA

Diffuse cerebral ischemia, by which is meant a level of blood flow insufficient to meet the metabolic needs of the brain but sufficient to prevent infarction, is very uncommon. Occasionally, with diffuse severe stenotic disease of the extracranial arteries, blood flow may fall to a level at which cerebral function is impaired and the patient shows evidence of slow cerebration. This situation may be relieved by vascular surgery.

A more frequent occurrence is the development of multiple small infarcts predominantly in the white matter with subsequent lacuna formation. This gives rise to impaired cerebral function and the type of dementia known as multi-infarct dementia (22). The patient shows loss of recent memory, periods of disorientation, and emotional lability, all of which develop in a patchy and stuttering fashion, with episodes of worsening and improvement superimposed on an overall downward course.

REFERENCES

1. Symon L, Lassen NA, Astrup J, Branston NM. Thresholds of ischaemia in brain cortex. *Adv Exper Med Biol* 94:775-782, 1977.
2. Marshall J. The natural history of transient ischaemic cerebrovascular attacks. *Quart J Med* 33:309-324 1964.
3. Kurtzke JF. *Epidemiology of Cerebrovascular Disease*. Springer-Verlag, New York, 1969.
4. Kurtzke JF. Epidemiology of cerebrovascular disease. In: National Institute of Neurological and Communicative Disorders and Stroke and National Heart and Lung Institute, *Cerebrovascular Survey Report for Joint Council Subcommittee on Cerebrovascular Disease* (Revised). Whiting Press, Rochester, MN, 1980, pp. 135-176.
5. Wolf PA, Dawber TR, Kannel WB. Heart disease as a precursor of stroke. *Adv. Neurol* 19-567-577, 1978.
6. Pearson TC, Wetherly-Mein G. Vascular occlusive episodes and venous haematocrit in primary proliferative polycythaemia. *Lancet* 2:1219-1222, 1978.
7. Kannel WB, Gordon T, Wolf PA, McNamara PM. Hemoglobin and risk of cerebral infarction: the Framingham study. *Stroke* 3:409-420, 1972.
8. Ross Russell RW. Observations on intracerebral aneurysms. *Brain* 86:425-442, 1963.
9. Acheson RM, Fairbairn, AS. Burden of cerebrobascular disease in the Oxford area in 1963 and 1964. *Br Med J* 2:621-626, 1970. 10.
10. Dalsgaard-Nielsen T. Some clinical experience in the treatment of cerebral apoplexy (1000 cases). *Acta Psychiat Scand Suppl* 108:101-119, 1956.
11. Denny-Brown D, Meyer JS. The cerebral collateral circulation, 2. Production of cerebral infarction by ischemic anoxia and its reversibility in early stages. *Neurology (Minneapolis)* 7:567-579, 1957.

12. Gunning AJ, Pickering GW, Robb-Smith AHT, Ross Russell R. Mural thrombosis of the internal carotid artery and subsequent embolism. *Quart J Med* 33:155-195, 1964.
13. Fisher CM. Observations on the fundus oculi in transient monocular blindness. *Neurology* (*Minneapolis*) 9:333-347, 1959.
14. Hutchinson EC, Stock JPP. Paroxysmal cerebral ischaemia in rheumatic heart disease. *Lancet* 2:653-656, 1963.
15. Cartlidge NEF, Whisnant JP, Elveback LR. Carotid and vertebral-basilar transient cerebral ischemic attacks. *Mayo Clinic Proc* 52:117-120, 1977.
16. Glynn AA. Vascular diseases of the nervous system. A series of 315 cases. *Br Med J* 2:1216-1219, 1956.
17. Torvik A, Jorgensen L. Thrombotic and embolic occlusions of the carotid arteries in an autopsy material, Part 1. Prevalence, location and associated diseases. *J Neurol Sci* 1:24-39, 1964.
18. Jorgensen L, Torvik A. Ischaemic cerebrovascular diseases in an autopsy series, Part 1. Prevalence, location and predisposing factors in verified thromboembolic occlusions, and their significance in the pathogenesis of cerebral infarction. *J Neurol Sci* 3:490-509, 1966.
19. Blackwood W, Hallpike JF, Kocen RS, Mair WGP. Atheromatous disease of the carotid arterial system and embolism from the heart in cerebral infarction: a morbid anatomical study. *Brain* 92:897-910, 1969.
20. Humphrey PRD, Harrison MJG. How often can an embolic stroke be diagnosed clinically? A clinicopathological correlation. *Postgrad Med J* 61: 1039-1042, 1985.
21. Wolf PA, Dawber TR, Thomas HE, Kannel WB. Epidemiologic assessment of chronic atrial fibrillation and risk of stroke: the Framingham study. *Neurology* 28:973-977, 1978.
22. Hachinski VC, Lassen NA, Marshall J. Multi-infarct dementia. A cause of mental deterioration in the elderly. *Lancet* 2:207-210, 1974.

2

Basic Mechanisms in Cerebral Ischemia

William Pearce
Loma Linda University School of Medicine, Loma Linda, California

Mark Fisher
University of Southern California School of Medicine, Los Angeles, California

I. INTRODUCTION

The study of cerebral ischemia is characterized by complexity, conflicting results, and differing opinions. Without doubt, this is due to the fact that there are several different types of cerebral ischemia, a wide variety of experimental approaches, and limited consensus concerning the clinical relevance of results. The purpose of this chapter is to briefly review the most important basic regulatory principles, and then to relate them to events that take place during and following an episode of cerebral ischemia.

II. BRAIN METABOLISM AND ITS RELATION TO BLOOD FLOW

Unlike the metabolism of skeletal or cardiac muscle, which is closely related to the output of mechanical work, the metabolism of the brain is related mainly to the electrochemical work associated with the maintenance of membrane ion gradients. The largest component of this work is a consequence of synaptic transmission and varies directly with electrocortical activity. A second, smaller, component of brain metabolism may be attributed to compensation for passive membrane ion leaks, and thus constitutes a relatively constant basal level of metabolism that is prerequisite for continued survival of brain paranchyma (1). Except in newborn, fasted, or diabetic individuals, brain metabolism is fueled almost exclusively by glucose, which, under normal conditions, easily traverses the blood-brain barrier by facilitated diffusion. Glucose is delivered to the brain in great excess, and only 10% of arterial blood glucose is normally extracted. However, up to 50% of arterial oxygen is normally extracted, which implies that as blood flow decreases, oxygen supply becomes deficient much more quickly than glucose supply. As a result, when arterial blood flow and oxygen supply become limiting, brain metabolism shifts to anaerobic glycolysis and maintains the critical membrane ion gradients at the expense of accumulating lactic acid (2).

In the brain, as in most tissues, total metabolic activity is closely related to the magnitude of blood flow. Although early studies suggested that both global cerebral blood flow and metabolism were relatively constant (3), more recent clinical measurements using inert gas clearance (4) and positron emission tomography methods (5) capable of measuring cerebral perfusion and metabolism with high degrees of temporal and spatial resolution have conclusively demonstrated that in humans both cerebral metabolism and blood flow change dramatically and simultaneously in response to well-defined tasks and physiological stimuli. These findings corroborate the results of autoradiographic studies in experimental animals and establish that cerebral perfusion and metabolism are tightly coupled (6). Of particular interest is the finding that despite a considerable heterogeneity of flow and metabolism among different brain areas, the ratio between flow and metabolism is remarkably uniform (7). The magnitude of this ratio can be altered by physiological influences such as systemic acidosis or norepinephrine administration, but the uniformity of the ratio among all brain structures persists, suggesting a very precise and efficient matching of cerebral metabolism and flow (8). The mechanisms responsible for this strong coupling, however, remain uncertain.

A. Metabolic Mechanisms

The oldest explanation of the link between brain blood flow and metabolism is the metabolic theory of Roy and Sherrington (9), which suggests that the tone of cerebral arteries is influenced directly by metabolic end products from the brain parenchyma. Without doubt, the main end product of cerebral metabolism, carbon dioxide, is one of the most powerful cerebral vasodilators known and as such has been considered a possible mediator of cerebrovascular regulation (3). However, the ability of topically applied bicarbonate to reverse hypercapnic vasodilation in pial arteries suggests that the effects of hypercapnia are mediated via decreases in extracellular pH (10). In turn, extracellular hydrogen ion, which is also an excellent vasodilator, has been considered a universal mediator of cerebrovascular regulation (10,11). Unfortunately, measurements of tissue pH during conditions of sustained vasodilatation or vasoconstriction do not exhibit changes large enough to explain the observed adjustments in cerebrovascular resistance (12,13). Thus, extracellular pH may be a particularly important influence on vascular tone during conditions such as lactic acidosis but probably is not the main mediator of the normal coupling between cerebral blood flow and metabolism.

Tissue potassium and adenosine have also been proposed as mediators of the link between cerebral perfusion and metabolism. Both agents are potent cerebral vasodilators whose interstitial concentrations rise during increased neuronal activity (14,15). However, when perivascular concentration of potassium are measured with ion-selective electrodes during hypoxia or seizures, the changes in local potassium activity are not sufficient or consistent enough to explain the associated vasodilatation (12,13). On the other hand, the results for adenosine are more convincing. Brain adenosine concentrations have been shown to rise dramatically during hypoxia (16), and inhibition of cellular uptake of adenosine has been shown to increase cerebral blood flow (17). Results obtained with inhibitors of adenosine deaminase, however, have been contradictory (18,19) and suggest that much additional work will be required to clearly define the role of adenosine.

Many other factors have also been suggested to play a role in the coupling of blood flow and metabolism, including prostaglandins (20), tissue osmolality (21), and glycolytic intermediates (18). However, no single factor yet examined can explain all facets of this coupling, which suggests that the relation between flow and metabolism may represent the integrated action of multiple metabolic factors. These factors may vary in importance in different brain regions, and changes in their concentrations may occur only within discrete anatomic compartments. Owing to the possible small size of such compartments, which may include glial cells immediately adjacent to arterioles (22), concentration changes in some factors may be detectable only with microhistochemical techniques (23). Equally important, the roles of some factors such as calcium(24) and free radicals (25) may change dramatically during ischemic conditions. Thus, a great deal of work remains to establish the mechanistic details of the metabolic theory, but it persists as an important concept for approaching an understanding of the coupling between brain blood flow and metabolism.

B. Vascular and Myogenic Mechanisms

With the metabolic hypothesis, the final target of all metabolic factors is the serosal surface of the cerebral arteries, which govern both cerbrovascular resistance and blood flow. In addition to these serosal influences, cerebral arteries are exposed to a variety of stimuli that arise from their luminal surface. Such stimuli include blood gases, perfusion pressure, and circulating transmitters and hormones. In general, cerebral arteries are protected from the action of most bloodborne compounds by the vascular endothelium, which in cerebral arteries contains high concentrations of degradative enzymes and, by virtue of tight junctions between adjacent cells, is highly impermeable to large polar molecules (26). This "blood-brain barrier" also contains a wide variety of specialized transport mechanisms to facilitate the transfer of many essential compounds between the bloodstream and the brain. Equally important, the vascular endothelium can have a direct effect on vascular tone through the release of endothelium-derived relaxing factor (EDRF) (27).

The discovery that vascular endothelium can directly influence vascular tone has stimulated new interest in its biochemistry, which now appears to be quite complex. The endothelium has an active arachadonic acid metabolism, contains both aminergic and cholinergic receptors, can produce vasodilatation through the synthesis and release of nitric oxide (NO), and has also been suggested to release vasoconstricting polypeptides (27-29). Although there have been relatively few studies of the physiological cardiovascular responses in which the endothelium participates, it is apparent that the endothelium strongly influences the regulation of vascular smooth muscle. In turn, recent studies of vascular smooth muscle biochemistry indicate that it also is highly complex and quite different from that of either skeletal or cardiac muscle. For example, the main calcium-binding protein of vascular smooth muscle is calmodulin, which, when bound to calcium, activates myosin light-chain kinase (30). Myosin light-chain kinase, in turn, phosphorylates myosin, which then binds actin to produce contraction. In addition to myosin light-chain kinase, other enzymes are also present in vascular smooth muscle that can affect the level of myosin phosphorylation and may mediate the vasoactive effects of certain compounds (31). In this manner, the generation of tension in vascular smooth muscle is governed dynamically by the ratio of phosphorylated to unphosphorylated myosin. Thus, the biochemistry of the endothelium/vascular smooth muscle unit is both unique and complex; owing to this complexity, derangements of this biochemistry and the associated metabolism may easily contribute to the pathology that accompanies cerebral ischemia.

One factor that may be particularly important for cerebral arterial function during ischemia is calcium. Under normal conditions, cerebral arteries contain less calcium than arteries of other vascular beds and are highly dependent on the entry of extracellular calcium to initiate and sustain contraction (32). Because their sarcoplasmic reticulum also is not extensive, cerebral arteries may be less able to regulate intracellular calcium during the conditions of calcium overload that commonly accompany ischemia (33). On the other hand, the importance of extracellular calcium in the contraction of cerebral arteries suggests that calcium entry blockers may be particularly efficacious in the cerebral circulation (34,25). Although the results obtained thus far concerning this possibility are inconsistent (36,37), these studies have stimulated new interest in mechanisms that influence intracellular calcium concentration (38) and in the membrane channels through which calcium enters smooth muscle cells (39-41).

At least two main calcium channels are recognized in vascular smooth muscle. Entry of extracellular calcium is increased by potential-operated channels as the smooth muscle membrane becomes depolarized, and by receptor-operated channels as a function of membrane receptor occupation. In addition, the existence of a third calcium channel that is resistant to blockade by organic calcium channel antagonists and increases its permeability to calcium when the vascular smooth muscle membrane is stretched has recently been demonstrated (42,43). This latter channel is particularly interesting, for, if confirmed, it may provide a mechanistic basis for the myogenic hypothesis that describes the well-known ability of cerebral vessels to contract in response to increased transmural pressure (44). On the organ level, the myogenic hypothesis has been employed to explain the phenomenon of autoregulation, which is defined as the ability to maintain a relatively constant blood flow through changes of vascular resistance in direct proportion to changes in perfusion pressure (45,46). The calcium channel data of Bevan and Hwa (42,43) together with the results of other studies (44,47) suggest that although autoregulation may be modulated by neurogenic (48) or metabolic (49) influences, the mechanistic basis for this phenomenon probably derives from local intrinsic properties of cerebrovascular smooth muscle. In turn, local conditions that interfere with the normal calcium metabolism of cerebral arteries, such as membrane depolarization or calcium overload induced by ischemia (33), may be expected to attenuate local autoregulatory function.

Another cerebrovascular response that may be mediated by local effects on vascular smooth muscle is the vasodilatation produced by hypoxia. For many years it has been known that hypoxia can relax isolated vascular smooth muscle (50,51), and recent results suggest that this effect may also involve the vascular endothelium (52). Other vascular mechanisms have also been suggested to play a role, including membrane hyperpolarization (53) and inhibition of calcium uptake (54). In contrast, attempts to demonstrate the participation of either metabolic or neurogenic mechanisms in this response have had only limited success

(55,55a). Thus, it appears likely that local vascular or endothelial damage, such as that produced by ischemia, may also interrupt cerebrovascular sensitivity to hypoxia.

C. Neurogenic Mechanisms

In addition to metabolic and vascular mechanisms, cerebrovascular smooth muscle is influenced by an abundant vascular innervation located between the adventitial and medial layers of the arteries that supply the brain. The most widely studied component of this innervation consists of norepinephrine-containing sympathetic fibers that arise mainly from the superior cervical ganglia and are distributed bilaterally to both arteries and veins (48,56,57). Although cerebral arteries are generally less sensitive to norepinephrine than systemic arteries (58,59), there is good evidence that sympathetic nerves participate in regulation of cerebrovascular resistance, particularly during hypertension; sympathetic nerves appear to extend the upper limit of autoregulation and sympathectomy aggravates increases in blood-brain permeability produced by hypertension (60,61). Sympathetic fibers also appear to play a trophic role in the development of maturation of cerebral arteries (62).

Evidence suggesting that cerebral arteries receive a serotonergic innervation has also been reported (63). This innervation appears to originate in the Raphe nuclei and is more dense in the larger cerebral arteries at the base of the brain in the pial arteries at the brain surface (64). Serotonin contracts cerebral arteries, but with much greater potency and efficacy than norepinephrine (63). Although the physiological importance of the serotonergic cerebrovascular innervation remains uncertain, it has been suggested to play a role in migraine, cerebral vasospasm, and ischemia (65).

The cerebrovascular innervation has also been suggested to contain a large number of polypeptides, including but not limited to avian pancreatic polypeptide, calcitonin gene-related peptide, cholecystokinin, gastrin-releasing peptide, neurokinin A, neuropeptide Y, neurotensin, peptide histidine isoleucine, somatostatin, substance P, and vasoactive intestinal polypeptide (66). Although the physiological importance of these peptides in cerebrovascular regulation remains largely unknown, recent attention has focused mainly on neuropeptide Y, substance P, and vasoactive intestinal polypeptide. Neuropeptide Y is a constrictor colocalized with norepinephrine in cerebrovascular sympathetic nerve terminals (67). Cerebrovascular nerve fibers originating in the trigeminal ganglion contain substance P (68,69), which may serve as a sensory transmitter in cerebral arteries (70). Substance P also produces a mild vasodilation of cerebral arteries (71) that is dependent on the endothelium (72) and is mediated via a specific receptor mechanism (73). Vasoactive intestinal polypeptide also acts in cerebral arteries via a specific receptor mechanism but, unlike substance P, is a highly potent vasodilator (74) and appears to be endothelium-independent

(72). The source of the fibers supplying vasoactive intestinal polypeptide to cerebral arteries, however, remains controversial (75-77). Clearly, the potential of a regulatory role for these peptides appears promising, but an assessment of their importance in cerebral ischemia must await extensive additional study.

Nerve fibers containing choline acetyl transferase, a marker specific for cholinergic neurons, also innervate cerebral arteries (78-80). The origin of these cholinergic fibers remains uncertain but has been suggested to be either the superifical petrosal ganglion (81) or, more recently, the sphenopalatine ganglion (77). The receptor mechanisms associated with this innervation exhibit significant regional differences in sensitivity to acetylcholine (82) but consistently produce relaxation that appears to be muscarinic in nature (80,83-85). Although in vitro attempts to assess the functional importance of this innervation have produced conflicting results (79,86-88), in vivo studies have consistently demonstrated that cholinergic agonists can increase cerebral blood flow (89-92) and suggest a possible role for a cholinergic innervation in the vasodilatation associated with EEG desynchronization (93).

Another possible role for the cholinergic innervation of cerebral arteries involves the cerebral vasodilation produced by stimulation of the cerebellar fastigial nucleus (94). This vasodilatation is not associated with an increase in cerebral metabolism and is not affected by sympathectomy or spinal cord transection (95) but can be inhibited by systemic administration of atropine (96). Equally important, lesions of the basal forebrain, which provides cholinergic fibers to the cortex, can also inhibit the response (97). Together, these results suggest the presence of an intrinsic neural system within the brain that involves cholinergic fibers and that can significantly influence the regulation of cerebral perfusion. If future studies can demonstrate an important role for this intrinsic system in the normal regulation of cerebral perfusion, then ischemic damage to the brain centers involved may logically be expected to compromise postischemic cerebrovascular regulation.

III. GLOBAL CEREBRAL ISCHEMIA

With the perspective provided by the preceding section, the discussion will now turn to the events associated with cerebral ischemia, of which there are two major categories: global ischemia, such as that associated with circulatory arrest or strangulation, and focal ischemia, which is typical of stroke and cerebral vasospasm (2,98). A third category of cerebral ischemia has also been proposed based on the damage associated with microemboli caused by gas bubbles or fat droplets (99,100), but this type of ischemia generally produces a more reversible pattern of metabolic changes and vasogenic edema dissimilar to that found in other types of ischemia (2) and thus will not be considered further here. Although the changes that occur during global ischemia are also quite different from those that occur during stroke, studies of global ischemia have provided much important information about the processes of ischemic damage that is worthy of consideration.

Following the onset of complete global ischemia, tissue NADH/NAD ratios rapidly increase, phosphocreatine decreases, and ATP levels begin to fall as local oxygen is depleted (23). With continued ischemia, dephosphorylation of ADP and AMP leads to the formation and release of significant quantities of tissue adenosine, which in turn decreases the tissue pool size of adenylate (101,102). Protein synthesis halts (103,104), and lipid breakdown ensues, releasing arachidonate and other free fatty acids (105). Tissue carbon dioxide accumulates, and pH falls daramatically to values of 6.5 or less (106). Aggravating this acidification of the parenchyma is the accumulation of lactic acid, which, during complete ischemia, can reach peak concentrations within 3 minutes (106). If, however, the ischemia is not complete and some residual blood flow persists, then tissue lactic acid levels can continue to increase throughout the duration of ischemia until tissue concentrations of 20-25 mM are attained that produce irreversible tissue damage and cell death (107). Because lactic acid is derived directly from blood glucose, hyperglycemia accelerates and hypoglycemia retards lactate accumulation.

Another consequence of the increased anaerobic metabolism that accompanies ischemia is the production and accumulation of osmotically active particles within the brain parenchyma (108). This increased tissue osmolality draws extracellular water into the cells and further complicates cell function. In the event of complete energy failure, the changes in tissue osmolality become even more pronounced as membrane gradients deteriorate and the cells rapidly lose potassium and gain both sodium and calcium. These changes, in turn, increase potassium and decrease calcium and sodium ion concentrations in the extracellular compartment (109-111), which draws water into the tissue and precipitates the development of cytotoxic edema (112). The extent of this edema is augmented during incomplete ischemia by a continued supply of blood, which provides additional water and ions for the formation of edema. Vascular permeability to proteins may also deteriorate over time and produce vasogenic edema (2,33,112). Overall, cerebral edema is a classic consequence of an ischemic insult and, due to tentorial herniation, constitutes a major cause of postischemic death (113).

Given the spectrum of changes in tissue composition that result from cerebral ischemia, it is not surprising that cerebral autoregulation and reactivity to carbon dioxide are often impaired in the postischemic brain (114,115). The lactic acidosis, local hypercapnia, and increased tissue concentrations of adenosine in ischemic regions act in concert to maximally vasodilate the vessels; thus, additional vasodilatory influences such as systemic hypotension or hypercapnia can be expected to have little effect (2). This apparent lack of reactivity may be reversible, however, if energy metabolism has not failed completely in the vascular smooth muscle. In such circumstances, postischemic reperfusion leads to hyperemia, which is a good indicator of potential for recovery (116). If, on the other hand, arterial energy metabolism has failed, all membrane ion gradients will be lost, perivascular neurotransmitters will be released, and the smooth muscle cells will be flooded with water and calcium (24,117). Under these latter conditions, the loss of vascular reactivity may become irreversible and lead to a condition known as "no reflow" in which cerebral perfusion does not recover during the potischemic period even after normal systemic cardiovascular parameters have been reestablished (118,119). Although the exact mechanisms that mediate "no reflow" remain uncertain, it is probable that an irreversible loss of vascular reactivity contributes to this pattern.

Whereas the "no reflow" phenomenon is immediately evident upon reperfusion of the postischemic brain, the delayed ischemic hypoperfusion syndrome appears only after several minutes or even hours of reperfusion (2,24). Cerebral autoregulation has been observed during postischemic hypoperfusion even though CO_2 reactivity is often depressed, suggesting that this syndrome is not due to a complete loss of vascular reactivity (116,120). Although relative importance of other factors such as partial uncoupling of oxidative metabolism, lactic acidosis, formation of vasogenic edema, and glial swelling remain uncertain (24, 121,122), some ischemic damage may require several hours or days to become evident. This characteristic pattern of postischemic change has been referred to as "maturation" by Ito et al. (123), which emphasizes that ischemic damage occurs not only during the period of ischemica but also during the reperfusion period immediately following.

One factor that may contribute to the delayed effects of ischemia is postischemic hypermetabolism (2,124). Cells that survive ischemia must resynthesize lost adenylate (101,102). Because NAD is unstable at acid pH values such as those attained during severe lactic acidosis (125), some new NAD may also be needed. Other catabolic repair processes are also undoubtedly stimulated (126). However, these increased demands come at a time when mitochondrial damage is prevalent (127), and the elevated levels of intracellular calcium typical of postischemic tissue further compromise mitochondrial function (128). Thus, postischemic hypermetabolism may promote additional damage, and inhibition of this increase in metabolism may be beneficial (129).

IV. FOCAL ISCHEMIA AND THRESHOLDS FOR ISCHEMIC DAMAGE

Although much of the preceding discussion has centered on changes associated with global ischemia, the pattern of changes associated with stroke are more closely related to those of focal cerebral ischemia (130). Clearly, the majority of changes that occur in the center of an ischemic focus are similar to those observed during global ischemia, but the cardiovascular instability, respiratory complications, and hypotension that often accompany global ischemia are less pronounced. A local ischemic focus is also surrounded by perfused tissue whose magnitude of blood flow is roughly proportional to the distance from the ischemic focus (131). This collateral circulation can provide needed oxygen but can also supply glucose for the formation of lactate and water for the formation of edema. Thus, a focal ischemic lesion may be viewed as an area of complete ischemia surrounded by areas of incomplete ischemia with varying degrees of severity. In each area, the extent of functional loss and damage is related to the ratio between oxygen delivery and demand. Systemic factors such as hypoxia and anemia, which reduce oxygen delivery, or cerebral conditions of seizure or hypermetabolism, which elevate demand, will reduce the supply/demand ratio and aggravate ischemic damage (1). The threshold values of the supply/demand ratio at which functional loss or damage first occurs, however, are not fixed and vary in relation to brain anatomy, the duration of ischemia, and the absolute levels of blood flow (132).

As cerebral perfusion approaches ischemic levels, the first obvious change in cerebral function is a loss of brain electrical activity. At a cerebral blood flow of approximately 20 ml/min per 100 g, evoked potential amplitudes begin to decrease. At 18 ml/min per 100 g, cortical unit activity ceases and EEG amplitude begins to decrease. At flows between 15 and 16 ml/min per 100 g, evoked potentials are completely suppressed and the EEG becomes isoelectric (1,2,98). With continued decreases in perfusion to approximately 10 ml/min per 100 g, membrane ion pumps begin to fail, which in turn radically alters water and ion distribution and initiates the beginning of irreversible tissue damage. The 10 ml/min per 100 g value of flow also appears to be the approximate threshold for infarction, which suggests that the damage caused by membrane ion pump failure is closely related to the development of infarction (33,132). Although these threshold flow values may vary somewhat in response to factors such as anesthesia and hematocrit that affect the oxygen supply/demand ratio (133), they are in general quite consistent and have been demonstrated in both primate and nonprimate species (1).

Of particular interest is the finding that loss of brain electrical activity occurs at higher levels of flow than those associated with irreversible damage. This suggests that the presence of EEG or evoked potentials may be a reliable indicator of reversible ischemic damage (130). In addition, this finding suggests the existence of an electrically quiet zone immediately surrounding the ischemic focus that is not irreversibly damaged. Histologically, such tissue is often characterized by capillary proliferation, inflammatory cells, and reactive changes in glial elements (134). Referred to as an ischemic penumbra (1) this zone may be particularly relevant clinically, as it represents threatened but still viable tissue that may survive with proper medical management.

V. SELECTIVE VULNERABILITY

Aside from the severity and duration of ischemia, a number of other factors also influence the extent of ischemic damage. Because the immature brain can utilize noncarbohydrate substrates that under anaerobic conditions do not obligatorily produce lactate as an end product, immaturity provides considerable resistance to ischemia (135). Conversely, aging tends to attenuate overall vascular reactivity and thus may also impair regulatory compensations during ischemia, worsening chances for recovery (136). At any given age, border zones between perfused territories appear most vulnerable to ischemia (137). In addition, the brain is quite heterogeneous in terms of its metabolism and blood flow; different functional groups of neurons may have different patterns of activity and thus different vulnerabilities to ischemia (129). For example, layers 3, 5, and 6 of the neocortex, small and medium-sized neurons of the striatum, the limbic system and in particular the CA 1 subfield of the hippocampus, cerebellar Purkinje cells, and neurons of the caudoputamen all appear to be more vulnerable to ischemia than other brain areas (129,138,139). On the other hand, white matter, which consists mainly of fiber tracts and has lower levels of blood flow than gray matter, appears to tolerate ischemia better than nerve cells (140) even though the pattern of metabolic changes is similar in both types of tissue (141). The reasons for these differences in vulnerability, however, are poorly understood but may involve the actions of excitatory neurotransmitters.

III. CEREBRAL INFARCTION AS A MANIFESTATION OF A PRETHROMBOTIC STATE

There is a consensus that the major mechanisms of cerebral ischemia in humans consist of thrombosis and embolism. For the past three or four decades, there has been considerable debate over the relative importance of these two processes. Funduscopic evidence for embolization from carotid artery atherosclerotic plaques has led to more emphasis on embolism as the major cause of cerebral infarction. Indeed, the current diagnostic work-up of the patient with suspected cerebral ischemia largely consists of a search for an embolic source. Any debate over the relative importance of thrombosis versus embolism can quickly degenerate into trivialities. It is thus with some trepidation that one suggests that, while the two processes are, of course, not mutually exclusive, thrombotic mechanisms are probably of greater importance in the pathogenesis of cerebral ischemia.

There are several arguments in favor of the importance of thrombotic mechanisms in stroke. First, etiological investigations of stroke patients regularly turn up substantial numbers of individuals in whom there is no identifiable embolic source (142-144). Second, when an embolic source, usually cardiac, is found, systemic (i.e., nonbrain) embolism is usually absent (145). Third, recent epidemiological evidence suggests that atrial fibrillation without valvular disease, the most common identifiable source of putative cardiac embolism, may not be associated with a significantly increased risk of stroke (146,147). Finally, the initial reports of transluminal angioplasty for carotid artery disease (Chapter 12) suggest that the brain is remarkably tolerant of the embolic fragments that almost certainly arise following in situ plaque compression.

Intravascular thrombosis is an attractive mechanism both as an alternative to embolization and as a potentiator of embolic phenomena. There is considerable indirect evidence suggesting the importance of intravascular thrombosis in cerebral ischemia. Perhaps the most important is the observation by Ishii et al. that thrombomodulin is absent from human brain endothelium (148). An appreciation of the importance of this observation requires an understanding of the role of vascular endothelium in anticoagulation (149). Briefly, vascular endothelium normally functions to prevent thrombus formation by one of two mechanisms: Heparin-like molecules on the endothelial surface bind with circulating antithrombin III to inactivate coagulation proteases; in addition, thrombomodulin, an endothelial-based protein interacts with thrombin in a way that results in altered function of the thrombin molecule. As a consequence, thrombin becomes less efficient in catalyzing clot formation and also acts a a powerful activator of the circulating anticoagulant protein C. In addition to these anticoagulant functions, vascular endothelium also functions as a platelet antiaggregant (by production of prostacyclin) and as a promoter of fibrinolysis (by production of tissue plasminogen activator).

The absence of thrombomodulin in brain capillaries leads to the hypothesis that the brain has an inherent predilection for thrombosis. Ishii and his co-workers have made the intriguing suggestion that absence of thrombomodulin may serve the useful function of providing protection from intracranial hemorrhage. It may be that such a phenomenon becomes dysfunctional with increasing age. The coagulation system changes with aging, as Bauer and colleagues (150) have demonstrated: fragment F (derived from the conversion of prothrombin to thrombin), fibrinopeptide A (produced during the formation of fibrin I monomer from fibrinogen), and protein C activation all increase in males with increasing age.

How do these observations relate to stroke? Coagulation studies in patients with cerebral ischemia suggest that increased platelet activation is found both acutely (within 3 days of symptom onset) and 2 months later (151). This is in contrast to fibrinopeptide A (elevated only acutely) and fibrinopeptide B beta 1-42 (a fibrin fragment released during fibrinolysis), which remains normal during both time periods (152). These data suggest the acute generation of fibrin superimposed on a background of increased platelet activation, with the latter likely preceding the acute event. Cerebral infarction can thus be conceptualized as a focal manifestation of a systemic prethrombotic state. The absence from the brain microcirculation of a critical endothelial-based anticoagulant (thrombomodulin) may explain why a systemic prethrombotic state could result in brain thrombosis in the absence of systemic thromboembolic phenomena.

VII. NEUROCHEMICAL ALTERATIONS IN CEREBRAL ISCHEMIA

Brain extraction of oxygen and glucose is, respectively, approximately 50% and 10%. Carbohydrate storage in the brain is rather limited compared to that in other organs and tends to be localized in glia rather than neurons (153). Anaerobic glycolysis thus becomes a key consideration in the neurochemistry of cerebral ischemia. The importance of glycolysis and lactate production tends to vary among different experimental models of stroke. These models induce either global or focal cerebral ischemia. In the former, cerebral ischemia is usually complete, meaning that cerebral blood flow is reduced to zero or negligible values prior to recirculation. Animal models of focal cerebral ischemia are usually "incomplete" in that at least a trickle of blood flow continues during the ischemic insult. Most studies indicate that, for equivalent duration of ischemia, brain injury is more extensive with incomplete than with complete ischemia (154).

The paradox of incomplete ischemia having more deleterious consequences may be explained by the concept that continued trickle flow provides glucose, with anaerobic glycolysis producing potentially toxic lactic acid (107,155). Moderate hyperglycemia (two or three times normal) in global cerebral ischemia can transform minor ischemic changes (limited to neuronal necrosis) into full-blown cerebral infarction, with irreversible damage to neurons, glia, and endothelium (156). There are several possible mechanisms for the effect of hyperglycemia. First, severe hyperglycemia is associated with reduced cerebral blood flow (157). Second, hyperglycemia may be associated with formation of the intracellular osmotic agent sorbitol, which can produce cellular swelling and rupture (158). A third and particularly intriguing possibility involves ferric ion, free radicals, and lipid peroxidation (158).

Most biochemical models of ischemic neuronal injury invoke lipid peroxidation as a critical process, usually the final common pathway of cell death. Lipid peroxidation, or autooxidation, is an oxygen-requiring chain reaction in which naturally occurring polyunsaturated fatty acids are converted into peroxides and hydroperoxides—compounds with the chemical configuration ROOR and ROOH, respectively. These compounds are somewhat unstable since the O–O bond is relatively weak (159); as a consequence, hydroperoxides act as both initiator and product of the lipid peroxidation process, a positive feedback system that is potentially devastating. The initiation of the lipid peroxodiation process requires a metal ion and free radicals; the latter are highly reactive molecules with an unpaired electron in their outer orbital (160). The requirement

77. Hara H, Hamill GS, Jacobowitz DM. Origin of cholinergic nerves to the rat major cerebral arteries: co-existence with vasoactive intestinal polypeptide. *Brain Res Bull* 14:179-188, 1985.
78. Florence VM, Bevan JA. Biochemical determinations of cholinergic innervation in cerebral arteries. *Circ Res* 45:212-218, 1979.
79. Duckles SP. Evidence for a functional cholinergic innervation of cerebral arteries. *J Pharmacol Exp Ther* 217:544-548, 1981.
80. Estrada C, Hamel E, Krause DN. Biochemical evidence for cholinergic innervation on intracerebral blood vessesl. *Brain Res* 266:261-270, 1983.
81. Chorobski J, Penfield W. Cerebral vasodilator nerves and their pathway from the medulla oblongata: with observations on pial and intracerebral vascular plexus. *Arch Neurol Psychiatry* 28:1257-1289, 1932.
82. Toda N. Acetylcholine-induced relaxation in isolated dog cerebral arteries. *J Pharmacol Exp Ther* 209:352-358, 1979.
83. Edvinsson L, Falck B. Owman C. Possibilities for a cholinergic action on smooth musculature and on sympathetic axons in brain vessels mediated by muscarinic and nicotinic receptors. *J Pharmacol Exp Ther* 200:117-126, 1977.
84. Harik SI, Sharma VK, Wetherbee JR, Warren RH, Banerjee SP. Adrenergic and cholinergic receptors of cerebral microvessels. *J Cereb Blood Flow Metab* 1:329-338, 1981.
85. Estrada C, Krause DN. Muscarinic cholinergic receptor sites in cerebral blood vessels. *J Pharmacol Exp Ther* 221:85-90, 1982.
86. Lee TJF. Direct evidence against acetylcholine as the dilator transmitter in the cat cerebral artery. *Eur J Pharmacol* 68;393–394, 1980.
87. Bevan JA, Buga GM, Florence VM, Gonsalves A, Snowden A. Distribution of choline acetyltransferase in cerebral and extracerebral cranial arteries of the cat: its relationship to neurogenic atropine-sensitive dilation. *Circ Res* 50:470-476, 1982.
88. Lee TJF, Saito A, Berezin I. Vasoactive intestinal polypeptide-like substance: the potential transmitter for cerebral vasodilatation. *Science* 224: 898-901, 1984.
89. Lowe RF, Gilboe DD. Canine cerebrovascular response to nitroglycerine, acetylcholine, 5-hydroxytryptamine and angiotensin. *Am J Physiol* 225: 1333-1338, 1973.
90. Matsuda M, Meyer JS, Deshmukh VD, Tagashira Y. Effect of acetylcholine on cerebral circulation. *J Neurosurg* 45:423-431, 1976.
91. D'Alecy LG, Rose CJ. Parasympathetic cholinergic control of cerebral blood flow in dogs. *Circ Res* 41:324-331, 1977.
92. Heistad DD, Marcus ML, Said SI, Gross PM. Effect of acetylcholine and vasoactive intestinal peptide on cerebral blood flow. *Am J Physiol* 239: H73-H80, 1980.
93. Pearce WJ, Scremin OU, Sonnenschein RR, Rubinstein EH. The electroencephalogram, blood flow, and oxygen uptake in rabbit cerebrum. *J Cereb Blood Flow Metab* 1:419-428, 1981.
94. Reis DJ, Iadecola C.Regulation by the brain of its blood flow and metab-

olism: role of intrinsic neuronal networks and circulating catecholamines. In: Owman C, Hardebo JE (Eds.), *Neural Regulation of Brain Circulation*, Elsevier, Amsterdam, 1986, pp. 129-145.

95. Reis DJ, Iadecola C, MacKenzie E, Mori M, Nakai M, Tucker L. Primary and metabolically coupled cerebrovascular dilation elicited by stimulation of two intrinsic systems in brain. In: Heistad DD, Marcus MM (Eds.), *Cerebral Blood Flow: Effects of Nerves and Neurotransmitters*. Elsevier, New York, 1982, pp. 475-484.
96. Iadecola C, Underwood MD, Reis DJ. Muscarinic cholinergic receptors mediate the cerebrovasodilation elicited by stimulation of the cerebellar fastigial nucleus in the rat. *Brain Res* 368:375-379, 1986.
97. Iadecola C, Mraovitch S, Meeley, MP, Reis DJ. Lesions of the basal forebrain in rat selectively impair the cortical vasodilation elicited from cerebellar fastigial nucleus. *Brain Res* 279:41-52, 1983.
98. Astrup J. Energy requiring functions in the ischemic brain. Their critical supply and possible inhibition in protective therapy. *J Neurosurg* 56: 482-497, 1982.
99. Furlow TW, Bass NH. Arachidonate-induced cerebrovascular occlusion in the rat. The role of platelets and aspirin in stroke. *Neurology* 56:482-497, 1982.
100. Meldrum BS, Papy JJ, Vigouroux RA. Intracarotid air embolism in the baboon: effects on cerebral blood flow and the electroencephalogram. *Brain Res* 25:301-315, 1971.
101. Kleihues P. Kobayashi K, Hossman KA. Purine nucleotide metabolism in the cat brain after one hour of complete ischemia. *J Neurochem* 23;417-425, 1974.
102. MacMillan V. Cerebral Na^+, K^+-ATPase activity during exposure to and recovery from acute ischemia. *J Cereb Blood Flow Metab* 2:457-465, 1982.
103. Cooper HK, Zalewska T, Kawakammi S. The effect of ischaemia and recirculation on protein synthesis in the rat brain. *J Neurochem* 28:929-934, 1977.
104. Dienel GA, Pulsinelli WA, Duffy TE. Regional protein synthesis in rat brain following acute hemispheric ischemia. *J Neurochem* 35:1216-1226, 1980.
105. Bazan NG. Effects of ischemia and electroconvulsive shock on free fatty acid pool in the brain. *Biochim Biophys Acta* 218:1-10, 1970.
106. Ljunggren B, Norberg K. Siesjo BK. Influence of tissue acidosis upon restitution of brain energy metabolism following total ischemia. *Brain Res* 77:173-186, 1974.
107. Rehncreona S, Rosen I, Siesjo BK. Brain lactic acidosis and ischemic cell damage: 1. Biochemistry and neurophysiology. *J Cereb Blood Flow Metab* 1:297-311, 1981.
108. Hossmann KA, Zimmermann V. Resuscitation of the monkey brain after 1 hour complete ischemia. I. Physiological and morphological observations. *Brain Res* 81:59-74, 1974.

109. Hansen AJ. The extracellular potassium concentration in brain cortex following ischemia in hypo- and hyperglycemic rats. *Acta Physiol Scand* 102:324-329, 1978.
110. Harris RJ, Symon L, Branston NM. Changes in extracellular calcium activity in cerebral ischemia. *J Cereb Blood Flow Metab* 1:203-209, 1981.
111. Siemkowicz E, Hansen AJ. Brain extracellular ion composition and EEG activity following 10 minutes ischemia in normo- and hyperglycemic rats. *Stroke* 12:236-240, 1981.
112. Klatzo I. Presidential address. Neuropathological aspects of brain edema. *J Neuropathol Exp Neurol* 26:1-14, 1967.
113. Katzman R, Clasen R, Klatzo I. Brain edema in stroke. Study group on brain edema in stroke. *Stroke* 8:512-540, 1977.
114. Shibata S, Hodge CP, Pappius HM. Effect of experimental ischemia on cerebral water and electrolytes. *J Neurosurg* 41:146-159, 1974.
115. Kagstrom E, Smith ML, Siesjo BK. Cerebral circulatory responses to hypercapnia and hypoxia in the recovery period following complete and incomplete ischemia in the rat. *Acta Physiol Scand* 118:281-291, 1983.
116. Hossman KA, Lechtaper-Gruter H. Hossman V. The role of cerebral blood flow for the recovery of the brain after prolonged ischemia. *Z Neurol* 204:281-299, 1973.
117. Wieloch T, Siesjo BK. Ischemic brain injury: the importance of calcium, lipolytic activities, and free fatty acids. *Pathol Biol* 30:269-277, 1982.
118. Ames A, Wright RL, Kowada M. Cerebral ischemia. II. The no-reflow phenomenon. *Am J Pathol* 52:437-453, 1968.
119. Fischer EG, Ames A, Lorenzo AV. Cerebral blood flow immediately following brief circulatory stasis. *Stroke* 10:423-427, 1979.
120. Nemoto EM, Snyder JV, Carroll RG, Morita H. Global ischemia in dogs: cerebrovascular CO_2 reactivity and autoregulation. *Stroke* 6:425-431, 1975.
121. Arsenio-Nunes ML, Hossman KA, Farkas-Bargeton E. Ultrastructural and histochemical investigation of the cerebral cortex of cat during and after complete ischaemia. *Acta Neuropathol* 26:329-344, 1973.
122. Hossman KA. Post-ischemic resuscitation of the brain: selective vulnerability versus global resistance. In: Kogure K, Hossman KA, Siesjo BK, Welsh FA (Eds.), *Progress in Brain Research* Vol. 63. Elsevier, Amsterdam, 1985, pp. 3-17.
123. Ito U, Spatz M, Walker JT, Klatzo I. Experimental cerebral ischemia in mongolian gerbils. I. Light microscopic observations. *Acta Neuropathol* 34:1-6, 1975.
124. Nemoto EM, Hossman KA, Cooper HK. Post-ischemic hypermetabolism in cat brain. *Stroke* 12:666-676, 1981.
125. Welsh FA. Regional evaluation of ischemic metabolic alterations. *J Cereb Blood Flow Metab* 4:309-316, 1984.
126. Levy DE, Duffy TE. Cerebral energy metabolism during transient ischemia and recovery in the gerbil. *J Neurochem* 28:63-70, 1977.

127. Rehncreona S, Mela L, Siesjo BK. Recovery of brain mitochondrial function in the rat after complete and incomplete cerebral ischemia. *Stroke* 10:437-446,1979.
128. Nicholls DG. A role for the mitochondrion in the protection of cells against calcium overload? In: Kogure K, Hossman KA, Siesjo BK, Welsh, FA (Eds.), *Progress in Brain Research* Vol. 63. Elsevier, Amsterdam, 1985, pp. 97-106.
129. Kirino T, Tamura A, Sano K. Selective vulnerability of the hippocampus to ischemia–reversible and irreversible types of ischemic cell damage. In: Kogure K, Hossman KA, Siesjo BK, Welsh FA (Eds.), *Progress in Brain Research* Vol 63. Elsevier, Amsterdam, 1985, pp. 39-58.
130. Garcia JH. Experimental ischemic stroke: a review. *Stroke* 15:5-14, 1984.
131. Symon L, Pasztor E, Branstom NM. The distribution and density of reduced cerebral blood flow following acute middle cerebral artery occlusion: an experimental study by the technique of hydrogen clearance in baboons. *Stroke* 5:355-364, 1974.
132. Heiss WD. Flow thresholds of functional and morphological damage of brain tissue. *Stroke* 14:329-331, 1983.
133. Michenfelder JD, Sundt TM, Fode N, Sharbrough FW. Isoflurane when compared to enflurance and halothane decreases the frequency of cerebral ischemia during carotid endarterectomy. *Anesthesiology* 67:336-340, 1987.
134. Garcia JH, Kamijyo Y. Cerebral infarction. Evolution of histopathological changes after occlusion of a middle cerebral artery in primates. *J Neuropathol Exp Neurol* 33:409-421, 1974.
135. Adolph EF. Regulations during survival without oxygen in infant mammals. *Respir Physiol* 7:356-368, 1969
136. Tomita M, Gotoh F, Maano T, Tanahashi N, Tanaka K. Low perfusion hyperemia following middle cerebral artery occlusion in cats of different age groups. *Stroke* 11:629-636, 1980.
137. Welsh FA. Role of vascular factors in regional ischemic injury. In: Kogure K, Hossman KA, Siesjo BK, Welsh, FA (Eds.), *Progress in Brain Research* Vol. 63. Elsevier, Amsterdam, 1985, pp. 19-28.
138. Brierley JB. Cerebral hypoxia. In: Blackwood W, Corsellis JAN (Eds.), *Greenfield's Neuropathology*, 3rd ed. Edward Arnold, London, 1976, pp. 43-85.
139. Kirino T. Delayed neuronal death in the gerbil hippocampus following ischemia. *Brain Res* 239:57-69, 1982.
140. Umbach C, Heiss WD, Traupe H. Effects of graded ischemia on functional coupling and components of somatosensory evoked potentials. *J Cereb Blood Flow Metab* 1 (Suppl 1):S198-S199, 1981.
141. Folbergrova J, Lowry OH, Passonneau JV. Changes in metabolites of energy reserves in individual layers of mouse cerebral cortex and subadjacent white matter during ischemia and anesthesia. *J Neurochem* 17: 1155-1162, 1970.
142. Pessin M, Lathi E, Cohen M, Kwan E, Hedges T, Caplan L. Clinical fea-

tures and mechanism of occipital infarction. *Ann Neurol* 21:290-299, 1900.
143. Caplan L, Hier D, D'Cruz I. Cerebral embolism in the Michael Reese Stroke Registry. *Stroke* 14:530-536, 1983.
144. Gross CR, Kase CS, Mohr J, et al. Stroke in South Alabama: incidence and diagnostic features–a population based study. *Stroke* 15:249-255, 1984.
145. Sherman D, Goldman L, Whiting R, Jurgensen K, Kaste M, Easton D. Thromboembolism in patients with atrial fibrillation. *Arch Neurol* 41:708-710, 1984.
146. Kopecky S, Gersh B, McGood M, et al. The natural history of lone atrial fibrillation. *N Engl J Med* 317:669-674, 1987.
147. Davis P, Dambrosia J, Schoenberg B, et al. Risk factors for ischemic stroke: a prospective study in Rochester, Minnesota. *Ann Neurol* 22:319-327, 1987.
148. Ishii H, Salem H, Bell C, Laposta E, Majerus P. Thrombomodulin, an endothelial anticoagulant protein, is absent from the human brain. *Blood* 67: 362-365, 1986.
149. Esmon C. The regulation of natural anticoagulant pathways. *Science* 235: 1348-1352, 1987.
150. Bauer K, Rosenberg R. The pathophysiology of the prethrombotic state in humans: insights gained from studies using markers of hemostatic system activation. *Blood* 70:343-350, 1987.
151. Fisher M. Platelet activation in patients with cerebral ischemia. *Ann Neurol* 22:115 1987.
152. Fisher M, Francis R. Altered coagulation in cerebral ischemia patients (abstract). *Thromb Haemost* 58:421, 1987.
153. Plum F. What causes infarction in ischemic brain. *Neurology* 33:222-233, 1983.
154. Hass W. The cerebral ischemic cascade. *Neurol. Clin* 1:345-353, 1983.
155. Kalimo H, Rehncrona S, Soderfeldt B, et al. Brain lactic acidosis and ischemic cell damage. 2. Histopathology. *J Cereb Blood Flow Metab* 1:313-327, 1981.
156. Pulsinelli W, Waldman S, Rawlinson D, Plum F. Moderate hyperglycemia augments ischemic brain damage: a neuropathologic study in the rat. *Neurology* 32:1230-1246, 1982.
157. Ginsberg M, Welsh F, Budd W. Deleterious effect of glucose pretreatment on recovery from diffuse cerebral ischemia in the cat. 1. Local cerebral blood flow and glucose utilization. *Stroke* 11:347-354, 1980.
158. Pulsinelli W, Kraig R, Plum F. Hyperglycemia, cerebral acidosis, and ischemic brain damage. In: Plum F, Pulsinelli W (Eds.), *Cerebrovascular Diseases*. Raven Press, New York, 1985, pp. 201–205.
159. Richards J, Cram D, Hammond G. *Elements of Organic Chemistry*. McGraw-Hill, New York, 1967, p. 66.
160. Murray R, Granner D, Mayes P. Rodwell V. *Harper's Biochemistry*. Appleton and Lange, Norwalk, CT, 1988, pp. 138-139.

161. McCord J. Oxygen-derived free radicals: a link between reperfusion injury and inflammation. *Fed Proc* 46:2402-2406, 1987.
162. Chan P, Fishman R. Free fatty acids, oxygen free radicals, and membrane alterations in brain ischemia and injury. In: Plum F, Pulsinelli W (Eds.), *Cerebrovascular Diseases*. Raven Press, New York, 1985, pp. 161-168.
163. Siesjo B, Wieloch T. Molecular mechanisms of ischemic brain damage: calcium-related events. In: Plum F, Pulsinelli W (Eds.), *Cerebrovascular Diseases*. Raven Press, New York, 1985, pp. 187-197.
164. Cotman C, Iversen L. Excitatory amino acids in the brain–focus on NMDA receptors. *Trends Neurosci* 10:263-265, 1987.
165. Benveniste H. Drejer J, Schousboe A, Diemer N. Elevation of the extracellular concentrations of glutamate and aspartate in rat hippocampus during transient cerebral ischemia monitored by intracerebral microdialysis. *J Neurochem* 43:1369-1374, 1984.
166. Simon R, Swan J, Griffiths T, Meldrum B. Blockade of *N*-methyl-*D*-aspartate receptors may protect against ischemic damage in the brain. *Science* 226:850-852, 1984.
167. Rothman S. Synaptic activity mediates death of hypoxic neurons. *Science* 220:536-537, 1983.
168. Globus M, Ginsberg M, Harik S, Busto R, Dietrich W. Role of dopamine in ischemic striatal injury: metabolic evidence. *Neurology* 37:1712-1719, 1987.

3

Hemorheological Aspects of Cerebral Ischemia

Mark Fisher and Herbert J. Meiselman
University of Southern California School of Medicine
Los Angeles, California

I. INTRODUCTION

Rheology is the science of the deformation and flow of materials; the terms "hemorheology" and "clinical hemorheology" are thus applied to studies of blood rheology and its clinical applications. In this chapter, we discuss some basic aspects of hemorheology and place them into the clinical context of the pathophysiology and treatment of cerebral vascular disease.

II. SOME BASIC SCIENCE CONSIDERATIONS IN HEMORHEOLOGY

Smooth fluid flow can be thought of as an infinite number of laminae sliding over each other. The properties of these laminae provide a definition of viscosity:

1. The force per unit area between adjacent laminae is termed shear stress.
2. The velocity gradient between adjacent laminae is the shear rate, which, in blood vessels of a given geometry, is directly proportional to velocity.
3. Viscosity, one of the major variables of clinical hemorheology (others include red cell aggregation and red cell deformability), is defined as the ratio of shear stress to shear rate.

Thus, viscosity is the "internal friction" exhibited by a fluid and is measured in either of two interchangeable units: the millipascal-second (mPas) or the centipoise (cP). Normal human blood is a non-Newtonian fluid, meaning that its viscosity is not constant with variation of shear rate; water, saline, and most plasmas are Newtonian. In vitro measurements, using mainly rotational viscometers, have demonstrated that at low rates of shear (less than 100-200/sec), the shear stress to shear rate ratio increases. Stated another way, the viscosity of normal blood (using rotational viscometers) increases with decreasing shear rates. In addition, a finite force (termed the "yield stress"), which increases as the third power of hematocrit and the square of fibrinogen concentration, is necessary to restart flow following a period of stasis. For whole blood or red cells in plasma, the non-Newtonian behavior and yield stress are due to fibrinogen-induced red blood cell (RBC) aggregation (i.e., rouleaux formation), an RBC-RBC interaction that is abolished at higher shear rates. At these higher rates of shear, blood viscosity tends to decrease with increasing shear rates up to approximately 1000/sec. This continued decrease in viscosity is attributed to increasing red cell deformation in this shear rate range (1) (Fig. 1).

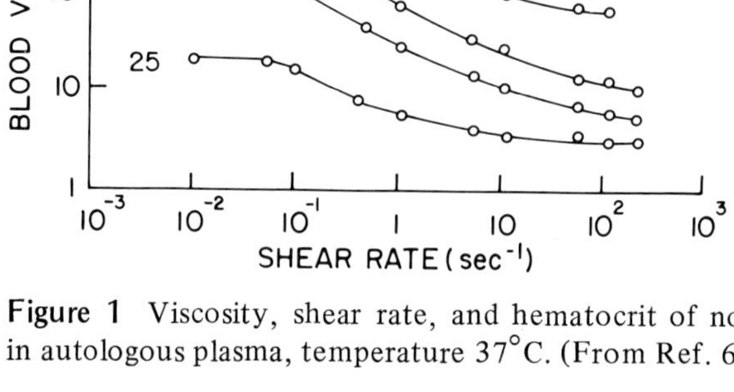

Figure 1 Viscosity, shear rate, and hematocrit of normal human erythrocytes in autologous plasma, temperature 37°C. (From Ref. 63).

Probably the most significant determinant of whole blood viscosity is hematocrit, with an approximately 4% increase in viscosity for each unit increase in hematocrit at shear rates above 10-50/sec. At lower shear rates, whole blood viscosity is even more sensitive to changes in hematocrit (e.g., a cubic function of hematocrit at very low rates of shear). Temperature is another variable affecting viscosity, with blood and plasma viscosity decreasing by 2-3% for each degree increase between 20°C and 37°C (1).

The above-mentioned "classic" description of the relationship between blood viscosity and shear rate is somewhat of an oversimplification, at least with respect to comparisons with in vivo phenomena. Blood samples examined by rotational viscometers are subjected to nearly uniform shear rates; in constrast, there is significant variation of shear rate within the vasculature and within a given blood vessel. For example, shear rate is maximal at the vessel wall; that is, the gradient between the velocity of the lamina of blood adjacent to the wall and the stationary wall itself is relatively high. At the center of the vessel (where blood flow velocity is maximal), adjacent lamina have rather similar velocities, resulting in a relatively small rate of shear. This variation of shear rate in blood vessels has the potential for causing migration of red cells toward the vessel center (where shear rate is lowest), thereby resulting in a cell-poor layer adjacent to the vessel wall. Under specific experimental conditions, measurements of blood viscosity in vertical tubes have demonstrated decreasing viscosity with diminishing shear rate; such an effect is due to increased axial migration of red cell aggregates and the formation of a low-viscosity layer at the tube wall (2).

As noted above, reversible RBC-RBC aggregation is a key phenomenon of hemorheology. Aggregation of red cells is due to adsorption of macromolecules to the surfaces of adjacent cells. Under normal physiological circumstances, fibrinogen molecules provide the major intercellular link; these interactions are rather weak and can be easily disrupted by increasing shear rates. This fibrinogen bridging does not appear to be receptor-mediated; the adsorption is nonspecific, lacks competitive inhibitors, and increases linearly with fibrinogen concentration. In addition to fibrinogen, other large molecules, including alpha$_2$ macroglobulin and immunoglobulins, may induce aggregation. In a suspending medium lacking these large proteins, macromolecules of appropriate size can also induce RBC aggregation; dextran is the most extensively studied substance in this experimental context (3).

The physiological significance of red cell aggregation is presently not completely clear. Aggregation may lead to erythrocyte migration away from the vessel wall, thereby increasing interactions between leukocytes or platelets and the endothelium. Additionally, red cell aggregates could block microcirculatory flow or alter RBC flux through a microcirculatory bed, particularly in the presence of hyperfibrinogenemia; increased fibrinogen levels produce red cell aggregates that are markedly shear rate resistant. Note, however, that in vivo experimental evidence to support these suggestions has yet to be demonstrated (4).

It is difficult to exactly ascertain the shear rates corresponding to in vivo blood flow, although venous flow has been characterized as having values below 50/sec. while arteries are felt to have values greater than 100/sec. In addition, shear rates may vary across vessel bifuractions or at other regions of irregular flow (i.e., near valves). Shear rates in the microcirculation are even more difficult to assess, since flow may be intermittent and the calculation of a true shear rate is difficult in capillary-size vessels (1).

Erythrocyte deformability, while difficult to precisely define, may be conceptualized as the resistance the cell offers to a change in its shape. Normal blood flow requires red cell deformation, since portions of the microcirculation contain blood vessels 3-4 μm in diameter, while the resting red cell diameter is 8 μm. In small-geometry systems (i.e., capillaries), RBC deformation permits red blood cells to enter and traverse these smaller vessels of the microcirculation. In large geometries (i.e., large vessels and in vitro viscometers), RBC deformation allows cells to become ellipsoid, with the major axis of the cells aligned with the flow, consequently reducing blood viscosity (5).

The deformation of erythrocytes depends on their intrinsic deformability as well as extrinsic deforming forces. The intrinsic deformability of an RBC is determined by three major factors: (1) geometric considerations, including the ratio of membrane surface area to cell volume (e.g., the decrease in surface/volume ratio induced by hypotonic media reduces deformability) and the shape of the erythrocyte (e.g., echinocytic or stomatocytic shape changes reduce deformability); (2) internal fluid viscosity, i.e., the viscosity of the hemoglobin-rich intracellular fluid; and (3) the viscoelastic mechanical properties of the membrane itself. The latter appears to be due, in large part, to the interconnected proteins spectrin (on the inner membrane surface) and glycophorin (spanning the entire membrane thickness). Extrinsic factors influencing erythrocyte deformation include interactions between the membrane and the surrounding media (i.e., the local shear stress), transmembrane pressure, and other physiochemical interactions (5).

While most hemorheological research has involved studies of RBC or blood rheology, there is increasing interest in the rheology of white blood cells (WBCs). In contrast to their appearance on dried blood smears, neutrophils in suspension have a diameter averaging 8.7 μm and thus have a size comparable to the resting diameter of the RBCs. The cell volume of neutrophils is, however, two to three times greater than that of the erythrocyte. Activation of granulocytes and pseudopod formation results in stiff WBCs, but even without activation, WBCs have a low deformability; the entry time of a neutrophil into a capillary is approximately three orders of magnitude greater than that of an RBC. Within a small vessel, leukocytes move more slowly than the RBCs; consequences of this slower movement include accumulation of erythrocytes proximal to granulocytes and the development of a distal cell-poor region. Granulocytes commonly attach to postcapillary venules, particularly when they are activated; as a consequence, activated granulocytes, especially those with large pseudopods, are not commonly encountered in the circulating blood (6).

III. BIORHEOLOGICAL FACTORS IN THE PATHOGENESIS OF CEREBRAL ISCHEMIA

In some respects, hemorheological investigation offers a unique opportunity for theory building in the field of cerebral vascular disease. While most experimental work in stroke has focused on the consequences of acute vascular occlusion, there has been far less attention focused on the underlying intravascular events that produce cerebral ischemia. The essential similarity between the neuropathology of experimental models of focal cerebral ischemia and human cerebral infarction is widely accepted, and justifiably so. It is far from clear, however, that acute occulsion of one or more vessels supplying the brain of an experimental animal represents an adequate analogy for vascular processes preceding human cerebral infarction.

Some of the most important rheological studies relevant to cerebral vascular disease are those that have examined scale models of arteries, particularly arterial bifurcations (7). One of the major findings of these studies is that the region immediately downstream (or distal) to a protrusion into the vessel lumen has a relatively stagnant "recirculation zone" where flow is irregular and both shear stresses and shear rates are low (Fig. 2) (7). This suggests that these regions are predisposed to intravascular thrombosis due to retarded convective transport of procoagulants (i.e., coagulation factors and platelets) away from this low-shear region. Placed into a clinical context, these findings suggest, for example, some underlying rheological similarities between "watershed" infarcts and infarction occurring in a more proximal arterial territory. Specifically, one can argue that the distal regions supplied by two or more major arteries (the watershed) are, when associated with an upstream hemodynamically significant stenosis, regions of particularly low shear rate and, consequently, areas at substantial risk for intravascular thrombosis. Thus, occlusion of these distal regions could occur without extensive arterial disease in the region of the watershed. In contrast, thrombotic occlusion of proximal arteries probably requires local arterial disease to create the recirculation zone that, from a hemorheological perspective, has some resemblance to the watershed.

Delineation of rheological features of arterial bifurcations also contributes importantly to an understanding of carotid atherogenesis. Scale models of the carotid bifurcation have demonstrated the recirculation zone of low shear rate and shear stress at the area opposite the arterial divider (8,9). The determinants

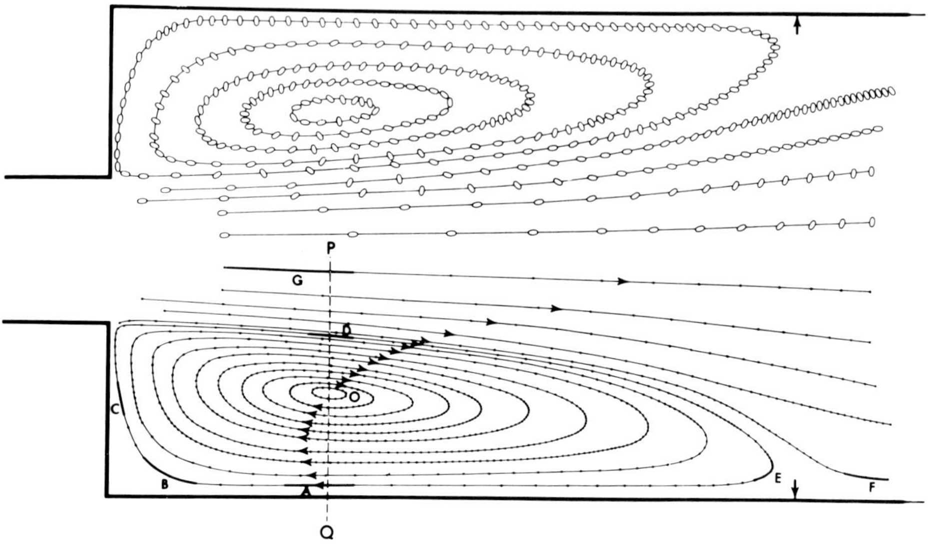

Figure 2 Stagnant recirculation zone (or vortex) just distal to protrusion into vascular lumen. Flow streamlines are shown in the lower half of the diagram (*PQ*) while red cell orientations are in the top half. Linear velocities increase in the sequence *O–A–B–C–D–E–F–G*. The mainstream is pushed away from the wall, in association with the vortex formation. Arrows demonstrate reattachment points of the mainstream. (From Ref. 7.)

of the recirculation zone consists of (1) the ratio of the diameter of the "daughter" to the "parent" artery, with a larger ratio associated with an increased recirculation zone; (2) the bifurcation angle (the angle between the two daughter arteries), with a larger angle associated with an increased recirculation zone; and (3) the radius of curvature of the outer wall of the artery, with a larger radius of curvature indicating a "gentle" bend of the artery and a smaller recirculation zone. The recirculation zone is consistently found on the lateral wall of the larger of the two daughter arteries (8,9) (Fig. 3). These rheological results accurately predict the pathological finding that early atherosclerotic lesions of the carotid bifurcation develop on the posterior wall of the internal carotid artery, i.e., the lateral wall of the larger of the two branches of the common carotid. An additional finding of interest involves tissue culture of endothelial cells, an experimental system in which it has been demonstrated that the rate of cell division is proportional to the variability in shear stresses to which cells are subjected (10). The recirculation zone is notable for these variations, and this experimental finding represents an additional explanation for the topography of carotid atherogenesis.

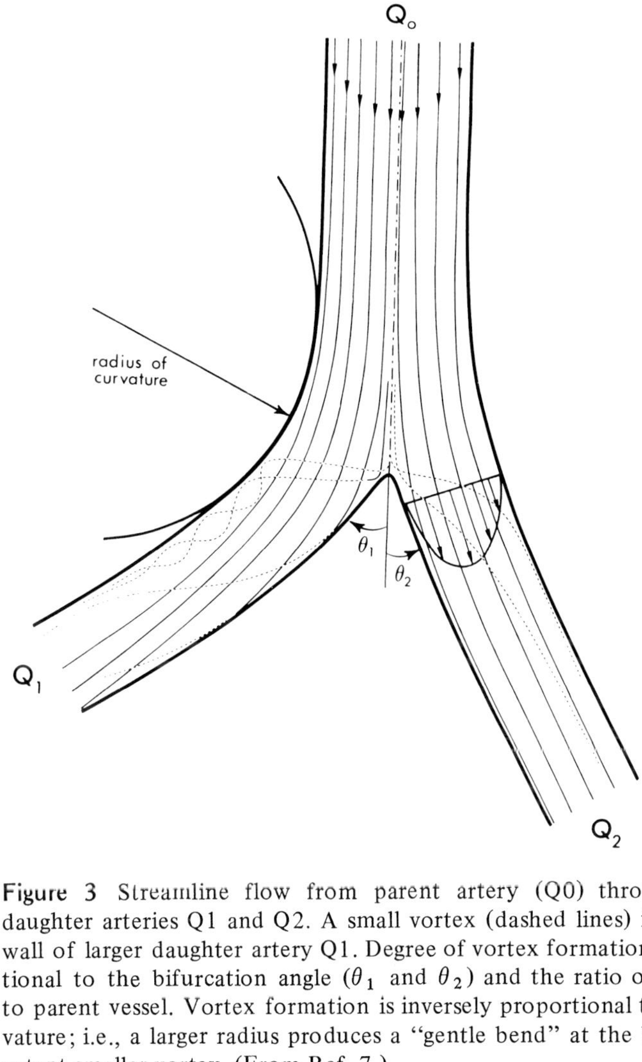

Figure 3 Streamline flow from parent artery (Q0) through bifurcation to daughter arteries Q1 and Q2. A small vortex (dashed lines) forms on the lateral wall of larger daughter artery Q1. Degree of vortex formation is directly proportional to the bifurcation angle (θ_1 and θ_2) and the ratio of areas of daughter to parent vessel. Vortex formation is inversely proportional to the radius of curvature; i.e., a larger radius produces a "gentle bend" at the bifurcation with resutant smaller vortex. (From Ref. 7.)

The significance of hemorheology in stroke appears to be closely related to another issue: the importance of thrombosis in the pathogenesis of human cerebral infarction. It seems likely that interactions between hemorheological and coagulation factors may lead to infarction. An observation favoring this scenario comes from the United Kingdom Aspirin Trial: Hemoglobin level did not predict cerebral infarction when the data analysis was performed on all patients at study entry. However, among the placebo group, high hemoglobin levels were significantly associated with an outcome of cerebral infarction, while no such association was found for the aspirin-treated patients (11). The implication seems clear: Cerebral infarction associated with hemorheological abnormalities is probably mediated through the coagulation system.

There is, in fact, a broad body of evidence indicating substantial interaction between the hemorheological and hemostasis systems. Perhaps the first piece of evidence in this regard was the observation that bleeding time increases in the presence of anemia (12). In addition, the structure of thrombi are dependent on shear rate: the "red thrombi" typical of veins, so called because they predominantly consist of erythrocytes in a fibrin network, are found in areas of low shear rate, whereas the "white thrombi," often noted in the arterial system, are dominated by platelets and contain far less fibrin and erythrocytes. Note that the work of Baumgartner and colleagues has demonstrated that high shear rates favor the formation of this latter kind of thrombus (13).

A number of experiments have focused on the rheological interactions between platelets and erythrocytes. During normal blood flow, erythrocytes tend to be concentrated at the vessel center, with the highest concentration of platelets at the periphery of the lumen. This minimizes the velocity of platelets in the blood stream, allowing greater potential interaction with the vessel wall (14). Platelet-vessel wall interactions are dependent, in part, on intercellular collisions between platelets (platelet-platelet) and between erythrocytes and platelets. Increasing hematocrit tends to increase diffusion of platelets toward the vessel wall, resulting in enhanced platelet-wall interactions (i.e., adhesion); the latter phenomenon is receptor-mediated and requires von Willebrand factor. Platelet adhesion also tends to increase as erythrocyte deformability decreases and as vessel shear rate and red cell size increase (14).

Reversible and irreversible platelet-platelet interactions (i.e., platelet aggregation) are also receptor-mediated, requiring the glycoprotein IIb-IIIa complex on the platelet surface. Fibrinogen is the major intercellular bridge between aggregated platelets, linking them at the receptor site. Thus, this fibrinogen effect represents another similarity with hemorheological phenomena, because, as noted above, the fibrinogen molecule also functions as a link for erythrocytes. Platelet aggregation, like adhesion, tends to increase with increasing shear rates. The most likely mechanism for this is shear-rate-dependent release of ADP from erythrocytes (14).

While the effects of altered blood viscosity and red cell aggregation are likely to be mediated via coagulation pathways, there remain other ways in which hemorheological factors may have pathogenic significance in cerebral ischemia. The most likely possibility involves capillary plugging by erythrocytes or leukocytes. Reduction of erythrocyte deformability can be thought of as primary or secondary; in this context, "primary" refers to deformability changes preceding ischemia, while secondary deformability changes are those occurring in association with an ischemic episode. Using the technique of centrifugal deformation (15), we have been unable to demonstrate reduction in erythrocyte deformability either acutely following a cerebral ischemic episode or 2 months later. Other studies of red cell deformability in stroke patients have used filtration devices: Lorient-Roudaut and colleagues reported diminished filterability of red cells but did not use an age- and sex-matched control group for data analysis (16); Pollock and Harrison, using such a control group, found no abnormalities in red cell filtration in stroke and TIA patients (17). It thus appears that primary changes in erythrocyte deformability are unlikely.

Erythrocyte deformability is reduced under ischemic conditions for reasons that are not entirely clear but probably include inactivation of an outward-directed "calcium pump" that uses ATP as an energy source and contributes to the low calcium concentration normally found in erythrocytes (18). A consequence of an increase in calcium ions within red cells is abnormal cross-linking of spectrin by a calcium-activated transaminase, thus most likely resulting in reduced erythrocyte deformability. Calcium channels of the erythrocyte membrane also regulate erythrocyte calcium concentration; flunarizine, a calcium channel antagonist, can inhibit the reduction of erythrocyte deformability induced by calcium ionophores in the presence of the calcium ion (19). It is of interest to note that nimodipine, another of the calcium channel blockers, has been shown to improve outcome in patients with aneurysmal subarachnoid hemorrhage, presumably by ameliorating the effects of cerebral vasospasm. In the landmark study on nimodipine and subarachnoid hemorrhage, average plasma concentrations of nimodipine were within one-quarter of the inhibitory concentration required for RBC calcium channel blockade (20). Thus, given interpatient variability of absorption and metabolism, it seems quite possible that plasma nimodipine concentrations capable of improving RBC deformability under ischemic conditions were achieved.

Recent investigations suggest that capillary plugging by leukocytes has profound importance in the pathogenesis of myocardial infarction (21). It is also quite likely that leukocyte rheology is of significant importance in the pathogenesis of cerebral infarction. In a series of experiments on myocardial ischemia, Schmid-Schonbein, Engler, and co-workers (21,22) have demonstrated that

1. The "no-reflow" phenomenon (i.e., impairment of postischemic reperfusion) can be due to capillary obstruction alone without involvement of larger vessels.
2. This obstruction is leukocytic, largely granulocytic, in origin.
3. Granulocytic influx and accumulation in capillaries continues during the first 3 hours following ischemia.
4. Erythrocytes accumulate proximal to the granulocyte plug, resulting in an increase in capillary hematocrit from the normal level of 20% up to 80%.

only limited relevance for the cerebral vasculature, which has a capacity for dilatation as part of the autoregulatory process. Despite the initial studies suggesting that whole blood viscosity and its determinants might substantially regulate cerebral blood flow (40,41), later investigations have demonstrated that neither whole blood nor plasma viscosity have major effects on cerebral blood flow. The low cerebral blood flow in polycythemia can be explained by the increased arterial oxygen content in that syndrome. Indeed, oxygen content, rather than viscosity, appears to have a major effect on cerebral blood flow regulation (42, 43).

V. HEMORHEOLOGY AND STROKE: EXPERIMENTAL AND CLINICAL INVESTIGATIONS

Experimental investigations of hemorheology and stroke have focused on two interrelated issues: (1) the relationship between blood viscosity and cerebral blood flow and (2) the relationship between blood viscosity and cerebral oxygen delivery. The first question has been addressed in far greater detail than the second. While there have been few studies that have directly measured viscosity in relation to cerebral blood flow, the overwhelming consensus is that there is an inverse relationship between "predictors" of viscosity, i.e., hematocrit and fibrinogen concentration, and cerebral blood flow in humans (2,41). These observations have been translated into therapeutic attempts to use hemodilution to increase blood flow associated with cerebral ischemia. A number of studies in experimental animals by Wood and colleagues have yielded the following results:

1. Following hypervolemic hemodilution with autologous plasma, there is an inverse correlation between cerebral blood flow and whole blood viscosity in both ischemic and nonischemic regions of the brain (44,45).
2. Intravascular volume expansion without hemodilution is not associated with increased blood flow (46).
3. Hypervolemic infusions of low molecular weight dextran can increase regional cerebral blood flow in areas of focal ischemia (47,48).
4. Infarct volume, following ligation of distal internal carotid and proximal middle cerebral arteries, may be reduced by as much as 60% if animals have plasma volume increased by 40% using low molecular weight dextran (47,48).

These and similar experimental findings have been extrapolated to the clinical setting, with the aim of reducing ischemic neurological injury by hemodilution following symptoms of stroke. A number of assumptions underlie such extrapolations. Before reviewing the clinical evidence to date, it may be useful to examine these assumptions:

1. Diminution of cerebral blood flow associated with ischemia is associated with focal increases in viscosity that contribute to further declines in regional blood flow.
2. Such a vicious cycle means that there is a progressive decline in blood flow, occurring over a sufficiently long period of time as to allow reversal by hemodilution.
3. Hemodilution will result in increased regional blood flow, which will in turn improve oxygen delivery to ischemic regions of the brain.
4. Most stroke patients have hematocrit that is "too high," so that reduction of hematocrit to an "optimal" range will improve brain oxygenation.

Careful analysis of these points raises a number of difficult questions. First, the consequences of low shear rate on blood viscosity in vivo are not necessarily those that follow from in vitro measurements (see above). Thus, it is by no means clear that the low shear rates associated with focal cerebral ischemia will consistently lead to focal increases in blood viscosity. Second, since the overwhelming majority of stroke patients present with nonprogressive symptoms, is it reasonable to assume that progressive diminution of cerebral blood flow in a substantial group of stroke patients? Third, even if hemodilution does increase cerebral blood flow, there is little evidence that this will increase brain oxygenation: Vasodilatory reserve is negligible under ischemic conditions, negating a potential compensatory mechanism for the reduced oxygen-carrying capacity associated with lowered hematocrit (2). Finally, the delineation of "optimal hematocrit" for stroke patients is highly controversial. Initial studies have suggested that the optimal hematocrit, i.e., the hematocrit at which oxygen delivery to the brain is maximal, is 33% (49,50). However, another investigation has suggested that the optimal hematocrit is 42% under normal conditions, and even higher during ischemia (51). If the latter study proves correct, it may be that, at least for purposes of oxygen delivery, the typical stroke patient (mean hematocrit = 42.0 ± 5.0%) (35) is already at an optimal hematocrit.

VI. CLINICAL TRIALS OF HEMORHEOLOGICAL THERAPY IN STROKE

Clinical trials of hemorheological therapy in stroke have used dextran, hemodilution, ancrod, and pentoxifylline, alone or in combination; the most commonly utilized agent is low-molecular-weight dextran (typically dextran 40 or Rheomacrodex). Dextran has been extensively studied for its hemorheological properties, which consist of a reduction of whole blood viscosity via expansion of plasma volume (i.e., decreased hematocrit) and decrease of red cell aggregation due to plasma dilution as well as to more specific effects (52). Matthews et al. (53) have reported a careful, single-blind study of dextran 40 in stroke patients, in which 100 patients were randomized to dextran or placebo within 48 hours of stroke onset; hemorrhagic stroke was ruled out by lumbar puncture, and follow-up was for up to 6 months. Intravenous therapy consisted of 500 ml of dextran 40 in 5% dextrose every 12 hours for a total of 72 hours; the placebo group received similar infusions of 5% dextrose. Data analysis revealed no benefit of dextran for the group of stroke patients taken as a whole. When the patients were divided into those with severe deficits and those with less severe deficits, there was a significant reduction in mortality for the dextran-treated group. However, the subgroup of dextran-treated survivors of severe stroke had severe neurological disability; only one of the 12 such survivors was functioning independently 6 months poststroke. There was no difference in the disability between dextran-treated and placebo-treated survivors of severe stroke. Note that the major limitations of this study were (1) the imprecision in excluding intracerebral hemorrhage (the study was performed before computerized tomography was routinely used); (2) the use of a hypotonic dextrose solution, which may have actually exacerbated cerebral edema, as the "placebo"; (3) the delay in instituting therapy for up to 48 hours poststroke; and (4) the lack of any measurements of hemorheology variables. These limitations notwithstanding, the study offers little encouragement for the use of dextran alone as a treatment for stroke.

Later studies have used dextran in combination with other therapies. Frei et al. (54) performed a randomized, double-blind trial of dextran and glycerol versus glycerol alone and versus placebo. Glycerol, a hyperosmolar agent with some antiedema qualities, has been shown by Bayer and co-workers (55) to reduce mortality (at 1 year, 58% for glycerol versus 77% for placebo) without affecting neurological morbidity in a group of elderly (mean age 78 years) stroke patients. However, in the study of Frei et al. (54), neither the dextran-glycerol combination nor glycerol alone was better than placebo; in this study, outcome was measured by neurological disability up to 24 weeks poststroke. In attempting to resolve the differences between the two studies (54,55), it is apparent that the Frei study evaluated a more "typical" group of stroke patients, with an average age approximately 10 years younger than the Bayer et al. study and a 6-month mortality of 16%. The Frei study is not without its own limitations, the most serious of which is that the exact time limit for initiation of therapy is unclear (probably 54 hours). Nevertheless, there is little support for the dextran-glycerol combination or glycerol alone.

The most ambitious study of hemorheological therapy in stroke comes from the Scandinavian Stroke Study Group (56), which, in a multicenter trial, randomized 373 patients to treatment with either hemodilution or placebo. Therapy began within 48 hours of stroke onset, and the hemodilution protocol consisted of venesection of 250-1000 ml of whole blood during the first 2 days of treatment and daily infusion of 500 ml of low-molecular-weight dextran over the first 5 days of therapy. There was no demonstrable benefit by hemodilution on morbidity or mortality at 3 months poststroke. Criticisms of this study, as the authors themselves readily concede, include the 48-hour window for entering patients, along with the relatively leisurely hemodilution protocol, with peak reduction of hematocrit (to 37.1%) at day 5 of the trial. Both points are debatable: 67% of all entered patients had treatment beginning within 24 hours of stroke onset, and the treated patients had more than twice as many cardiac complications attributable to volume overload than the placebo group had. While perhaps not definitive, this study offers no encouragement for hemodilution therapy.

Two additional hemodilution studies have not provided encouragement for the use of hemodilution monotherapy. The Italian Acute Stroke Study Group evaluated isovolemic hemodilution (venesection with dextran 40 infusion) in stroke patients within 12 hours of stroke onset. 1266 patients were randomized to a control or a hemodilution group, the latter having mean hematocrit decreased from 43% to 37% after 48 hours. After 6 months, there was no significant difference in morbidity and mortality between the two groups (57). A more aggressive protocol used hypervolemic hemodilution with pentastarch to lower hematocrit rapidly to 33%. Patients with under 24 hours of acute ischemic stroke were randomized to this hemodilution protocol or a control group. There was a trend toward improved morbidity in the treatment group, but this was not statistically significant. However, the treatment group had increased mortality associated with cerebral edema (58).

Three additional clinical trials are worthy of note here. Hossman et al. (59) studied the viper venom enzyme ancrod, an enzyme that degrades fibrinogen. A group of 30 patients with cerebral infarction were randomly allocated to 5 days of treatment consisting of subcutaneous ancrod plus low-molecular-weight dextran plus mannitol or dextran plus mannitol alone. While the small number of patients made it difficult to reach a statistically significant conclusion, there was a trend toward faster recovery and reduced mortality at 12 months in the ancrod-treated group. Ancrod was capable of safely reducing whole blood viscosity by 30% in conjunction with a reduction of fibrinogen concentration from 267 to 100 mg/dl; this provocative study was followed by a study of 20 patients randomized to ancrod or placebo. While the initial ancrod study followed patients admitted to a hospital up to 48 hours poststroke, this latter study evaluated patients treated within 12 hours of stroke onset. The treated patients had a significantly better neurological outcome at 3 months (60). Finally, pentoxifyllin, a purported hemorheological agent that perhaps reduces erythrocyte deformability, was demonstrably ineffective in a double-blind, placebo-controlled trial of 297 patients with cerebral infarction in which therapy began within 15 hours poststroke (61).

Viewed collectively, the above-mentioned trials do not support the routine use of hemorheological therapy as a monotherapy for stroke. However, several points emerge from these studies that should be and are being taken into consideration for current and future investigations. First, low-molecular-weight dextran should be eliminated from hemorheology protocols: there is ample evidence that it is ineffective, and, in addition, experimental observations suggest that repeated infusions of low-molecular-weight dextran may result in increased plasma viscosity due to the retention of higher-molecular-weight dextrans (62). Second, stroke protocols should probably focus on those subsets of stroke patients who are more likely to respond to hemorheological therapy. These subsets include stroke-in-evolution patients (where progressive diminution of cerebral blood flow is suspected). Third, the lag time for therapeutic intervention should be kept to less than 24 hours from the time of stroke onset, and probably to less than 12 hours. Fourth, hemorheological therapy needs to be studied in combination with other stroke therapies to determine if a synergistic effect may be present; such therapies include recanalization attempts (i.e., fibrinolysis or angioplasty) and calcium channel antagonists.

VII. CONCLUSIONS

The science of hemorheology provides information from which useful theories can be derived regarding the pathogenesis of cerebral vascular disease. For example, hemorheological factors help to explain the topography of carotid atherogenesis. Most important, interactions between hemorheology and the coagulation system may explain such diverse phenomena as the efficacy of aspirin in stroke prevention an the pathophysiology of watershed infarcts. In contrast, the importance of hemorheology in the regulation of cerebral blood flow has probably been overestimated. The most important remaining question regarding hemorheology and stroke is the issue of hemorheological therapy. While initial clinical trials of hemorheological monotherapy have not, with the exception of ancrod, been encouraging, hope persists that combination (i.e., hemorheological plus another) therapy for suitable subgroups of cerebral infarction patients will prove efficacious.

Supported in part by Teacher-Investigator Development Award K07 NS 884 (Fisher) and NIH research grants NS20989, HL15722, and HL15162.

REFERENCES

1. Stuart J, Kenny M. Blood rheology. *J Clin Pathol* 33:417-429, 1980.
2. Gaehtgens P, Marx P. Hemorheological aspects of the pathophysiology of cerebral ischemia. *J Cereb Blood Flow* 7:259–265, 1987.
3. Meiselman H, Merrill E, Salzman E, et al. The effect of dextran on the rheology of human blood. *J Appl Physiol* 22:480-486, 1967.

4. Brooks D, Evans E. Rheology of blood cells. In: Chien S, Dormandy J, Ernst E, Matrai A (Eds.), *Clinical Hemorheology*. Martinus Nijhoff, Dordrecht, 1987, pp. 73-96.
5. Chien S. Principles and techniques for assessing erythrocyte deformability. *Blood Cells* 3:71-99, 1977.
6. Schmid-Schonbein G. Capillary plugging by granulocytes and the no-reflow phenomenon in the microcirculation. *Fed Proc* 46:2397-2401, 1987.
7. Goldsmith H, Turitto V. Rheologic aspects of thrombosis and haemostasis: basic principles and applications. *Thromb Haemost* 55:415-435, 1986.
8. Zarins C, Giddens D, Bharadvaj B, Scottiural V, Mabon R, Glagov S. Carotid bifurcation atherosclerosis: quantitative correlation of plaque localization with flow velocity profiles and wall shear stress. *Circ Res* 53:502-514, 1983.
9. Karino T, Goldsmith H. Particle flow behavior in models of branching vessels: effects of branching angle and diameter ratio on flow patterns. *Biorheology* 22:87-104, 1985.
10. Davies P, Gimbrone M, Gordon E, Remuzzi A, Dewey C. Structural and functional responses of vascular endothelial cells to shear flow in vitro. *Biorheology* 23:195, 1987.
11. Thomas DJ. The influence of hematocrit on the cerebral circulation in man. *Clin Hemorheol* 7(Suppl):346S, 1987.
12. Duke W. The relation of blood platelets to haemorrhagic disease. *JAMA* 60:1185-1192, 1910.
13. Baumgartner H. The role of blood flow in platelet adhesion, fibrin deposition, and formation of mural thrombi. *Microvasc Res* 5:167-179, 1973.
14. Lowe G. Thrombosis and hemorheology. In: Chien S, Dormandy J. Ernst E, Matrai A (Eds.), *Clinical Hemorheology*. Martinus Nijhoff, Dordrecht, 1987, pp. 194-226.
15. Corry W, Meiselman H. Centrifugal method of determining red cell deformability. *Blood* 51:693-701, 1978.
16. Loreint-Roudaut M, Manuau J, Bricaud H, Boisseau M. Filterability and cerebro-vascular thrombosis. *Scand J Clin Lab Invest* 41(Suppl 156):203-208, 1981.
17. Pollock S, Harrison M. Red cell deformability is not an independent risk factor in stroke. *J Neurol Neurosurg Psychiatry* 45:369-371, 1982.
18. Van Neuten J, DeClerck F. Vascular reactivity and calcium entry blockers. *Adv Cyclic Nucl Protein Phosph Res* 17:575-583, 1984.
19. Striessnij J, Zernig G, Glossman H. Human red blood cell Ca-antagonist binding sites. *Eur J Biochem* 150:67-77, 1985.
20. Allen G, Ahn H, Preziosi T. Cerebral arterial spasm in a controlled trial of nimodipine in patients with subarachnoid hemorrhage. *N Engl J Med* 308: 619-624, 1983.
21. Engler R, Schmid-Schonbein G, Pavelec R. Leukocyte capillary plugging in myocardial ischemia and reperfusion in the dog. *Am J Pathol* 111:98-111, 1983.

22. Engler R. Consequences of activation and adenosine-mediated inhibition of granulocytes during myocardial ischemia. *Fed Proc* 46:2407-2412, 1987.
23. Hallenbeck J. Dutka A, Tanishima T, et al. Polymorphonuclear leukocyte accumulation in brain regions with low blood flow during the early post-ischemic period. *Stroke* 17:246-253, 1986.
24. Kochanek P, Dutka A, Hallenbeck J. Indomethacin, prostacyclin, and heparin improve postischemic cerebral blood flow without affecting early post-ischemic granulocyte accumulation. *Stroke* 18:634-637, 1987.
25. Kannel W, Gordon T, Wolf P, et al. Hemoglobin and the risk of cerebral infarction: the Framingham study. *Stroke* 3:409-419, 1972.
26. Tohgi H, Yamanouchi H, Murakami M, Kameyama M. Importance of the hematocrit as a risk factor in cerebral infarction. *Stroke* 9:369-374, 1978.
27. Kiyohara Y, Ueda K, Hasuo Y, et al. Hematocrit as a risk factor of cerebral infarction: long-term prospective population survey in a Japanese rural community. *Stroke* 17:687-692, 1986.
28. Welin L, Svardsudd K. Wilhelmsen L, Larsson B, Tibblin G. Analysis of risk factors for stroke in a cohort of men born in 1913. *N Engl J Med* 317:521-526, 1987.
29. Wade JPH, Taylor DW, Barnett HJM, Hachinski VC. Hemoglobin concentration and prognosis in symptomatic obstructive cerebrovascular disease. *Stroke* 18:68-71, 1987.
30. Wilhelmsen L, Svardsudd K, Korsan-Bengtsen K, Larsson B, Welin L, Tibblin C. Fibrinogen as a risk factor for stroke and myocardial infarction. *N Engl J Med* 311:501-505, 1984.
31. Prentice RL, Szatrowski TP, Kato H, Mason MW. Leukocyte counts and cerebrovascular disease. *J Chronic Dis* 35:703-714, 1982.
32. Eisenberg S. Blood viscosity and fibrinogen following cerebral infarction. *Circulation* 33(Suppl II):10-14, 1966.
33. Lechner H, Ott E, Ossama N, Fazekas F. Follow-up studies of the haemorheologic profile in acute ischaemic stroke. *Clin Hemorheol* 6:3-9, 1986.
34. Coull B, Beamer N, Seaman G. Physiochemical risk factors in stroke. *Clin Hemorheol* 6:17-33, 1986.
35. Fisher M, Meiselman H. Hemorheological abnormalities in acute cerebral ischemia. In: Hartmann A, Kuschinsky W (Eds.), *Cerebral Ischemia and Hemorheology*. Springer-Verlag, New York, 1987, pp. 445-451.
36. Ionescu D, Ghitescu M, Marcu I, Xenakis A. Erythrocyte rheology in acute cerebral thrombosis: Effects of ABO blood groups. *Blut* 39:351-357, 1979.
37. Pouzzilli C, Lenzi G, Argentino C, Bozzao L, et al. Peripheral white blood cell count in cerebral ischemic infarction. *Acta Neurol Scand* 71:396-400, 1985.
38. Lowe G, Jaap A, Forbes C. Relation of atrial fibrillation and high haematocrit to mortality in acute stroke. *Lancet* 1:784-786, 1983.
39. Thomas D, Du Boulay G, Marshall J, et al. Cerebral blood flow in polycythemia. *Lancet* 2:161-163, 1977.

40. Thomas D, Du Boulay G, Marshall J, et al. Effect of haematocrit on cerebral blood flow in man. *Lancet* 2:941-943, 1977.
41. Grotta J, Ackerman R, Correia J, Fallick G, Chang J. Whole blood viscosity parameters and cerebral blood flow. *Stroke* 13:296-301, 1982.
42. Brown M, Wade J, Marshall J. Fundamental importance of oxygen content in the regulation of cerebral blood flow in man. *Brain* 108:81-93, 1985.
43. Brown M, Marshall J. Regulation of cerebral blood flow in response to changes in blood viscosity. *Lancet* 1:604-609, 1985.
44. Wood J, Simeone F, Kron R, Synder L. Experimental hypervolemic hemodilution: Physiological correlations of cortical blood flow, cardiac output, and intracranial pressure with fresh blood viscosity and plasma volume. *Neuorsurgery* 14:709-723, 1984.
45. Kee D, Wood J. Influence of blood rheology on cerebral circulation. In: Wood J (Ed.), *Cerebral Blood Flow: Physiologic and Clinical Aspects*. McGraw-Hill, New York, 1987, pp. 173-185.
46. Wood J, Simeone F, Synder L. Failure of intravascular volume expansion without hemodilution to elevate cortical blood flow in region of experimental focal ischemia. *J Neurosurg* 56:80-91, 1982.
47. Wood J, Simeone F, Fink E, Golden M. Hypervolemic hemodilution in experimental focal cerebral ischemia: elevations of cardiac output, regional cortical blood flow, and ICP after intravascular volume expansion with low molecular weight dextran. *J Neurosurg* 59:500-509, 1983.
48. Wood J, Simeone F, Fink E, Golden M. Correlative aspects of hypervolemic hemodilution with low-molecular weight dextran after experimental cerebral arterial occlusion. *Neurology* 34:24-34, 1984.
49. Messmer K, Gornandt L, Jesch F, Sinagowitz E, Sunder-Plassmann L, Kessler M. Oxygen transport and tissue oxygenation during hemodilution with dextran. *Adv Exp Med Biol* 37:669-680, 1980.
50. Gottstein U. Normovolemic and hypervolemic hemodilution in cerebrovascular ischemia. *Bibl Haematol* 47:127-138, 1981.
51. Gaehtgens P, Kreutz F, Albrecht K. Optimal hematocrit for canine skeletal muscle during rhythmic isotonic exercise. *Eur J Appl Physiol* 41:27-39, 1979.
52. Gelin L-E, Ingleman B. Rheomacrodex–a new dextran solution for rheological treatment of impaired capillary flow. *Acta Chir Scand* 122:294-302, 1961.
53. Matthews W, Oxbury J, Grainger K, Greenhall R. A blind controlled trial of dextran 40 in the treatment of ischemic stroke. *Brain* 99:193-206, 1976.
54. Frei A, Cottier C, Wunderlich P, Ludin E. Glycerol and dextran combined in the therapy of ischemic stroke. *Stroke* 18:373-379, 1987.
55. Bayer A, Pathy M, Newcombe R. Double-blind randomized trial of intravenous glycerol in acute stroke. *Lancet* 1:405-408, 1987.
56. Scandinavian Stroke Study Group. Multicenter trial of hemodilution in acute ischemic stroke. *Stroke* 18:691–699, 1987.
57. Italian Acute Stroke Study Group. The Italian hemodilution trial in acute stroke. *Stroke* 19:145, 1988.

58. Hemodilution in Stroke Study Group. Effect of hypervolemic hemodilution treatment of acute stroke. *Stroke* 19:150, 1988.
59. Hossman V, Heiss WD, Beivermeyer H, Wiedemann G. Controlled trial of ancrod in ischemic stroke. *Arch Neurol* 40:803-808, 1983.
60. Olinger C, Brott T, Barsan W, Hedges J, Glas-Greenwalt P, Pollak V. Double blind, randomized placebo controlled study of ancrod as therapy for acute cerebral infarction. *Stroke* 19:133, 1988.
61. Pentoxifylline Study Group. Pentoxifylline (PTX) in acute ischemic stroke. *Stroke* 18:298, 1987.
62. Hass A, Kroemer H, Jager H, Oest A, Schimrigk K. Similar and opposite hemorheological effects of dextran 40 and hydroxyethyl starch in hemodilution therapy for stroke. In: Hartmann A, Kuschinsky W (Eds.), *Cerebral Ischemia and Hemorheology*. Springer-Verlag, New York, 1987, pp. 487-495.
63. Chein S. Biophysical behavior of red cells in suspension. In: Surgenor DM (Ed.), *The Red Blood Cell.* Academic, New York, 1975, pp. 1031-1033.

4

Anticoagulation in Cerebral Ischemia

J. Donald Easton
Brown University–Rhode Island Hospital, Providence, Rhode Island

I. INTRODUCTION

Anticoagulation is widely used, relatively poorly studied, and substantially of unproven value in the management of cerebral vascular disease. Even after 30 years of use there is major controversy over its value in preventing infarction in patients with transient ischemic attack, in arresting progression in evolving stroke, and in preventing cerebral reinfarction. Nevertheless, most clinicians

posterior circulation do so (16-18). Consequently, evolving stroke is common.

Even though heparin appears to be the preferred treatment for evolving stroke (and crescendo TIA), the data that support its efficacy in this situation are meager. The belief is that patients with these disorders have, or may have, an ongoing thrombosis and that heparin will prevent the formation of large, red thrombi. The data supporting heparin's efficacy in this situation come largely from old and limited studies.

In 1961, Whisnant reported that heparin's effect was dramatic in preventing stroke progression in patients with acute brainstem ischemia; 9% of the heparinized group died, while 59% of a similar untreated group died (19). He also pointed out that the criteria used for diagnosing progressing vertebrobasilar stroke are extremely important if one is to predict the natural history of the event with accuracy.

Subsequently, several other randomized and nonrandomized studies were conducted (9).The patients were generally heparinized at the time of diagnosis and then switched over to a coumarin anticoagulant for several weeks or months thereafter. The data in aggregate suggest, but do not prove, that heparin reduces the risk of progression in evolving stroke. Based in part on the single report by Whisnant, it seems that most clinicians are more inclined to agree on the use of heparin for progressing brainstem ischemia than in those with carotid ischemia.

Duke et al. conducted a randomized, controlled trial of heparin for the prevention of stroke progression in acute partial thrombotic stroke (18). They studied 225 patients. Of the heparin-treated patients, 15.2% progressed in the first week compared to 19.5% of the placebo-treated patients. There were no major hemorrhagic complications. They concluded that "This study does not support the use of heparin in 'acute partial stable' stroke." I cannot entirely disagree, but 19.5% to 15.2% is a 22% reduction. A 22% benefit of heparin may be clinically significant in this very common, disabling, and sometimes lethal disorder.

In view of the large number of stroke patients and the high percentage that experience progression of their infarction (16,17), it is astounding that a carefully controlled, short-term study of heparin for unstable TIA and evolving stroke has not been conducted.

C. Completed Stroke

There are no data to support the use of heparin for completed stroke when the infarct is not cardioembolic in origin (see review in Ref. 12). This is true even though the probability of recurrence may be as high as 9 or 10% per year subsequently (20). Nevertheless, we use heparin for all patients with a *minor* carotid distribution stroke that occurred within the previous 24-48 hours, because 20% or more will turn out to have evolving, rather than completed, strokes. If a minor vertebrobasilar stroke has occurred within the previous 3 or 4 days, we use heparin throughout the first week.

The bleeding complication rate for 7 days of heparin is about 10%, with a serious bleed rate of about 2%.

D. Cardioembolic Stroke

The data supporting the use of anticoagulation in patients who are at risk of imminent embolization of thrombi from the left heart are more convincing (13,14). The discussion of anticoagulation in cardioembolic stroke is best divided into prevention of recurrence and prevention of the first embolus.

1. Prevention of Recurrence

Grouped data from several recent studies indicate that approximately 15-20% of patients with a cardioembolic stroke will experience a second embolism within 2 weeks if they are not treated (14). Three-fourths of these emboli will go to the brain, and one-fourth to a systemic or peripheral site. (All types of heart disease causing nonseptic emboli have a similar rate of recurrent stroke, about 1% daily for the first 2 weeks.) Emboli arising from the atrial or ventricular wall, as opposed to those arising from native or prosthetic valves, tend to be large and cause large infarcts. Consequently, they are very well worth preventing.

Anticoagulation has been shown to prevent embolic recurrence. In rheumatic heart disease, nonrheumatic atrial fibrillation, and acute myocardial infarction, the natural recurrence rate is reduced to approximately one-third to one-half in the high-risk period of the first few weeks. Thereafter, anticoagulation is no longer necessary following myocardial infarction. The benefit in long-term prevention persists in rheumatic heart disease and in patients with prosthetic valves (14). Long-term anticoagulation has not been studied in nonrheumatic atrial fibrillation.

While the evidence indicates that early heparinization substantially reduces the chance of early recurrent embolism, many clinicians fear brain hemorrhage. It is well known that cardioembolic infarcts are commonly hemorrhagic, and there is concern that anticoagulation will worsen the bleeding and increase the morbidity and mortality. Additionally, there is some morbidity associated with systemic hemorrhage.

The risks and benefits of immediate anticoagulation of patients with cardioembolic stroke have been reviewed by Hart et al. (14). Although the conversion of brain petechiae into purpura is probably common, major hemorrhage is not. The evidence overall suggests that immediate anticoagulation is beneficial, except in patients with CT scan evidence of blood, substantial arterial hypertension, or a large infarct. Patients with these abnormalities appear to be at higher risk of developing clinically important hemorrhagic transformation of their infarct.

2. Prevention of the First Embolus

Emboli arising from the wall of the left heart tend to produce large infarcts, and they are not usually heralded by warning TIAs. Since many potential sources of cardiac emboli are identifiable prior to stroke, emphasis recently has properly centered on prevention of the first embolus. In this situation the data are very limited.

Anticoagulation prevents stroke in patients with prosthetic heart valves (14, 21). It almost certainly also does so in patients with severe rheumatic heart disease, i.e., those with mitral stenosis, an enlarged left atrium, atrial fibrillation, and congestive heart failure (14). Most cardiologists prophylactically anticoagulate such patients. On the other hand, most do not anticoagulate the young patient with minimal rheumatic heart disease. The issue is where along the spectrum of severity one should decide to treat. Data do not exist to guide us in this regard.

Patients with nonvalvular, or nonrheumatic, atrial fibrillation (NVAF) have a five to six times higher likelihood of experiencing a stroke each year than their age-matched counterparts without NVAF (14,22,23). This is a stroke risk factor of the same magnitude as new-onset TIA. Identification of subgroups of individuals with NVAF has not been accomplished, except that atrial fibrillation within 1 year of onset carries an increased risk of stroke (24-26). NVAF affects 3-5% of the elderly and is the most common cause of cardioembolic stroke in America. It is not known whether prophylactic anticoagulation is beneficial for these stroke-threatened individuals. Two multicenter trials are under way in the United States to study this issue. One study compares low-level anticoagulation using warfarin with placebo. The other is a three-arm trial comparing low-level anticoagulation using warfarin, 325 mg aspirin daily, and placebo.

About 3% of patients with acute myocardial infarction experience an ischemic stroke within 4 weeks (14). The embolic etiology of the majority of these strokes is supported by their striking relationship to the presence of left ventricular thrombi. A minority are attributable to atrial thrombi or other causes. About 90% of these strokes occur in patients with transmural infarctions. Left ventricular mural thrombi are present in about 35% of patients with a transmural anterior myocardial infarction (MI), and they are largely confined to areas of wall dyskinesis (28-30). Consequently, it appears that the combination of an ECG and two-dimensional echocardiography can identify the 20-25% of patients with an acute MI who have a transmural anteroapical infarct with wall dyskinesis (14). This is the group at special risk for cardioembolic stroke. The two-dimensional echocardiogram may also demonstrate thrombus.

Several reports, old and recent, indicate that anticoagulation substantially reduces the incidence of stroke in patients with MI (13; 14, pp. 61-63; 31-33). If anticoagulation is restricted to the "at risk" patients noted above, it is very likely that treatment is indicated and that it should be continued for 3 or 4 months.

Cerebral embolism following MI recurs in one-fourth to one-third of patients, and two-thirds of the recurrences take place within 2 weeks. It is for this reason that any patient with an acute MI who suffers an arterial embolism should be heparinized immediately unless the infarct is large or there are contraindications to anticoagulation.

Persistent left ventricular dyskinesis in healed myocardial infarction can be a source of cardioembolic stroke. Surgical, echocardiographic, and autopsy studies demonstrate mural thrombi in about 50% of ventricular aneurysms late after infarction. However, only about 5% of such patients experience a stroke. When a ventricular aneurysm is found late after myocardial infarction, with or without a mural thrombus and in the absence of embolism, chronic anticoagulation does not appear to be indicated routinely (14).

There are no data about the efficacy of anticoagulant or platelet antiaggregation therapy in the secondary prevention of embolism, but chronic anticoagulation is generally recommended empirically for patients with a ventricular aneurysm who embolize once.

Patients with cardiomyopathies of all etiologies are also at risk for systemic embolism, especially if there is associated congestive heart failure. Mural thrombi are found at autopsy in 35-100% of patients who die with cardiomyopathy (34-36). Consequently, long-term anticoagulation is recommended for patients with substantial cardiomyopathies.

E. Cervicocerebral Arterial Dissections

Dissections of arteries supplying the brain occur when blood extrudes into the wall of the artery (37-40). The intramural hematoma causes a dilatation in the wall, called a pseudoaneurysm, and more or less compresses the lumen. In addition, an intralumenal thrombus forms: This may occlude the lumen or produce emboli that obstruct distal arteries. Dissections may result from major or trivial head and neck trauma, or they may occur spontaneously.

While the initial event in the arterial wall is hemorrhage, the consequence of concern is thrombosis and embolism with brain infarction. This concern is based on observations at angiography, surgery, and autopsy. The treatments usually recommended are anticoagulation, surgery to open or bypass the obstruction, or nothing (37,38).

Anecdotal reports (38-44) of the use of heparin in arterial dissection are encouraging, but no definitive studies have been reported. Approximately 90% of patients with extracranial carotid and vertebral artery dissections do well without any treatment. It would therefore require a very large randomized study to show a convincing benefit for anticoagulation. Nevertheless, it is the 10% of patients who do poorly because of arterial thrombosis that lead to the recommendation to treat.

Dissection of intracranial arteries appears to be less common, but the consequences are more severe. Massive stroke at the outset of the dissection is common. Additionally, rupture of the external arterial wall with subarachnoid bleeding often occurs. For these reasons, the opportunity to treat is limited, and anticoagulation seems less rational. The decision regarding anticoagulation is especially difficult because intracranial dissections are most often confused with arterial obstruction from an embolus, for which the treatment is typically heparin.

IV. MANAGEMENT RECOMMENDATIONS

A. Initiating, Maintaining, and Discontinuing Anticoagulation

The methods of initiating and maintaining treatment with heparin and warfarin are described in Section II.

Recommendations vary on how the changeover from heparin to coumarin therapy should be accomplished. Some clinicians give warfarin in an initial dose of 30-40 mg along with heparin at the time of the decision to anticoagulate. In most cases this brings the prothrombin time to about twice the control value by 48 hours, at which time heparin is discontinued. Others recommend that warfarin be started at 10-15 mg daily, concomitant with the initiation of heparin therapy, and that heparin be continued for 5-10 days thereafter. The heparin is then tapered off over 1 or 2 days. Those who recommend a short overlap period for heparin and warfarin suggest a minimum of 7-10 days of heparin. A reasonable overall recommendation is to begin with heparin. If the decision is made to continue anticoagulation beyond 7-10 days, warfarin is started in a dose of 10 mg daily. The heparin should be maintained for 2 or 3 days after the prothrombin time is therapeutic; then it is tapered off over 1 or 2 days.

There is controversy over how anticoagulation should be discontinued. The existence of a "rebound hypercoagulable state" after cessation of both warfarin and heparin has been suggested. Several anecdotal observations of an unduly high stroke incidence in the period following immediate cessation of anticoagulation have been reported (45-47). Study of rebound hypercoagulability has been undertaken for patients with prosthetic heart valves in whom warfarin was stopped briefly for elective surgery (48,49). No untoward effects resulted. The duration of cessation averaged 2-6 days, a period during which some anticoagulant effect is known to persist, and a small number of patients were involved. Others have reported several patients who experienced stroke 5-7 days after discontinuing warfarin (45).

A recent study was reported on the withdrawal of heparin in patients treated for TIA or ischemic stroke (47). Those who were not started on aspirin or warfarin before heparin was stopped had five times as many episodes of clinical deterioration over the subsequent 24 hours as those who were. The rapidity of heparin withdrawal was not discussed.

B. Specific Recommendations

We presently have limited treatments to offer the large number of people who arrive at our hospitals with progressing cerebral infarction. We heparinize many of them, even though it has not been proved that we are benefiting them.

Although the data supporting coumarin anticoagulation for prevention of stroke are limited and are largely derived from nonrandomized studies, the limited evidence that is available supports the use of anticoagulation in certain stroke-threatened patients.

Patients with TIA and appropriate carotid artery lesions are usually treated with carotid endarterectomy or aspirin. Those with surgically inaccessible lesions and those who remain symptomatic on aspirin are generally treated with anticoagulation. Since the risk of stroke is highest in the early weeks and months following the onset of TIA, and since the hemorrhagic complications of coumarin anticoagulation accumulate arithmetically over time, it seems prudent to recommend that anticoagulation be used infrequently for TIA after the first 3-4 months. Some experts use long-term anticoagulation in patients with a tight, inoperable stenosis. Overall, warfarin is not widely used in North America for stroke prevention in patients with TIA because there are few studies supporting its efficacy.

Patients with crescendo TIA and evolving stroke should generally be heparinized as soon as possible. Heparin should usually be continued for 5-7 days. A decision can then be made about the appropriateness of angiography, surgery, aspirin, or coumarin anticoagulation.

Patients with completed stroke should not generally be heparinized. However, an apparently completed stroke must be viewed as potentially progressing until at least 2 or 3 days have passed since onset. Consequently, we treat most partial strokes with heparin for several days if we see them within the first 24-48 hours after onset. We realize that 60-80% of them will be treated unnecessarily, since they are not destined to progress. Nevertheless, we cannot identify those that will progress until they actually worsen, and short-term heparin is quite safe compared to the damage done by the progression of ischemia.

All in all, our general procedure is to heparinize patients with evolving stroke, crescendo TIA, recent-onset TIA, and recent partial stroke. The first two groups are treated with enthusiasm, the latter two with some reluctance. We look forward to studies that will provide definitive information regarding the risks and benefits of heparin in these situations.

Heparin is used regularly in cardioembolic stroke from most causes. If the stroke is mild or the deficit is rapidly resolving and no contraindications exist, the patient is heparinized immediately to avoid recurrent embolism. In patients with moderate-sized infarcts, a CT scan is obtained after 24 hours to identify the 5% of patients with early spontaneous hemorrhagic infarction. Anticoagulation is delayed for several days in these patients and in those with large infarcts or a blood pressure higher than about 180/100 mmHg.

Individuals with nonvalvular atrial fibrillation who have not had transient or permanent cerebral ischemic episodes are a therapeutic problem. Although the presence of nonvalvular atrial fibrillation identifies a population at considerable risk of large, unheralded ischemic stroke, there are no data regarding stroke prevention in these individuals. Aspirin or prophylactic anticoagulation at a relatively low level (prothrombin time 1.3-1.8 times the control value), should be considered, especially in those with recent onset of atrial fibrillation.

REFERENCES

1. O.Reilly RA. Anticoagulant, antithrombotic, and thrombolytic drugs. In: Gilman AG, Goodman LS, Gilman A (Eds.) *The Pharmacological Basis of Therapeutics*, 6th ed.Macmillan, New York, 1980, pp. 1347-1360.
2. Hirsh J. Anticoagulant and platelet antiaggregant agents. In: Barnett HJM, Mohr JP, Stein BM, Yatsu FM (Eds.), *Stroke: Pathophysiology, Diagnosis and Management*. Churchill, Livingstone, New York, 1986, pp. 925-966.
3. Schafer AI. The hypercoagulable states. *Ann Intern Med* 102:814-828, 1985.
4. Koch-Weser J, Sellers EM. Drug interactions with coumarin anticoagulants. *N Engl J Med* 285:487–498, 547-558, 1971.
5. Report of the Veterans Administration. Cooperative Study of Atherosclerosis, Neurology Section. An evaluation of anticoagulant therapy in the treatment of cerebrovascular disease. *Neurology* 11:132-138, 1961.
6. Baker RN, Broward JA, Fang HC, et al. Anticoagulant therapy in cerebral infarction. *Neurology* 12:823-835, 1962.
7. Pierce JMS, Gubbay SS, Walton JN. Long-term anticoagulant therapy in transient cerebral attacks. *Lancet* 1:6-9, 1965.
8. Baker RN, Schwartz W, Rose AS. Transient ischemic attacks–a report of a study of anticoagulant treatment. *Neurology* 16:841-847, 1966.
9. Easton JD, Hart RG, Sherman DG, Kaste M. Diagnosis and management of ischemic stroke. Part I. Threatened stroke and its management. *Curr Probl Cardiol* 8:1-76, 1983.
10. Olsson JE, Brechter C, Backlund H, et al. Anticoagulant vs. anti-platelet therapy as prophylaxis against cerebral infarction in transient ischemic attacks. *Stroke* 11:4-9, 1980.
11. Buren A, Ygge J. Treatment program and comparison between anticoagulants and platelet aggregation inhibitors after transient ischemic attack. *Stroke* 12:578-580, 1981.

12. Byer JA, Easton JD. Therapy of ischemic cerebrovascular disease. *Ann Intern Med* 93:742--756, 1980.
13. Easton JD, Sherman DG. Management of cerebral embolism of cardiac origin. *Stroke* 11:433-442, 1980.
14. Hart RG, Sherman DG, Miller VT, Easton JD. Diagnosis and management of ischemic stroke. Part II. Selected controversies. *Curr Probl Cardiol* 8:1-80, 1983.
15. Putman SF, Adams HP Jr. Usefulness of heparin in initial management of patients with recent transient ischemic attacks. *Arch Neurol* 42:960-962 1985.
16. Jones HR, Millikan CH, Sandok BA. Temporal profile (clinical course) of acute vertebrobasilar system cerebral infarction. *Stroke* 11:173-177, 1980.
17. Jones HR, Millikan CH. Temporal profile (clinical course) of acute carotid system cerebral infarction. *Stroke* 7:64-71, 1976.
18. Duke, RJ, Bloch RF, Turpie AGG, Trebilcock R, Bayer N. Intravenous heparin for the prevention of stroke progression in acute partial stable stroke: a randomized controlled trial. *Ann Intern Med* 105:825-828, 1986.
19. Whisnant JP. Discussion of progressing stroke: anticoagulant therapy. In: Millikan CH, Siekert RH, Whisnant JP (Eds.), *Cerebral Vascular Diseases.* Third Princeton Conference. Grune & Stratton, New York, 1961, pp. 182-183.
20. Marquardsen J. The natural history of acute cerebrovascular disease. A retrospective study of 769 patients. *Acta Neurol Scand* 45(Suppl 38):1-192, 1969.
21. Chesebro JH, Fuster V, Pumphrey CW, et al. Combined warfarin-platelet inhibitor antithrombotic therapy in prosthetic heart valve replacement. *Circulation* 64(Suppl IV):IV76, 1981.
22. Beer DT, Ghitman B. Embolization from the atria in arteriosclerotic heart disease. *JAMA* 177:287-291, 1961.
23. Wolf PA, Dawber TR, Thomas HE, et al. Epidemiologic assessment of chronic atrial fibrillation and risk of stroke: the Framingham study. *Neurology* 28:973-977 1978.
24. Bharucha NE, Wolf PA, Kannel WB, et al. Epidemiological study of cerebral embolism: the Framingham study, *Ann Neurol* 10:105, 1981.
25. Wolf PA, Kannel WB, McGee DL, Meeks SL, Bharucha NE, McNamara PA. Duration of atrial fibrillation and imminence of stroke: the Framingham study. *Stroke* 14:664-667, 1983.
26. Hart RG, Easton JD, Sherman DG. Duration of nonvalvular atrial fibrillation and stroke. *Stroke* 14:827, 1983.
27. Bean WB. Infarction of the heart. III. Clinical course and morphological findings. *Ann Intern Med* 12:71-94, 1938.
28. Friedman MJ, Carlson K, Marcus FI, et al. Clinical correlation in patients with acute myocardial infarction and left ventricular thrombus detected by two-dimensional echocardiography. *Am J Med* 72:894-898, 1982.
29. Asinger RW, Mikell FL, Elsperger J, et al. Incidence of left ventricular thrombosis after acute transmural myocardial infarction. *N Engl J Med* 305:297-302, 1981.

30. McEntee CW, Van Reet RE, Winters WL, et al. Incidence and natural history of mural thrombi in acute myocardial infarction by two-dimensional echocardiography. *Circulation* 64(Suppl IV):IV93, 1981.
31. Meltzer RS, et al. Intracardiac thrombi and systemic embolisation. *Ann Intern Med* 104:689, 1986.
32. Resnekov L, et al. Antithrombotic agents in coronary artery disease. *Chest* 89(2):54S, 1986.
33. VA Hospital investigators. Anticoagulants in acute myocardial infarction. *JAMA* 225:724, 1973.
34. Demakis JG, Proskey A, Rahimatoola SH, et al. The natural course of alcoholic cardiomyopathy. *Ann Intern Med* 80:293-297, 1974.
35. McDonald CD, Burch GE, Walsh JJ. Prolonged bedrest in the treatment of idiopathic cardiomyopathy. *Am J Med* 52:41-50, 1972.
36. Vost A, Wolochow DA, Howell DA. Incidence of infarcts of the brain in heart disease. *J Pathol Bacteriol* 88:463-470, 1964.
37. Hart RG, Easton JD. Dissections and trauma of cervicocerebral arteries. In: Barnett HJM, Mohr JP, Stein BM, Yatsu FM (Eds.), *Stroke: Pathophysiology, Diagnosis and Management*. Churchill, Livingstone, New York, 1986, pp. 775-788.
38. Mokri B, Sundt TM Jr, Houser OW, Piepgras DG. Spontaneous dissection of the cervical internal carotid artery. *Ann Neurol* 19:126-138, 1986.
39. Biller J, Hingtgen WL, Adams HP Jr, Smoker WRK, Gogersky JC, Toffol GL. Cervicocephalic arterial dissections. A ten year experience. *Arch Neurol* 43:1234-1238, 1986.
40. Bogousslavsky J, Despland P-A, Regli F. Spontaneous carotid dissection with acute stroke. *Arch Neurol* 44:137-140, 1987.
41. Chapleau CE, Robertson JT. Spontaneous cervical carotid artery dissection: outpatient treatment with continuous heparin infusion using a totally implantable infusion device. *Neurosurgery* 8:83, 1981.
42. Fisher CM, Ojemann RG, Robertson GH. Spontaneous dissection of cervicocerebral arteries. *Can J Neurol Sci* 5:9, 1978.
43. McNeill DH Jr, Dreisback J, Marsden RJ. Spontaneous dissection of the internal carotid artery: its conservative management with heparin sodium. *Arch Neurol* 37:54, 1980.
44. Sherman DG, Hart RG, Easton JD. Abrupt change in head position and cerebral infarction. *Stroke* 12:2, 1981.
45. Hart RG, Coull BM. Hypercoagulability following coumadin withdrawal. *Am Heart J* 106:169-170, 1983.
46. Hart RG, Coull BM, Miller VT. Rebound hypercoagulability. *Stroke* 13:527, 1982.
47. Slivka AP, Levy DE. Risk associated with heparin withdrawal in ischemic cerebrovascular disease (abstract). *Stroke* 18:298, 1987.
48. Tinker JH, Tarnahan S. Discontinuing anticoagulant therapy in surgical patients with cardiac valve prostheses. *JAMA* 239:738-739, 1978.
49. Katholi RE, Nolan SP, McGuire LB. The management of anticoagulation during noncardiac operations in patients with prosthetic heart valves. *Am Heart J* 96:163-165, 1978.

5

Antiplatelet Therapy in Cerebral Ischemia

Chung Y. Hsu and Edward L. Hogan
Medical University of South Carolina, Charleston, South Carolina

IV. THE ROLES OF PLATELETS IN CEREBRAL ISCHEMIA

A. Participation in Atherosclerosis

Platelets are involved in the development of atherosclerosis (see Ref. 24). Atherosclerotic lesions develop at sites (orifices or bifurcations) where disturbed flow favors platelet accumulation (25,26). Mural thrombi composed of platelets and fibrin on the atherosclerotic lesions are incorporated into the vessel wall. The release of platelet-derived growth factor, which stimulates proliferation of smooth muscle cells, results in mural thickening (27). Platelets also release serotonin and thromboxane A_2. Both cause vasoconstriction and may lead to endothelial cell contraction with exposure of the thrombogenic subendothelium (24). Impaired platelet function due to thrombocytopenia or von Willebrand's disease (a genetic defect in platelet surface interaction) is noted to slow the atherosclerotic process (24). Atherosclerotic arteries produce less PGI_2 than normal (28, 29), perhaps as a result of accumulation of lipid peroxides in the vessel wall (9). Lipid peroxides may shift the balance of TXA_2 and PGI_2 to favor thrombus formation by inhibiting vascular PGI_2 synthetase (9). In regions of arterial stenosis with intact endothelium, PGI_2 production may be increased, probably due to stimulation by abnormal blood flow (30) or increased platelet-vessel wall interaction (23). This is thought to be a protective mechanism preventing platelet adhesion, aggregation, and thrombosis that may occur at sites of disordered flow (23,30). It is noteworthy that high-density lipoproteins that protect against ischemic heart disease stimulate PGI_2 (31,32); the low-density lipoproteins, a risk factor in atherosclerosis, reduce PGI_2 output (31).

B. Involvement in Thromboembolic Events

The major sites of arterial thrombi are atherosclerotic bifurcations and stenoses. Artery-to-artery embolism has emerged as a major mechanism of TIA and thromboembolic strokes (33). Atherosclerotic disease in the neck and in the large intracranial arteries is a major source of emboli. Platelet emboli have been observed in retinal vessels during attacks of transient monocular blindness (33). Platelet thrombi have been found in atherosclerotic plaques removed by carotid endarterectomy (34,35). Emboli of cardiac origin originating from valvular disease with small lesions (e.g., mitral valve prolapse) may contain largely platelets and fibrin (36). The induction of platelet-fibrin thrombi by experimental injury of vessels is inhibited by aspirin and NSAIDs; this suggests that platelet aggregation mediated by TXA_2 plays a major role in thrombus generation (37,38). Platelet activation reflected by an increase in platelet aggregates in blood, shortened platelet half-life, and an enhanced aggregation in response to stimulatory agents has been found in patients who had a stroke or are at risk of developing one (40-44). The direct role of platelets in causing cerebral ischemia has not been fully established; that enhanced platelet activity may be a risk factor is suggested by the increased incidence of stroke occurring with thrombocytosis (45).

C. Vasospasm

Because TXA_2 and PGI_2 have potent effects on vascular tone, a TXA_2-PGI_2 imbalance in favor of thrombotic process may also cause vasospasm. In coronary artery disease, increased TXA_2 formation with intravascular platelet aggregation and resulting vasospasm has been implicated as one of the causes of sudden death and unstable angina (46). Although the role of vasospasm in cerebral ischemia has not been established, focal vasospasm is thought to be one of the rare causes of TIA (33). In stroke patients without a cardiac source of emboli or angiographic evidence of arterial occlusion, and in patients with severe and complicated migraine, vasospasm is among the possible mechanisms of cerebral ischemia.

D. Contribution to Postischemic Injury

Delayed postischemic hypoperfusion (47) or no-reflow phenomenon may follow a period of ischemia (48). Arachidonic acid released during ischemia is converted to eicosanoids, and free radicals are generated during reperfusion (6). Free radicals may inhibit PGI_2 synthesis (9) and cause endothelial injury with resultant TXA_2-PGI_2 imbalance (6). Increased urinary levels of TX metabolites occur with stroke (49). Platelets accumulate in ischemic brain in animal models of stroke (50-52). The altered platelet-vessel wall interaction fostered by the TXA_2-PGI_2 imbalance may lead to platelet aggregation, vasospasm, and in turn postischemic hypoperfusion (47) or microvascular stasis (48) even if ischemia is only temporary or collateral circulation distal to the occlusion can be established.

V. ANTIPLATELET DRUGS—AN OVERVIEW

The term "antiplatelet drug" has a broad definition and applies to any drug that interferes with platelet release mechanism, aggregation, adhesion, or platelet-induced thrombus formation (53). The laboratory hallmarks of antiplatelet agents are prolonged bleeding time and platelet survival in vivo. The determination of platelet TX formation and serum and urinary levels of TXA_2 metabolites have been used to measure the potency of antiplatelet agents (54). Their relevance to the efficacy of antiplatelet therapy has not yet been established. The antiplatelet drugs available in the United States include aspirin, NSAIDs, sulfinpyrazone (Anturane) and dipyridamole (Persantine) (13,53). Ticlopidine is a new antiplatelet drug undergoing clinical trials for its efficacy in stroke prevention (55). Synthetic PGI_2 has also been studied in acute ischemic stroke (see Secs. VII.A.2 and VII.B).

Antiplatelet drugs can be tentatively classified according to their presumed mechanism of action. There are other effects of these drugs, but their relevance to antiplatelet function and thromboembolic events remain to be determined (13). Aspirin, other NSAIDs, and sulfinpyrazone are inhibitors of cyclo-oxygenase. Dipyridamole and PGI_2 increase cyclic-AMP levels in platelets by inhibiting cyclic-AMP phosphodiesterase and stimulating adenyl cyclase, respectively. The mechanism of action of ticlopidine is not clear but may involve interference with fibrinogen binding to platelets (13). Several other potential therapeutic agents affecting cerebral ischemia discussed in this book also share antiplatelet activity. These include dextran (56), pentoxifylline (57), and calcium entry blockers (58).

VI. ANTIPLATELET DRUGS IN STROKE PREVENTION

A. Aspirin

Aspirin (acetylsalicylic acid) is one of the world's oldest and most widely used drugs. It prolongs bleeding time (59,60) and inhibits platelet aggregation (61). Aspirin inhibits prostaglandin synthesis (62,63) by irreversibly acetylating cyclo-oxygenase (64) and prevents the conversion of platelet AA to TXA_2 (12). Since platelets cannot synthesize protein, the inactivation of cyclo-oxygenase by aspirin affects platelets permanently. Inhibition by other NSAIDs and sulfinpyrazone, however, is reversible (65). Delineation of platelet involvement in thromboembolic disorders and identification of the antiplatelet effects of aspirin have prompted extensive clinical trials to determine its efficacy in prevention of occlusive vascular disease including stroke (66). To date, six trials have included aspirin in the regimens examined for stroke prevention. In two double-blind randomized studies, aspirin reduced the risk of stroke and death for men but not women with TIAs (1,67), while in a third trial aspirin reduced death or cerebral infarction in patients with multiple TIAs and appropriate carotid lesions (2). Strokes that do occur may be less severe when patients have been treated with aspirin (68). In cerebral occlusive events (TIA 16%, completed stroke 84%), aspirin reduced the incidence of later cerebral infarction in one trial (3) but not in another (69). The sixth trial compared the effect of aspirin alone and in combination with dipyridamole (see Sec. VI.C). Taken overall, aspirin appears to have a real but moderate action to prevent stroke and death in TIA and minor stroke. The effect of aspirin in TIA is complemented by its efficacy in the prevention of other thrombotic disorders (66). It should be noted that these studies of stroke prevention in TIA were conducted before the basic facts of AA metabolism and aspirin in pharmacology were established, and many questions remain regarding the use of aspirin for stroke prophylaxis. A few important clinical issues will be discussed here.

1. Aspirin Dose: How Much, How Often, and When?

Aspirin inhibits formation of PGI_2 in blood vessels as well as TXA_2 in platelets, constituting what can be termed the "aspirin dilemma" (70). One widely held solution to this is based on the following: Platelet cyclo-oxygenase is more sensitive to aspirin inhibition than its vascular counterpart (71,72), and the inhibition of the platelet enzyme is permanent (64) while that of the endothelial enzyme is reversible (73). Thus smaller and less frequent doses have been advocated in an effort to spare the beneficial endothelial PGI_2 production. Short-term pharmacokinetic studies and ex vivo measurement of cyclo-oxygenase activity indicate that a daily dose of as little as 20-40 mg (approximately 0.5 mg/kg) acts in a cumulative manner, with maximal inhibition of platelet cyclo-oxygenase within 6-12 days (65). Aspirin 20-40 mg/day produced partial inhibition of PGI_2 formation (65). Complete sparing of vascular PGI_2 inhibition has not been achieved by adjusting aspirin dose alone. It may be that intermittent dosing will lessen the cumulative effect of aspirin on vascular PGI_2 production. An effective lower dose of aspirin also reduces incidence of side effects, especially gastric irritation and renal injury (74). Most of the aspirin trials in TIA were begun before the aspirin effect on PGI_2 formation was known, and relatively large doses of aspirin (900-1300 mg/day) were used. In clinical trials in other vascular disorders, lower doses of aspirin have been found effective. A 50% or greater reduction in thrombotic events was found in trials of one-a-day dosing amounting to 325 mg in men with unstable angina (75) and 100 mg in patients undergoing aorto-coronary bypass (76).

The UK-TIA aspirin trial for secondary stroke prevention evaluated the effectiveness of aspirin in daily doses of 300 mg and 1200 mg (77). Use of aspirin was associated with an 18% reduction of nonfatal myocardial infarction, nonfatal major stroke, vascular death, or nonvascular death; there was no significant difference between the effects of the 300-mg and 1200-mg dose, with the exception that there were fewer gastrointestinal side effects with the lower dose (77). The issue of primary prevention of stroke by aspirin has been evaluated in two trials of healthy male physicians. An American trial of 325 mg aspirin every other day reported a nonsignificant 15% increase in stroke, compared to placebo, among those receiving aspirin (78). A British study of 500 mg aspirin daily showed a significant reduction in TIA compared to placebo but, disturbingly, also demonstrated a nonsignificant increase in stroke (79). One can tentatively conclude from these studies that the optimal daily dose of aspirin for secondary stroke prevention is 5 grains daily or one adult aspirin, which can be enteric-coated if necessary. Aspirin appears to have no role in primary stroke prevention among healthy individuals.

2. Is Aspirin Effective in Women?

Two trials of aspirin in TIA (1,68) and a study of aspirin prophylaxis on venous thromboembolism after total hip replacement showed a lack of effect in women

(80). Animal experiments also showed a reduced effect of aspirin in the female (81,82). The sex difference in aspirin protection is difficult to explain on the basis of known aspects of arachidonic acid metabolism (83) and has not been found in other clinical trials (2,3). The validity of the claim in the Canadian and American trials of aspirin in TIA has also been questioned because of the small number of female patients enrolled and the relatively benign natural course of atherosclerosis in women (84). The UK-TIA aspirin trial demonstrated no significant gender differences in response to aspirin (77). We continue to prescribe aspirin as indicated regardless of sex.

3. Is It Advantageous and Safe to Combine Aspirin and Anticoagulant Therapy?
Thrombin-induced platelet aggregation involves at least two distinct mechanisms: the AA pathway and a second, unknown, mechanism. Thus, thrombin may stimulate platelet aggregation in the presence of cyclo-oxygenase inhibitors (aspirin or other NSAIDs) (85). Anticoagulants (heparin and oral anticoagulants) inhibit either the production or the activity of thrombin and hence may be expected to inhibit platelet behavior that is thrombin-mediated (53).

The combination of aspirin and anticoagulant offers a theoretic advantage in thrombosis prevention but also entails a higher risk of bleeding because of the inhibition of two components of hemostasis, platelet aggregation and coagulation. No study addressing this issue in stroke prevention has been done. Two clinical trials have shown that the combination of aspirin and oral anticoagulant were more effective than anticoagulant alone in reducing thromboembolic complications of prosthetic heart valves (86,87). However, the addition of aspirin at 1000 mg/day (86) or 500 mg/day (88) increased the frequency of gastrointestinal bleeding to a prohibitive level (88). Thus the combination of aspirin and anticoagulant for stroke prevention cannot be recommended unless its benefit outweighs the risk of bleeding (89). A combination of oral anticoagulant and dipyridamole may be a safer regimen (see Sec. VI.C).

B. Sulfinpyrazone

Sulfinpyrazone, a pyrazolidine derivative with a potent uricosuric effect, inhibits cyclo-oxygenase. It is less potent than aspirin, and the inhibition is reversible. The antiplatelet effect of sulfinpyrazone may be due to its metabolites (90). In the Canadian Cooperative Group study of TIA, no benefit of sulfinpyrazone in prevention of stroke and death was noted. The combination of sulfinpyrazone with aspirin offered no significant advantage over aspirin alone (1). Another Canadian multicenter trial of aspirin, sulfinpyrazone, or both (in unstable angina) reached the same conclusion. No benefit of sulfinpyrazone alone or in combination with aspirin was found in the prevention of myocardial infarction or death (91). The efficacy of sulfinpyrazone in other studies remains controversial (66). Pharmacologically there is no advantage in using two drugs acting on the same enzyme (cyclo-oxygenase). The rationale for combining aspirin and sulfinpyrazone in previous trials (1,91) was not clear, and the failure of sulfinpyrazone to potentiate the antiplatelet effect of aspirin is not surprising (92). On the basis of available data, sulfinpyrazone cannot be recommended for stroke prevention.

C. Dipyridamole

Dipyridamole is an inhibitor of cyclic nucleotide phosphodiesterase (93). Its antiplatelet effect is due to elevation of levels of cyclic AMP, which is inhibitory to platelet aggregation (53,93). Another action is to block the uptake of adenosine into red blood cells. Adenosine inhibits platelet aggregation (95) probably due to its stimulation of adenyl cyclase (96), which catalyzes the formation of cyclic AMP. Dipyridamole potentiates anticoagulant action to reduce thromboembolic proclivity in patients with artificial heart valves (97,98). The combined regimen does not increase the bleeding tendency as in the case of aspirin-anticoagulant therapy (86,88). Unfortunately, the addition of dipyridamole to aspirin has been of no definite value in trials of stroke prophylaxis (3,99) and prevention of myocardial reinfarction (100). While dipyridamole has been studied extensively in combination with aspirin (3,99-103), its efficacy when administered alone has not been carefully evaluated (66). Thus its usefulness as a substitute for aspirin in patients with aspirin intolerance and in women remains unknown. Its cost, substantially higher than that of aspirin, is a consideration in prescribing this drug with doubtful efficacy for stroke prevention.

D. Ticlopidine

Two multi-institutional studies of ticlopidine in ischemic stroke have been completed. One study (Ticlopidine Aspirin Stroke Study) entered over 3000 patients with TIA or minor ischemic stroke. Patients were given 1300 mg aspirin or 500 mg ticlopidine and followed for up to nearly 6 years. The ticlopidine-treated patients had a 21% reduction in fatal or nonfatal strokes compared with aspirin-treated patients. This protective effect appeared to be even greater for women than for men. The second study (Canadian-American Ticlopidine Study) randomized over 1000 patients with recent cerebral infarction to receive either ticlopidine or placebo. Among the ticlopidine-treated patients, there was an approximately 30% reduction of stroke, myocardial infarction, and vascular death. These promising preliminary results are somewhat tempered by side effects of ticlopidine, including dermatitis, diarrhea, and rarely, neutropenia (Syntex Research, unpublished observations). The exact role of ticlopidine in stroke prevention remains to be determined.

The moderate effect of aspirin and lack of efficacy of drugs such as sulfinpyrazone or dipyridamole suggests that stroke prevention should be directed

A. Modification of Fatty Acid Precursors—Influence of Diet

Essential fatty acids such as DHLA and EPA in the diet might prevent thrombosis by competing with AA for cyclo-oxygenase by conversion to the less potent TX analogues TXA_1 and TXA_3, respectively. EPA is also a source of PGI_3, a potent vasodilator and aggregation inhibitor. The low incidence of myocardial infarction in Greenland Eskomos has been attributed to their high dietary EPA and low AA (123). In Holland, an inverse relationship was found between fish consumption in 1960 and death from coronary heart disease in the subsequent two decades (124). In human volunteers, an EPA-rich diet (mackerel) decreased platelet aggregation and TXB_2 formation (125). Experimental brain infarcts are smaller in cats fed a diet rich in fish oil (126). EPA-rich diets prevent postischemic hypoperfusion and reduce brain edema after bilateral carotid occlusion in gerbils (127). In addition to benefiting platelet-vessel wall interactions, polyunsaturated fatty acids in fish may prevent atherosclerosis by lowering plasma triglycerides, cholesterol, and very-low-density lipoproteins (128), and they inhibit invasion of monocytes and neutrophils, which participate in atherosclerosis (129). Thus a diet rich in fish fatty acids may prevent atherosclerotic disorders, serve for stroke prophylaxis, and reduce brain damage when acute cerebral ischemia develops. The effects of fish oil in preventing atherosclerotic complications including ischemic stroke in humans have not been examined adequately.

B. Restoration of TXA_2-PGI_2 Balance

To improve TXA_2-PGI_2 balance, a specific TX synthetase inhibitor would be more useful than the cyclo-oxygenase inhibitors that reduce PGI_2 production as well. Specific inhibition of TXA_2 leads to accumulation of PGH_2, which is also a precursor for PGI_2 or PGD_2, both antiaggregatory. Shunting of PGH_2 from platelet to vascular endothelium for PGI_2 production (Fig. 2) has been reported (130,131). However, PGH_2 itself, like TXA_2, is a potent platelet aggregator and causes vasoconstriction. Thus inhibition of TX synthetase alone may results in mixed effects that are not clearly in favor of platelet inhibition. Platelet aggregation did not occur despite inhibition of TXA_2 formation by TX synthetase inhibitors (14). So far, clinical trials with TX synthetase inhibitors have been disappointing (118). The possible answer to this dilemma is the addition of a TXA_2 antagonist (118), PGI_2 or its analogues (118), or a small dose of aspirin (132), which result in far superior antiplatelet effects than TX synthetase inhibitor alone in in vitro studies. The efficacy of the combined regimen in thromboembolic disorders in humans should be examined.

C. Modulation of LT Metabolism

LTB4 is a potent chemotactant (133). LTs increase vascular permeability and contribute to vasogenic brain edema (134). Moreover, an increase in the synthesis of compounds resembling LTC4 and LTD4 has been reported to accompany postischemic reperfusion (135). Both lipoxygenase inhibitors that inhibit LT synthesis and LT receptor antagonists are now available (121). The potential therapeutic efficacy of these agents in the postischemic vasogenic edema, hypoperfusion, and leukocyte-mediated damage offers another promising avenue for clinical study. LTBs in the 5-series derived from EPA in fish oil are less potent biologically than those in the 4-series from AA. Thus dietary modification in the fashion described earlier may also be beneficial by reducing the potency of LTs.

D. Inhibition of Platelet-Activating Factor

A phospholipid mediator of platelet activation, platelet-activating factor (PAF), has recently been identified as the third pathway leading to platelet aggregation (the other two pathways are AA and ADP). PAF is generated by platelets, leukocytes, and endothelial cells. Its formation has been linked to activation of phospholipase A_2 and release of AA during activation of these cells (122). PAF generation is stimulated by LTC4 and LTD4 (136) and inhibited by PGI_2 (137). PAF has been implicated in the platelet-leukocyte-endothelium interaction and thus provides a cellular and molecular basis of potent mechanisms amplifying injurious events in vascular disorder (122). PAF inhibitors are now available (138,139). The elucidation of the role of PAF in platelet-vessel wall interaction and ischemic cerebral injury undoubtedly will lead to additional therapeutic options.

ACKNOWLEDGMENTS

We appreciate the critical review and comments of Drs. John A. Gross, Jerome Kurent, Michael Malone, Jackson Pickett III, and Reid Taylor. We thank Mrs. Elaine Tidwell for preparation of the manuscript. The authors are supported by Public Health Service Grants NS-11066, NS-12044, NS-25545, South Carolina Heart Association, and MUSC Research Fund. Dr. Hsu is a recipient of a Teacher Investigator Development Award from NINCDS (NS-00792).

REFERENCES

1. The Canadian Cooperative Study Group. A randomized trial of aspirin and sulfinpyrazone in threatened stroke. *N Engl J Med* 299:53, 1978.
2. Fields WS, Lemak NA, Frankowski RF, Hardy RJ. Controlled trial of aspirin in cerebral ischemia. *Stroke* 8:301, 1977.
3. Bousser MG, Eschswege E, Haguenau M, et al. "AICLA" controlled trial of aspirin and dipyridaprole in the secondary prevention of athero-thrombotic cerebral ischemia. *Stroke* 14:5, 1983.
4. Farber JL, Chien KR, Mittnacht S Jr. The pathogenesis of irreversible cell injury in ischemia. *Am J Pathol* 102:271, 1981.

5. Rehncrona S, Westerberg E, Akesson B, Siesjo BK. Brain cortical fatty acid and phosphoipids during and following complete and severe incomplete ischemia. *J Neurochem* 38:84, 1982.
6. Chen ST, Hsu CY, Hogan EL, et al. Thomboxane, prostacyclin and leukotrienes in cerebral ischemia. *Neurology* 36:466, 1986.
7. Blackwell GJ, Flower RJ. Inhibition of phospholipase. *Br Med Bull* 39:260, 1983.
8. Wolfe LS. Eicosanoids: prostaglandins, thromboxanes, leukotrienes, and other derivatives of carbon-20 unsaturated fatty acids. *J Neurochem* 38:1, 1982.
9. Moncada S, Vane JR. Pharmacology and endogenous roles of prostaglandin endoperoxides, thomboxane A_2 and prostacyclin. *Pharmacol Rev* 30:293, 1979.
10. Samuelsson B. Leukotrienes: mediators of immediate hypersensitivity reactions and inflammation. *Science* 220:568, 1983.
11. Taylor GW, Morris HR. Lipoxygenase pathways. *Br Med Bull* 39:219, 1983.
12. Mondaca S, Vane JR. Arachidonic acid metabolites and interactions between platelets and blood vessel walls. *N Engl J Med* 300:1142, 1979.
13. de Gaetano G, Cerletti C, Dejana E, Vermylen J. Current issues in thrombosis prevention with antiplatelet drugs. *Drugs* 31:517, 1986.
14. Grimm L, Knapp DL, Halushka PV. 7-(1-Imidazolyl) heptanoic acid: dissociation of platelet thrombosis inhibition from aggregation. *Thromb Res* 24:307, 1981.
15. Mondada S. Biological importance of prostacyclin. *Br J Pharmacol* 76:3, 1982.
16. Higgs EA, Moncada S, Vane JR. Effect of PGI_2 on platelet adhesion to rabbit arterial subendothelium. *Prostaglandins* 16:17, 1978.
17. Mills DC, Smith JB. The influence on platelet aggregation of drugs that affect the accumulation of adenosine 3′:5′-cyclic monophosphate in platelets. *Biochem J* 121:185, 1971.
18. Ellis EF, Nies AS, Oates JA. Cerebral arterial smooth muscle contraction by thromboxane A_2. *Stroke* 8:480, 1977.
19. Von Holst H, Granstrom E, Hammarstrom S, Samuelsson B, Steiner L. Effects of leukotrienes C_3, D_4, prostacyclin and thromboxane A_2 on isolated human cerebral arteries. *Acta Neurochir* (*Wien*) 62:177, 1982.
20. Silver MJ. Mechanisms of hemostasis and therapy of thrombosis: new concept based on metabolism of arachidonic acid by platelets and endothelial cells. *Adv Pharmacol Chermother* 18:2, 1981.
21. Wu KK. Microvascular thrombosis: pathophysiology and new strategies. *Hosp Pract* 47, May 15, 1985.
22. Halushka PV, Dollery CT, MacDermot J. Thromboxane and prostacyclin in disease: a review. *Quart J Med* 208:461, 1983.
23. Fitzgerald GA, Smith B, Pedersen AK, Brash AR. Increased prostacyclin biosynthesis in patients with severe atherosclerosis and platelet activation. *N Engl J Med* 310:1065, 1984.

24. Packham MA, Mustard JF. The role of platelets in the development and complications of atherosclerosis. *Sem Hematol* 23:8, 1986.
25. Mustard JF, Murphy EA, Rowsell HC. Factors influencing thrombus formation in vivo. *Am J Med* 33:621, 1962.
26. Lewis JK, Kohke BA. Endothelial damage and thrombocyte adhesion in pigeon atherosclerosis. *Science* 196:1007, 1977.
27. Ross R, Glomset J, Kariya B, et al. A platelet dependent serum factor that stimulates the proliferation of arterial smooth muscle. *Proc Natl Acad Sci USA* 71:1207, 1974.
28. D'Angelo V, Villa S, Myslixies M, Donati MB, de Gaetano G. Defective fibrinolytic and prostacyclin-like activity in human atheromatous plaques. *Thromb Haemost* 39:535, 1978.
29. Sinzinger H, Silberbauer K, Feigl W, Wagner O, Winter M, Auerswald W. Prostacyclin activity is diminished in different types of morphologically controlled human atherosclerotic lesions. *Thromb Haemost* 42:803, 1979.
30. Qvarfordt PG, Reilly LM, Lusby RJ, et al. Prostacyclin production in regions of arterial stenosis. *Surgery* 98:484, 1985.
31. Beitz J, Foster W. Influence of human low density and high density lipoprotein cholesterol on the in vitro prostaglandin I synthetase. *Acta Biochem Biophys* 620:352, 1980.
32. Fleischer LN, Tall AR, Whitte LD, Miller RW, Cannon PJ. Stimulation of arterial endothelial cell prostacyclin synthesis by high density lipoproteins. *J Biol Chem* 257:6653, 1982.
33. Barnett HJM. Progress towards stroke prevention: Robert Wartenberg Lecture. *Neurology* 30:1212, 1980.
34. Gunning AJ, Pickering GW, Robb-Smith AHT, et al. Mural thrombosis of the internal carotid artery and subsequent embolism. *Quart J Med* 33:155, 1964.
35. Harrison MJG, Marshall J. The finding of thrombus at carotid endarterectomy and its relationship to the timing of surgery. *Br J Surg* 64:511-512, 1977.
36. Chesler E, King RA, Edwards JE. The myxomatous mitral valve and sudden death. *Circulation* 67:632, 1983.
37. Folts JD, Crowell EB, Jr, Rowe GG. Platelet aggregation in partially obstructed vessels and its elimination with aspirin. *Circulation* 54:365, 1976.
38. Folts JD, Gallagher K, Rowe GG. Blood flow in stenosed canine coronary arteries: vasospasm or platelet aggregation? *Circulation* 65:248, 1982.
39. Wu KK, Hoak JC. Increased platelet aggregates in patients with transient ischemic attacks. *Stroke* 6:521, 1975.
40. Dougherty JH, Jr. Levy DE, Weksler BB. Platelet activation in acute cerebral ischemia. *Lancet* 1:821, 1977.
41. Al-Mefty O, Marano G, Rajaraman S, Nugent GR, Rodman N. Transient acute cerebral ischemia. *Lancet* 1:821, 1977.
42. Hamberg M, Svensson J, Blomback M, Mettinger KL. Shortened megakaryocyte-platelet regeneration time in patients with ischemic cerebrovascular disease. *Thromb Res* 21:675, 1981.

43. Mettinger KL, Egberg N. A study of hemostasis in ischemic cerebrovascular disease. II. Abnormalities in platelet ADP release, platelet cyclooxygenase regeneration time and platelet factor 3 availability. *Thromb Res* 26:193, 1982.
44. Uchiyama S, Takeuchi M, Osawa M, et al. Platelet function tests in thrombotic cerebrovascular disease. *Stroke* 14:511, 1983.
45. Wu KK. Platelet hyper-aggregability and thrombosis in patients with thrombocythemia. *Ann Intern Med* 88:7, 1978.
46. Del Zoppo GJ, Harker LA. Blood/vessel interaction in coronary disease. *Hosp Pract Mag* 163, 1984.
47. Levy DE, Uitert RL, Pike CL. Delayed postischemic hypoperfusion: a potentially damaging consequence of stroke. *Neurology* 29:1245, 1979.
48. Ames A, Wright RL, Kowada M, et al. Cerebral ischemia: II. The no-reflow phenomenon. *Am J Pathol* 52:437, 1968.
49. Fisher M, Zipser R. Increased excretion of immunoreactive thromboxane B_2 in cerebral ischemia. *Stroke* 16:10, 1985.
50. Waltz AG, Sundt TM, Jr. The microvasculature and microcirculation of the cerebral cortex after arterial occlusion. *Brain* 90:681, 1967.
51. Petito C. Platelet thrombi in experimental cerebral infarction. *Stroke* 10: 192, 1979.
52. Obrenovitch TP, Kumaro KK, Hallenbeck JM. Autographic detection of ^{111}indium-labelled platelets in brain tissue sections. *Stroke* 15:1029, 1984.
53. Weiss HJ. *Platelets: Pathophysiology and Antiplatelet Drug Therapy*. Alan R. Liss, New York, 1982.
54. Fitzgerald GA, Pederson AK, Patrono C. Analysis of prostacyclin and thromboxane A_2 biosynthesis in cardiovascular disease. *Circulation* 67: 1174, 1983.
55. Mass WK, Kamm B. The North American ticlopidine aspirin stroke study: structure, stratification variables and patient characteristics. *Agents Actions* Suppl 15:273, 1984.
56. Bygdenman S, Eliasson R. Effects of dextrans on platelet adehesiveness and aggregation. *Scan J Clin Lab Invest* 20:17, 1967.
57. Weithmann KU. Pentoxifylline, its influence on interaction between blood vessel wall and platelets. *IRCS Med Sci* 8:293, 1980.
58. Takahara K, Kuroiwa A, Matsushima T, Nakashima Y, Takasugi M. Effects of nifedipine on platelet function. *Am Heart J* 109:4, 1985.
59. Gast LF. Influence of aspirin on hemostasis parameters. *Ann Rheum Dis* 23:500, 1964.
60. Quick AJ. Salicylates and bleeding: the aspirin tolerance test. *Am J Med Sci* 252:265, 1967.
61. Weiss HJ, Aledort LM. Impaired platelet/connective tissue reaction in man after aspirin ingestion. *Lancet* 2:495, 1967.
62. Smith JG, Willis AL. Aspirin selectively inhibits prostaglandin production in human platelets. *Nature* 231:235, 1971.
63. Vane JR. Inhibition of prostaglandin biosynthesis as a mechanism of action of aspirin-like drugss. *Nature* 231:232, 1971.

64. Roth CJ, Majerus PW. The mechanism of the effect of aspirin on human platelets. I. Acetylation of a particular fraction protein. *J Clin Invest* 56: 624, 1975.
65. Patrono C, Ciabattoni G, Patrignani P, et al. Clinical pharmacology of platelet cyclooxygenase inhibition. *Circulation* 72:1177, 1985.
66. Harker LA. Clinical trials evaluating platelet-modifying drugs in patients with atherosclerotic cardiovascular disease and thrombosis. *Circulation* 73: 206, 1986.
67. Grotta JC, Lemak NA, Gary H, Fields WS, Vital D. Does platelet antiaggregant therapy lessen the severity of stroke? *Neurology* 35:632, 1985.
68. Candelise L, Landi G, Perrone P, Bracchi M, Brambilla G. A randomized trial of aspirin and sulfinpyrazone in patients with TIA. *Stroke* 13:175, 1982.
69. Sorensen PS, Pedersen H, Marquardsen J, et al. Acetylsalicylic acid in the prevention of stroke in patients with reversible cerebral ischemic attacks: a Danish cooperative study. *Stroke* 14:15, 1983.
70. Marcus AJ. Aspirin and thromboembolism: a possible dilemma. *N Engl J Med* 297:1284, 1977.
71. Burch JM, Baenziger NL, Stanford N, Majerus PW. Selective cumulative inhibition of platelet thromboxane production by low-dose aspirin in healthy subjects. *Proc Natl Acad Sci USA* 75:5181, 1985.
72. Weksler BB, Pett SB, Alonso D, et al. Differential synthesis in atherosclerotic patients. *N Engl J Med* 308:800, 1983.
73. Jaffe EA, Weksler BB. Recovery of endothelial cell prostacyclin production after inhibition by low dose aspirin. *J Clin Invest* 63:532, 1979.
74. Hirsh J. Progress review: the relationship between dose of aspirin, side effects and antithrombotic effectiveness. *Stroke* 16:1, 1985.
75. Lewis HD Jr, Davis JW, Archibald DG, et al. Protective effects of aspirin against acute myocardial infarction and death in men and unstable angina. *N Engl J Med* 309:396, 1983.
76. Lorenz R, Weber M, Kotzur J, et al. Improved aorto-coronary bypass patency by low dose aspirin (100 mg daily). Effects on platelet aggregation and thromboxane formation. *Lancet* 1:1261, 1984.
77. UK-TIA Study Group: United Kingdom transient ischaemic attack (UK-TIA) aspirin trial: Interim results. *Brit Med J* 296:316, 1988.
78. Steering Committee of the Physicians' Health Study Research Group: Preliminary report: Findings from the aspirin component of the ongoing physicians' health study. *N Engl J Med* 318,262, 1988.
79. Peto R, Gray R, Collins R, et al. Randomized trial of prophylactic daily aspirin in British male doctors. *Brit Med J* 296:313, 1988.
80. Harris WH, Salzman EN, Athanasoulis CA, Waltman AC, DeSanctis RW. Aspirin prophylaxis of venous thromboembolism after total hip replacement. *N Engl J Med* 297:1246, 1977.
81. Kelton JG, Hirsh J, Carter J, Buchanan MR. Sex difference in the antithrombotic effects of aspirin. *Blood* 52:1072, 1978.

117. Hsu CY, Faught RE, Furlan AJ, et al. Intravenous prostacyclin in acute nonhemorrhagic stroke. *Stroke* 18:352, 1987.
118. Fitzgerald GA, Reilly IR, Pedersen AK. The biochemical pharmacology of thromboxane synthase inhibition in man. *Circulation* 72:1194, 1985.
119. Saussy DL, Mais DE, Knapp DR, Halushka PV. Thromboxane A_2 and prostaglandin endoperoxide receptors in platelets and vascular smooth muscle. *Circulation* 72:1202, 1985.
120. Whittle BJR, Moncada S. Platelet actions of stable analogues of prostacyclin. *Circulation* 72:1219, 1985.
121. Taylor GW, Clarke SR. The leukotriene biosynthetic pathway: a target for pharmacological attack. *Trends Pharmacol Sci* 7:95, 1986.
122. Benveniste J, Chignard M. A role for PAF-acether (platelet-activating factor) in platelet-dependent vascular disease? *Circulation* 72:713, 1985.
123. Dyerberg J, Bang HO. Hemostatic function and platelet polyunsaturated fatty acid in Eskimos. *Lancet* 2:433, 1979.
124. Kromhout D, Bosschieter EB, Coulander CL. The inverse relation between fish consumption and 20-year mortality from coronary heart disease. *N Engl J Med* 312:1205, 1985.
125. Siess W, Roth P, Scherer B, Kurzmann I, Bohlig B, Weber PC. Platelet membrane fatty acids, platelet aggregation and thromboxane formation during a mackerel diet. *Lancet* 1:441, 1980.
126. Black KL, Culp B, Madison P, Randall OS, Lands WEM. The protective effects of dietary fish oil on focal cerebral infarction. *Prostaglandins Med* 3:257, 1979.
127. Black KL, Hoff JT, Radin NS, Deshmukh GD. Eicosapentaenoic acid: effect on brain prostaglandins, cerebral blood flow and edema in ischemic gerbils. *Stroke* 15:65, 1984.
128. Philipson BE, Rothrock DW, Connor WE, Harris WS, Illingworth DG. Reduction of plasma lipids, lipoproteins, and apoproteins by dietary fish oils in patients with hypertriglyceridemia. *N Engl J Med* 312:1210, 1985.
129. Lee TH, Hoover RL, Williams JD, et al. Effect of dietary enrichment with eicosapentaenoic and docosahexaenoic acids on in vitro neutrophil and monocyte leukotriene generation and neutrophil function. *N Engl J Med* 312:1217, 1985.
130. Needleman P. Prostacyclin and blood vessel platelet interactions. Perspectives and questions. *Nature* 279:14, 1979.
131. Marcus AJ, Weksler BB, Jaffe EA, Broekman MJ. Synthesis of prostacyclin from platelet derived endoperoxides by cultured human endothelial cells. *J Clin Invest* 66:979, 1980.
132. Bertele V, Falanga A, Tomasiak M, Dejana E, Cerletti C, de Gaetano G. Platelets thromboxane synthetase inhibitors with low doses of aspirin: possible resolution of the "aspirin dilemma." *Science* 220:517, 1983.
133. Ford-Hutchinson AW, Bray MA, Doig MV, Shipley ME, Smith MJH. Leukotriene B, a potent chemokinetic and aggregation substance released from polymorphonuclear leukocytes. *Nature* 286:264, 1980.
134. Black KL, Hoff JT. Leukotrienes increase blood-brain barrier perme-

ability following intraparenchymal injections in rats. *Ann Neurol* 18:349, 1985.

135. Moskowitz MA, Kiwak KJ, Hekimian K, Levine L. Synthesis of compounds with properties of leukotrienes C_4 and D_4 in gerbil brains after ischemia and reperfusion. *Science* 224:896, 1984.
136. McIntyre TM, Zimmerman GA, Prescott SM. Leukotrienes C_4 and D_4 stimulate human endothelial cells to synthesize platelet-activating factor and bind neutrophils. *Proc Natl Acad Sci USA* 83:2204, 1986.
137. Zimmerman GA, McIntyre TM, Prescott SM. Production of platelet activating factor by human vascular endothelial cells: evidence for a requirement for specific agonists and modulation by prostacyclin. *Circulation* 72: 718, 1985.
138. Huang S-B, Lam M-H, Biftu T, Beattie TR, Shen TY. Trans-2,5-bis(3,4,5-trimethoxyphenyl)tetrahydrofuran: an orally active specific and competitive receptor antagonist of platelet activating factor (PAF). *J Biol Chem* 260:15-39, 1985.
139. Handley DA, Van Valen RG, Saunders RN. Vascular responses of platelet-activating factor in the *Cebus apella* primate and inhibitory profiles of antagonists SRI 63-072 and SRI 63-199. *Immunopharmacology* 11:175, 1986.

6

Fibrinolysis and Stroke: Implications for Pathogenesis and Therapy

Robert B. Francis, Jr.
University of Southern California School of Medicine and Coagulation Laboratory, University of Southern California Medical Center, Los Angeles, California

I. ENDOGENOUS PLASMIN-DEPENDENT FIBRINOLYSIS

When vascular damage occurs, fibrin formation is critically important for effective repair of the injured vessel. As healing progresses, fibrin must be removed in order for adequate blood flow to be restored. The endogenous plasmin-dependent fibrinolytic pathway serves to generate the fibrinolytic enzyme plasmin in the proper locations and at the proper rate for effective wound healing. By means of a series of activation and inhibition steps, plasmin is generated selectively in the fibrin clot and not in the systemic circulation. The degradation of fibrin proceeds at a carefully regulated pace, avoiding both hemorrhage due to premature removal of fibrin and thrombosis due to a pathological accumulation or persistence of fibrin.

Fibrinolysis is initiated by the release from endothelium of tissue-type plasminogen activator (tPA) (1). This serine protease is capable of activating a circulating zymogen, plasminogen, to plasmin. Little activation of plasmin takes place in the free circulation, however. Instead, both tPA and plasminogen bind to lysine residues in the fibrin clot, thereby resulting in activation of plasmin on the fibrin surface.

Fibrinolysis is inhibited at two levels. Platelets and endothelium produce a specific inhibitor of tPA (endothelial plasminogen activator inhibitor, or PAI-1) (2). A rapid, specific inhibitor of plasmin, alpha$_2$ plasmin inhibitor (a2PI), is present in blood and is bound into the developing fibrin clot by the fibrin cross-linking enzyme, factor XIII (3). PAI-1 and a2PI form 1:1 complexes with their respective enzyme substrates, resulting in irreversible inhibition. PAI-1 thus regulates the rate of activation of plasmin, whereas a2PI inhibits plasmin itself, both in the systemic circulation ("free plasmin") and in the fibrin clot.

The ability of endothelium to produce both tPA and PAI-1 means that the relative rate of production of these two fibrinolytic components by endothelium is a crucial determinant of the level of endogenous fibrinolytic activity (4). Although the regulation of endothelial production of tPA and PAI-1 is not completely understood, several possible physiological modulators have been described. One possible mechanism whereby clot formation could result in activation of fibrinolysis involves thrombin and the protein C anticoagulant system. Thrombin has been shown to stimulate endothelium to produce both tPA and PAI-1, resulting in no net free tPA activity (5). Thrombin bound to the endothelial cell-surface molecule thrombomodulin also activates protein C, however, and activated protein C inhibits PAI-1 (6). According to this model, then, thrombin formed in an area of vascular damage would stimulate the adjacent intact endothelium to release both tPA and PAI-1. The PAI-1 would be inhibited by activated protein C produced simultaneously, and the net result would be production of free tPA capable of binding to the fibrin clot and initiating fibrinolysis.

Plasmin is capable of degrading not only fibrin but also fibrinogen, procoagulant factors V and VIII, and the platelet receptor for the von Willebrand factor. These nonfibrinolytic effects of plasmin are collectively called "fibrinogenolysis." Two features of the endogenous fibrinolytic pathway prevent significant fibrinogenolysis under normal conditions. First, tPA and plasminogen interact only when bound to fibrin, so that very little free plasmin is produced in the systemic circulation. Second, any free plasmin that might form is rapidly inhibited by a2PI. As described below, fibrinogenolysis does occur during administration of supraphysiological amounts of plasminogen activators for purposes of therapeutic thrombolysis and may increase the risk of hemorrhage in subjects undergoing thrombolytic therapy.

Pathologically increased fibrinolysis can cause severe bleeding. Individuals with homozygous a2PI deficiency (no detectable a2PI activity), a very rare inherited disorder, have a severe bleeding diathesis caused by excessively rapid removal of hemostatically useful fibrin (7). The bleeding pattern mimics that seen in persons with severe hemophilia and is treatable with the synthetic fibrinolytic inhibitor ε-aminocaproic acid (EACA). Interestingly, these individuals have no fibrinogenolysis (8), demonstrating that the specificity of tPA for fibrin is sufficient to prevent fibrinogenolysis even in the complete absence of a2PI. Individuals with congenitally high levels of tPA activity causing a similar bleeding diathesis have also been described (9). Insufficient studies have been done to determine whether the high tPA activity is due to low levels of PAI-1 or to excessive endothelial production of tPA. Both homozygous a2PI deficiency and congenitally increased tPA activity have been reported to cause spontaneous, fatal intracranial hemorrhage. Acquired increased fibrinolytic activity with bleeding is sometimes seen in individuals with liver cirrhosis (10) or with amyloidosis (11). A possible association between increased fibrinolysis in liver cirrhosis and increased risk of intracranial hemorrhage has been suggested (10).

Abnormally reduced fibrinolytic activity has been implicated in the pathogenesis of arterial and venous thrombosis. Hereditary deficiency of endothelial tPA secretion has been described in several kindreds with recurrent venous thromboembolism (12,13), although abnormally high PAI-1 production has not been excluded as the cause of reduced fibrinolysis in these individuals. Decreased fibrinolysis may contribute to the development of idiopathic (14) and postoperative (15) venous thrombosis, as well as coronary artery disease (16). As discussed further below, impaired fibrinolysis has also been linked to the pathogenesis of thrombotic stroke by some investigators.

II. ROLE OF ABNORMAL FIBRINOLYSIS IN THE PATHOGENESIS OF STROKE

Congenital abnormalities of fibrinolysis leading to pathologically increased fibrinolytic activity predispose to the development of cerebral hemorrhage (7,9), presumably due to abnormally rapid removal of fibrin from sites of subclinical intracranial vascular damage. Patients with increased fibrinolysis due to liver cirrhosis may also be at increased risk of cerebral hemorrhage (10).

High alcohol consumption has also been associated with an increased risk of cerebral hemorrhage (17). A possible role for increased fibrinolysis in these subjects is suggested by the findings that ethanol increases tPA production by cultured endothelium (18) and that persons who drink heavily have greater fibrinolytic activity than persons who do not drink (19). The possible role of increased fibrinolysis in the pathogenesis of cerebral hemorrhage in heavy alcohol drinkers thus deserves further study.

Several studies have suggested an association between abnormally low fibrinolytic activity and development of thrombotic cerebral infarction. Pilgeram et al. (20) studied 10 potential risk factors in 406 subjects with ischemic thrombotic cerebrovascular disease and found reduced fibrinolytic activity (as measured by therapy for thrombotic stroke (43,44), but these have not produced clinically significant sequelae. Balanced against the risk of postreperfusion bleeding is the generally favorable clinical effect of reperfusion so far reported in patients with acute thrombotic stroke (43-47). Zeumer et al. (44) achieved recanalization of occluded carotid or vertebrobasilar arteries in 19 of 29 patients treated with local intra-arterial urokinase. Most patients in whom early reperfusion was achieved had either no neurological deficit or moderate deficit. Del Zoppo et al. (43) reported successful reperfusion in 12 of 17 patients with acute middle cerebral artery thrombosis. Four patients had no neurological deficit, and seven improved. In contrast, none of the patients in whom reperfusion was not achieved improved, and two died. Similar benefits for early reperfusion of thrombosed cerebral vessels have been reported in two other very small uncontrolled trials (46,47).

Benefits for neurological function of prompt thrombolysis of cerebral thrombosis or thromboembolism have also been shown in controlled trials in animal models (48,49). Del Zoppo et al. (48) studied the effect of intracarotid urokinase on baboons with experimental thrombotic occlusion of the middle cerebral artery. Neurological function was better, and infarct size smaller, in five treated animals than in six untreated control animals. Zivin et al. (49) studied the effect of intravenous tPA on rabbits previously given an intracarotid injection of multiple small thrombi. Treated rabbits had significantly less neurological damage and better survival than untreated control animals.

The true risks and benefits of thrombolytic therapy for thrombotic stroke are not yet established. Large, randomized trials employing careful selection criteria and a uniform treatment protocol are essential to establishing the true benefits and risks of this form of therapy. At present thrombolytic therapy represents a potentially attractive approach to treatment of carefully selected patients during the early phase of thromboembolic cerebrovascular occlusion.

REFERENCES

1. Collen D. The regulation and control of fibrinolysis. *Thromb Haemost* 43: 77-89, 1980.
2. Sprengers ED, Kluft C. Plasminogen activator inhibitors. *Blood* 69:381-387, 1987.
3. Sakata Y, Aoki N. Significance of cross-linking of alpha-2 plasmin inhibitor to fibrin in inhibition of fibrinolysis and in hemostasis. *J Clin Invest* 69:536-542, 1982.
4. Loskutoff DJ. The fibrinolytic system of cultured endothelial cells: deciphering the balance between plasminogen activation and inhibition. *Prog Fibrinolysis Thrombolysis* 7:15-22, 1985.
5. Gelehrter TD, Sznycer-Laszuk R. Thrombin induction of plasminogen activator-inhibitor in cultured human endothelial cells. *J Clin Invest* 77:165-169, 1986.

6. van Hinsbergh VWM, Bertina RM, van Wijngaarden A, van Tilburg NH, Emeis JJ, Haverkate F. Activated protein C decreases plasminogen activator-inhibitor activity in endothelial cell-conditioned medium. *Blood* 65:444-451, 1985.
7. Aoki N, Saito H, Kamiya T. Koie K, Sakata Y, Kobakura M. Congenital deficiency of alpha-2 plasmin inhibitor associated with severe hemorrhagic tendency. *J Clin Invest* 63:877-884, 1979.
8. Aoki N, Sakata Y, Matsuda M, Tateno K. Fibrinolytic states in a patient with congenital deficiency of alpha-2 plasmin inhibitor. *Blood* 55:483-488, 1980.
9. Booth NA, Bennett B, Wijngaards G, Grieve JHK. A new life-long hemorrhagic disorder due to excess plasminogen activator. *Blood* 61:267-275, 1983.
10. Francis RB Jr, Feinstein DI. Clinical significance of accelerated fibrinolysis in liver disease. *Haemostasis* 14:460-465, 1984.
11. Liebman H, Chinowsky M, Valdin J, Kenoyer G, Feinstein DI. Increased fibrinolysis and amloidosis. *Arch Inter Med* 143:678-682, 1983.
12. Stead NW, Bauer KA, Kinney TR, Lewis JG, Campbell EE, Shifman MA, Rosenberg RD, Pizzo SV. Venous thrombosis in a family with defective release of vascular plasminogen activator and elevated plasma factor VIII/von Willdebrand's factor. *Am J Med* 74:33-39, 1983.
13. Johansson L, Hedner U, Nilsson IM. A family with thromboembolic disease associated with deficient fibrinolytic activity in vessel wall. *Acta Med Scand* 203:477-480, 1978.
14. Wiman B, Ljungberg R, Chmielewska J, Urden G, Blomback M, Johnsson H. The role of the fibrinolytic system in deep vein thrombosis. *J Lab Clin Med* 105:265-270, 1985.
15. Comp PC, Jacocks RM, Taylor FB. The dilute whole blood clot lysis assay: a screening method for identifying postoperative patients with a high incidence of deep venous thrombosis. *J Lab Clin Med* 93:120-127, 1979.
16. Hamsten A, Wiman B, de Faire U, Blomback M. Increased levels of a rapid inhibitor of tissue plasminogen activator in young survivors of myocardial infarction. *N Engl J Med* 313:1557-1563, 1985.
17. Gorelick PB. Alcohol and stroke, In: Caplan ER (Ed.), *Current Concepts of Cerebrovascular Disease–Stroke*. American Heart Assoc., Dallas, Texas, 1986, pp. 21-25.
18. Laug WE. Ethyl alcohol enhances plasminogen activator secretion by endothelial cells. *JAMA* 250:772-776, 1983.
19. Meade TW, Chakrabarti R, Haines AP, North WRS, Stirling Y. Characteristics affecting fibrinolytic activity and plasma fibrinogen concentrations. *Br Med J* 1:153-156, 1979.
20. Pilgeram LO, Chee AN, von dem Bussche G. Evidence for abnormalities in clotting and thrombolysis as a risk factor for stroke. *Stroke* 4:643-657, 1973.
21. Mettinger KL, Nyman D, Kjellin KG, Siden A, Soderstrom CE. Factor VIII related antigen, antithrombin III, spontaneous platelet aggregation and plas-

cannot be revived, it may be similarly true that ischemically impaired tissue that displays functional deficits, such as hemiparesis for motor cortex ischemia, can be restored. It is hoped that high technology instruments will accurately delineate reversible ischemia and also identify factors accounting for heterogeneous susceptibility of brain cells (1).

The second problem relates to factors resulting from ischemia as well as from reperfusion and the uncertain contribution of "toxic" substances. These latter factors relate to the release of excitatory neurotransmitters, free radicals, and intracellular lactic acidosis with the apparent step-function loss of tissue function (2,3). The monumental task in preserving ischemic brain tissue is to optimize the supply of substrates, such as oxygen and glucose, while minimizing untoward secondary effects resulting from either ischemia or reperfusion. Since ischemic brain injury probably reflects a host of metabolic derangements, future therapies of ischemic tissue will likely be a "cocktail" of drugs aimed at correcting the various cellular and vascular alterations that conspire to provoke neuronal death.

Barbiturates are among the drugs that may have an important role in such a combination chemotherapy approach to the treatment of acute cerebral ischemia. Barbiturate therapy has been proposed for use in both global and focal cerebral ischemia. Recent clinical studies on the use of barbiturates are contradictory, but overall the data are provocative and warrant continued investigative attention, both experimentally and clinically. The indiscriminate use of "barbiturate coma" following cardiopulmonary arrest or stroke, on the pretext of saving brain tissue, should be avoided (4). However, beneficial effects have been reported with barbiturate pretreatment in averting cerebral ischemic complications associated with open heart surgery (5,6).

II. STUDIES ON BARBITURATE PROTECTION IN STROKE

A variety of experimental studies in animals have been undertaken to simulate human stroke (7). Because of their differing pathological alterations, earlier investigations on anoxia alone are not relevant, nor are models of global cerebral ischemia (8). Animal models most closely simulating human stroke are those in which cerebral arteries are either occluded, embolized, or occluded and then reperfused. The basic rationale in expecting pharmacological agents to avert irreversible ischemic brain damage has to do with the existence of brain tissue receiving critically reduced but sustaining blood flow; this perfusion is insufficient to cause infarction or lactic acidosis. The hope is that pharmacological manipulations can reduce metabolic demands of the ischemic tissue and thereby prolong viability until the timely delivery of substrates is provided. This shadowy or tenuous area of reduced blood flow has been popularized as the "ischemic penumbra" by Astrup et al. (9), but definitive evidence supporting its anticipated yield of functioning brain tissue remains to be demonstrated. "Ischemic penumbra" specifically refers to blood flow that is reduced from the normal of approximately 55-60 ml per 100 g of brain tissue per minute to below 25% of normal, or approximately 12-15 ml per 100 g per minute. Although pharmacological agents, by virtue of their anesthetic effect, might be expected to convey protection by reducing the metabolic rate, this assumption has not been borne out by experimental studies of the underlying neurochemical mechanisms (10).

In a variety of animal models for stroke using intermediate-acting barbiturates, such as pentobarbital and thiopental, treatment either before or after induction of infarction has yielded generally favorable results. Results have depended on dosing, timing, and the stroke model used. For example, the doses of pentobarbital and thiopental have been enormous compared to those given humans–such as 90-120 mg/kg or 60 mg/kg doses, respectively, for the two barbiturates in experimental studies. Similarly, pretreatment has been beneficial in reducing ischemic impairment, but this procedure has limited applicability, except perhaps in patients undergoing surgical procedures associated with cerebral emboli. Barbiturate therapy begun beyond 3 hours postischemia has been generally unsuccessful, and models of stroke in which occlusion of a cerebral artery is followed by reperfusion have had no benefit demonstrated. It is likely that reperfusion initiated destructive effects such as free radical formation (11-14).

One of the first clinical reports on the use of pharmacological protection with barbiturates in stroke was by Agnoli and his colleagues (15). Thirty-five patients with ischemic strokes were divided into "conventional therapy" and thiopental treatment. In the former group, 24 patients received glycerol and low molecular weight dextran, while the latter received 2.0 g of thiopental every 8 hours for a total dose of 10 g. Of the 24 control strokes, 19 died, while 5 of the 11 thiopental stroke victims died. The authors suggest that barbiturates averted certain death in some patients. However, the question of "quality of survival" remains uncertain in this group of patients. In addition, complications with cardiac arrhythmias and respiratory depression necessitated intensive care monitoring. Although this study was not convincing with respect to the value of using barbiturates with ischemic stroke, it nonetheless provided a framework for the design of later studies concerned with pharmacological protection of the brain.

In anecdotal surgical experience, Rockoff et al. (16) reported the uncertainty and even catastrophic aspects of barbiturate therapy when cerebral arteries require intraoperative ligation. They describe four patients who had proximal middle cerebral or anterior cerebral artery ligation during aneurysm surgery. In the hope of averting ischemic brain injury, patients were treated with 3-5 mg/kg of pentobarbital, sufficient to maintain a serum level of 2.5-4.0 mg/dl and produce anesthesia. Hypotension was avoided, and the intracranial pressure was kept at less than 20 mmHg. When the barbiturates were later discontinued, all patients experienced fatal rises in intracranial pressure. Whether the ischemic injury was sufficiently massive to preclude any hopes of interventional therapy is problematic, but in these cases the enormous rise in intracranial pressure was likely a reflection of massive cerebral edema that accompanied brain infarction. It is not possible to conclude that the barbiturates hastened the patients' infarction, since multiple factors conspire to aggravate the cerebral ischemia in patients with cerebral aneurysms. Nonetheless, this report cautions against the indiscriminate use of barbiturates under circumstances of cerebral ischemia.

In a double-blind prospective study on the value of phenobarbital in ischemic stroke, we studied the feasibility of using anticonvulsant doses (60-100 mg phenobarbital three times daily) for 2 days in 26 patients within 24 hours of stroke onset (17). Low-dose phenobarbital was chosen, since Crane et al. (18) suggest that significant reductions in brain metabolism can be achieved by a proportionately smaller dose of barbiturates. For example, one-fifth to one-tenth the narcotizing dose of barbiturates will reduce the metabolic rate by one-half. Furthermore, we were reluctant to impair or markedly reduce a patient's sensorium with high doses of barbiturates, since this requires intensive care monitoring and may obscure important clues on the clinical status of the patient. With the use of a weighted neurological examination, the patients who received phenobarbital did slightly better, but no statistically significant benefit was demonstrated. A study with a larger number of patients would be necessary to definitely establish benefit or lack thereof. Although this is a negative study, it appears that low-dose phenobarbital can be given safely to patients with acute cerebral infarction. In addition, this and other studies on acute ischemic stroke suggest that the therapeutic "window" is relatively narrow; enlisting patients with strokes of 12-24 hours duration may only recruit those with irreversible neurological deficits.

In a well-designed and rigorously implemented study orchestrated by Safar, the value of thiopental loading was evaluated in comatose survivors of cardiac arrest (19). A total of 262 patients were randomly assigned to either standard intensive care therapy or this plus a single loading dose of thiopental (30 mg/kg weight) within 50 minutes of circulatory restoration. The two groups were similar in demographics, and at the end of the one year follow-up no significant differences were detected with thiopental loading. Eighty percent of the control group died, compared to 77% in the thiopental group, and the occurrence of "good" and "bad" recovery was identical. On the basis of experimental studies and these preliminary data, this negative result is discouraging for any attempts to stem the onslaught of anoxic/ischemic brain injury after the fact (8). However, the nearly 20% survivorship in both groups provides a clue that factors exist that avert lethal brain damage, but more research is needed to explore and identify what these factors might be and how they could be "normalized."

There are suggestions that use of calcium channel blockade and free radical scavengers might operate as adjunctive therapies to reduce the damaging effects produced by the intracellular rush of calcium and of free radical production with reperfusion (20). It might be predicated that in the future a "cocktail" of drugs and maneuvers might be used to minimize irreversible brain tissue damage and optimize recovery.

In the most promising study on the value of barbiturates with cerebral ischemia, Nussmeier et al. (6) reported on the dramatically improved outcome for neurological dysfunction with thiopental pretreatment in patients undergoing open heart surgery and requiring cardiopulmonary bypass. Prior experience indicated an increased incidence of cerebral emboli in patients undergoing open ventricle operations. In this study, 89 patients received an average thiopental dose of nearly 40 mg/kg, sufficient to maintain the EEG isoelectric from the time of atrial cannulation to termination of cardiopulmonary bypass. The 93 control patients received no pentobarbital but only fentanyl. On the first postoperative day, five thiopental (nearly 6%) and eight controls (nearly 9%) displayed neuropsychiatric impairment; by the tenth postoperative day, none of the thiopental patients displayed any abnormalities, while seven (or nearly 8%) of the control group did, for a statistically significant difference in outcome. The neuropsychiatric dysfunctions were believed to be primarily from emboli and were associated with the valve replaced (aortic), the status of the valve (calcified), the age of the patient, and the duration of bypass; the dysfunctions were not associated with the reduction of blood pressure during the bypass.

Close scrutiny of this study indicates that patient selection and evaluation were reasonable and included the standard neurological evaluation along with psychological assessments such as the two-part Trail Making Test. The goal of thiopental administration was to create an isoelectric EEG, and this was accomplished by administering 100-500 mg increments of thiopental initially followed by continuous infusion beginning at a rate of 500 μg/kg/min. This was adjusted to maintain a burst suppression pattern on EEG with more than 60 seconds between bursts. Other aspects of the care, operation, exclusions, and postoperative care were standard, including intra-aortic balloon counterpulsation. The postoperative evaluation was "blinded" by an individual without knowledge of the intraoperative therapy. The population of patients, as noted above, were similar for demographic features; for example, the average age was in the mid-50s, with males accounting for approximately two-thirds of each group. Other features such as the duration of cardiopulmonary bypass, type of valvular replacement, its calcification, lowest flow duration during bypass, and hypotension were similar. Also identical were the neuropsychiatric complications immediately postoperatively. The 10-day difference is striking, with none in the thiopental group and nearly 8% persisting deficits in the "untreated" group. The exact nature of the neuropsychiatric deficits and long-term follow-up would be welcome information to fully assess the outcome data, especially since the incidence of postoperative complications is relatively high. While the scientific method requires replication of these studies, the enthusiastic reception of this paper reflects a long-awaited hope that pharmacological protection against ischemic brain damage is feasible.

III. CONCLUSIONS

The use of barbiturate coma as monotherapy following either cardiopulmonary arrest or ischemic stroke should be abandoned. However, clinical and basic investigations assessing various means to reduce ischemic brain damage promise that this goal can be met. Clinical investigators committed to this challenge must continue to develop and implement rigorous protocols to develop criteria for patient entry, objective evaluations of outcome, use of high technology instrumentation, and, likely, multimodel interventional therapies to preserve ischemically impaired brain. The challenge to minimize acute ischemic stroke damage is frustrating and difficult, but the payoff will be great, and current clues from pathophysiological studies give substantial support that pharmacological protection of the brain can become a reality in the clinical setting.

ACKNOWLEDGMENTS

This work was supported in part by the Cullen Trust for Health Care, Houston, Texas.

REFERENCES

1. Wise RJS, Bernardi S, Frackowiak RSJ, Legg NJ, Jones T. Serial observations on the pathophysiology of acute stroke. *Brain* 106:197-222, 1983.
2. Siesjo BK. Cell damage in the brain: a speculative synthesis. *J Cereb Blood Flow Metab* 2:155-185, 1981.
3. Yatsu FM, McKenzie J, Lockwood AH. Cardiopulmonary arrest and glucose infusion. *Emergency Med* in press.
4. Yatsu FM. Cardiopulmonary-cerebral resuscitation. *N Engl J Med* 314:440-441, 1986.
5. Michenfelder JD. A valid demonstration of barbiturate-induced brain protection in man—at last. *Anesthesiology* 64:140-141, 1986.
6. Nussmeier NA, Arlund C, Slogoff S. Neuropsychiatric complications after cardiopulmonary bypass: cerebral protection by a barbiturate. *Anesthesiology* 64:165-170, 1986.
7. Yatsu FM. Pharmacologic protection against ischemic brain damage. *Neurol Clin* 1:37-53, 1983.

8. Yatsu FM, Diamond I, Graziano C, et al. Experimental brain ischemia: protection from irreversible damage with a rapid-acting barbiturate (methohexital). *Stroke* 3:726-731, 1972.
9. Astrup J, Siesjo BK, Symon L. Thresholds in cerebral ischemia—the ischemic penumbra. *Stroke* 12:723-725, 1981.
10. Michenfelder JD, Nukde JH. Influence of anesthetics on metabolic, functional and pathological responses to regional cerebral ischemia. *Stroke* 6: 405, 1975.
11. Hoff JT, Smith AL, Hankinson HL, Nielsen SL. Barbiturate protection from cerebral infarction in primates. *Stroke* 6:28-33, 1975.
12. Corkill G, Sivalingam S, Reitan JA, et al. Dose dependency of the post-insult protective effect of pentobarbital in the canine experimental stroke model. *Stroke* 9:10-12, 1978.
13. Michenfelder JD, Milde JH, Sundt TM. Cerebral protection by barbiturate anesthesia. Use of middle cerebral artery occlusion in Java monkey. *Arch Neurol* 33:345-350, 1976.
14. Smith AL, Hoff JT, Nielsen SL, Larson CP. Barbiturate protection in acute focal cerebral ischemia. *Stroke* 5:1-7, 1974.
15. Agnoli A, Palesse N, Ruggieri S, et al. Barbiturate treatment of acute stroke. *Adv Neurol* 25:269, 1979.
16. Rockoff MA, Marshall LF, Shapiro HM. High-dose barbiturate therapy in humans: a clinical review of 60 patients. *Ann Neurol* 6:194-199, 1979.
17. Yatsu FM, Coull BM. Pharmacological protection against ischemic stroke: feasibility of low-dose phenobarbital in acute stroke (in preparation).
18. Crane PD, Braun LD, Cornford EM, et al. Dose dependent reduction of glucose utilization by pentobarbital in rat brain. *Stroke* 9:12-17, 1978.
19. Brain Resuscitation Clinical Trial I Study Group. *N Engl J Med* 314:397-403, 1986.
20. Steen PA, Gisvold SE, Milde JH, et al. Nimodipine improves outcome when given after complete cerebral ischemia in primates. *Anesthesiology* 62:406–414, 1982.

8

Antihypertensive Therapy in Stroke

Thomas Brott and E. Paul MacCarthy
University of Cincinnati College of Medicine, Cincinnati, Ohio

I. INTRODUCTION

Blood pressure reduction is one of the most common therapies provided in the setting of acute stroke. However, too frequently blood pressure is reduced too rapidly, with little attention to the patient's prior blood pressure status or to the end organ at greatest risk, the brain. Controlled clinical trials addressing the role of blood pressure reduction in this setting are lacking, but data from experimental and clinical studies can provide tentative guidelines for the blood pressure management decisions faced daily by physicians caring for stroke patients.

II. RELATIONSHIP OF BLOOD PRESSURE TO CEREBRAL BLOOD FLOW

Cerebral blood flow (CBF) is proportional to mean arterial blood pressure minus intracranial pressure (with mean arterial blood pressure defined as the diastolic pressure plus one-third the pulse pressure). CBF is inversely proportional to cerebral vascular resistance (1). Studies in animals and humans have established an autoregulatory relationship among these variables whereby moderate increases or decreases in blood pressure are compensated by changes in resistance so that cerebral blood flow remains constant over a wide range (2). In young, healthy human subjects, this autoregulatory range for mean arterial pressure is thought to span from a lower limit of 50-70 mmHg to an upper limit of 150 mmHg (2,3).

In the setting of chronic hypertension, the autoregulatory curve is shifted to the right (3). The precise lower and upper limits have not been well studied in humans. In baboons, chronic hypertension results in a shift toward the right of the upper autoregulatory limit from a mean arterial pressure of approximately 120-150 mmHg to 150-170 mmHg (4). The human data available suggest that the lower autoregulatory limit may change from approximately 50-70 mmHg to 85-150 mmHg (3,5,6). The clinical consequence of this hypertensive autoregulatory adaptation is that rapid reduction of blood pressure to "normal" levels in the hypertensive stroke patients may result in significant reduction in cerebral blood flow (6).

Autoregulation in the elderly stroke population is even less predictable from patient to patient and is probably less reliable (7). Orthostatic light-headedness and other symptoms suggestive of autoregulatory failure are common and are often precipitated by the introduction of antihypertensive medications. Measurements of cerebral blood flow in seven elderly patients with symptomatic postural hypotension (8) documented a significant decline in CBF after modest tilt-table-induced blood pressure reduction (i.e., to blood pressures still above the presumed lower limit of autoregulation). Four additional patients with asymptomatic postural hypotension (8) did not show any significant decline in CBF, nor did the single elderly control patient. Systemic autoregulation in the elderly is also impaired. Blunted baroreceptor-mediated cardioacceleration in response to hypotensive stimuli such as upright posture (9) or nitroprusside infusions (10) have been well documented in healthy elderly subjects. Control of systolic blood pressure is also more fragile in the elderly; in a recent careful study of 20 nursing home residents, a standard breakfast lowered the systolic blood pressure a mean 25 mmHg (11). In elderly patients with risk factors for stroke, the impairment in autoregulation may be amplified by an already lower baseline regional cerebral blood flow (12); in diabetics, it may be amplified by the autoregulatory blunting commonly resulting from that disorder (13).

Autoregulation is also affected by acute ischemic infarction. In the infarction core and in the penumbra, vascular reactivity is often severely impaired or even abolished (14). Cerebral infarction-related changes in autoregulation may be prominent in the larger hemispheric infarctions and in brainstem infarction (15). These changes may persist for several weeks (15).

Changes in intracranial pressure (ICP) have not been shown to influence cerebral blood flow except at very high levels (16). Because an increase in systemic blood pressure frequently parallels increases in ICP, the independent CBF effects of increases in ICP have not been determined in humans (17).

III. BLOOD PRESSURE IN ACUTE STROKE

Approximately 50% of patients with acute ischemic stroke will present with a history of prior hypertension (18-20). With intracerebral hemorrhage, approximately 60% will have a history of prior hypertension (21). Wallace and Levy studied the course of blood pressure in 334 consecutive patients with acute ischemic stroke or intracerebral hemorrhage (18). At the time of admission, the blood pressure was elevated in 84%. The elevations were most pronounced for patients with intracerebral hemorrhage, but elevations were seen for all categories of stroke (patients with subarachnoid hemorrhage were excluded). A history of prior hypertension was elicited in 48% of the patients, implying that the acute blood pressure elevations were secondary to the acute stroke event for many of the patients. Britton and colleagues recently reported on the natural course of blood pressure after emergency hospitalization in 209 consecutive stroke patients and a similar number of age- and sex-matched controls (20). Histories of hypertension were more common among patients than among controls (46% vs. 26%), and 69% of the stroke group and 36% of the controls had blood pressure higher than 170/100 mmHg on admission to the hospital. In the first 4 days of hospitalization there was a spontaneous blood pressure deline that was greater the higher the initial values.

The mechanism for secondary blood pressure elevation in acute stroke likely involves an increase in peripheral vascular resistance, as increases in sympathetic tone have been found acutely in stroke (22,23) while increases in cardiac output have not been documented (22,24). This phenomenon of acute blood pressure elevation could be part of a general homeostatic response to acute injury, or it could relate to a more specific and as yet ill-defined response to acute brain injury. Whatever the mechanism(s) for acute blood pressure elevation, the increase is usually temporary. Wallace and Levy found that during the first 10 days after stroke, the systolic pressure spontaneously fell an average of 20 mmHg and the diastolic pressure fell an average of 10 mmHg without specific antihypertensive therapy. The fall was documented for all of the categories of stroke but was quite variable for the patients with intracerebral hemorrhage (18). The blood pressure remained elevated after 10 days in only one-third of the patients. The decline documented by Britton et al. was quantitatively similar (20).

IV. COMPLICATIONS OF ACUTE HYPERTENSION

The complications of sustained hypertension are summarized in Table 1 and may be divided into atherosclerotic or hypertensive.

Table 1 Complications of Hypertension

Target organ	Atherosclerotic	Hypertensive
Brain	Transient ischemic attacks Infarction	Encephalopathy Hemorrhage Lacunar infarction
Eye	Vascular accidents	Arteriolar constriction sclerosis Papilledema Retinopathy
Heart	Angina pectoris Myocardial infarction Sudden death	Congestive heart failure Left ventricular hypertrophy
Kidney	Renal artery disease	Nephrosclerosis
Peripheral arteries	Arteriosclerosis obliterans Intermittent claudication	Aortic dissection

A. Nonneurological Complications

A sudden severe increase in blood pressure may result in the following nonneurological complications: retinal hemorrhages and exudates, papilledema, left ventricular failure with acute pulmonary edema, acute myocardial ischemia or infarction, aortic dissection, acute oliguric renal failure, microangiopathic hemolytic anemia, and an increased likelihood of a bleeding complication in the perioperative period or during anticoagulant therapy.

Acute left ventricular failure is a well-reorganized complication of severe hypertension. In patients with pre-existing myocardial dysfunction from any cause, even mildly elevated blood pressure may decompensate the left ventricle. Immediate reduction in the systemic vascular resistance will decrease the afterload on the failing myocardium and increase cardiac output. Prompt reduction of blood pressure with an afterload-reducing agent is indicated in this situation.

Systemic hypertension increases myocardial oxygen consumption. Therefore, the patient with ischemic heart disease and severe hypertension should benefit from a lowering of the blood pressure. Reduction of blood pressure reduces the cardiac work, wall tension, and oxygen demand and may therefore be a rational approach to limit the extent of any myocardial ischemic damage.

Systemic hypertension plays an important role in the pathogenesis of acute aortic dissection. Antihypertensive treatment should be instituted immediately in this situation to reduce the risk of aortic rupture and to limit the extent of the disssection.

Renal function may deteriorate rapidly as a complication of severe hypertension and may progress to an irreversible stage within days to weeks if blood pressure is not controlled.

Moderate to severe postoperative hypertension, especially following cardiac or vascular surgery, considerably increases the risk of bleeding problems and should also be treated promptly.

B. Neurological Complications

Despite the common belief that severe hypertension with acute stroke will often result in neurological deterioration, convincing supporting data are lacking (18,25,26). The variable natural history of acute infarction makes any relationship of severe hypertension to outcome difficult to demonstrate. Experimentally, massive diffuse or focal brain edema or acute infarction may occur as a result of severe acute hypertension (27,28). However, in the Wallace and Levy study of 334 stroke patients, no systemic or neurological complications of severe hypertension were reported (18). The study of 209 stroke patients by Britton and his colleagues likewise does not mention complications of acute hypertension, and the 35 patients who died had pressures similar to those of the survivors (20). Somewhat paradoxically, Wise and his co-workers reported improvement in

5 of 13 normotensive acute stroke patients treated with pharmacological blood pressure elevation (29).

Theoretically, severe hypertension could be detrimental, as autoreregulation is often lost in the core and penumbra of infarction. With restoration of flow, excess perfusion pressure could increase the tendency for hemorrhagic change (14) or could augment acute edema formation (30). Spence and Maestro have proposed that the danger of acute edema formation is an important reason for early antihypertensive therapy (31). However, edema formation cannot be demonstrated for at least several hours by MRI (32) and does not result in detectable mass effect by computerized tomography for 24-48 hours (33), usually following the peak of acute hypertension (18,20). That is, by the time mass effect from edema begins to develop, the spontaneous gradual declines in blood pressure documented by Wallace and Levy and Britton et al. have already begun. Therefore, emergency blood pressure reduction instituted immediately after the onset of stroke may not affect later edema formation.

C. Complications of Antihypertensive Therapy

Hypotension, usually as a result of overly aggressive antihypertensive therapy, can be particularly hazardous. In the areas of brain parenchyma where autoregulation has been abolished or significantly impaired, blood flow is passively dependent on the level of blood pressure (26). "Normotensive" levels in the 120/80 range may be disastrous if therapy is begun at initially elevated levels in the 170-190/90-110 range, particularly if the lower pressures are attained within 30-120 minutes (34,35). Certain groups of patients are at particular risk for cerebral ischemia or infarction during an acute lowering of blood pressure. These include patients with malignant hypertension (36,37), hypertensive encephalopathy, advanced age (38,39), or carotid artery stenosis (40).

In addition to producing cerebral ischemia or infarction, an excessive acute lowering of blood pressure with antihypertensive drugs may also result in myocardial ischemia (41), renal failure (42), or blindness or paraplegia (43,44). The angiotensin-converting enzyme inhibitors captopril and enalapril may also produce acute renal failure if administered to patients with bilateral renal artery stenosis or renal artery stenosis in a solitary functioning kidney (45). The direct-acting arteriolar vasodilators hydralazine, diazoxide, and minoxidil reflexly increase heart rate, cardiac output, and myocardial oxygen consumption and may cause a deterioration in clinical status if administered to patients with underlying coronary artery disease or aortic dissection.

V. PATIENT ASSESSMENT

An integral part of the assessment of any patient with hypertension (regardless of severity) is a complete history and physical examination. Specific objectives of the initial evaluation include (1) an assessment of the degree of target organ involvement, (2) detection of other major system diseases that may influence therapy, and (3) identification of any underlying secondary causes of hypertension. The history should include details of previous hypertension, renal disease, and cardiac disease and a precise history of drug therapy. Recent therapy with medications that may adversely influence blood pressure and contribute to neurological catastrophes, e.g., nasal decongestants, anorectic agents (46), nonsteroidal anti-inflammatory drugs, oral contraceptives, antidepressants, sympathomimetics, and corticosteroids, should be documented. Abrupt discontinuation of certain antihypertensive drugs, in particular clonidine and guanabenz, may precipitate a catecholamine excess-like state.

Symptoms that suggest target organ involvement should be thoroughly evaluated. Chest pain, dyspnea, edema, and palpitations may indicate cardiac involvement. Renal involvement is suggested by nocturia, urinary frequency, peripheral edema, and weakness.

The physical examination should include careful assessment of the optic fundi for vascular changes, hemorrhages, exudates, and papilledema. Cardiovascular abnormalities such as extra heart sounds or murmurs should be sought, and one should check that bilateral peripheral arterial pulsations are equal in order to detect an underlying aortic dissection that may be painless and present as an acute neurological syndrome (47). Blood pressure measurements should be made in both arms with a cuff of appropriate size as recommended by the American Heart Association guidelines (48). If the patient is hemiplegic, subsequent blood pressure measurements should be made using the nonparalyzed arm (49). Because of the high prevalence of auscultatory gaps in the elderly and the frequent difficulty in hearing Korotkoff sounds (11,50), palpation should be used liberally as a cross-check of the auscultatory method of measurement.

The timing of blood pressure measurements should be flexible. Adherence to a 4-hour schedule may miss early blood pressure fluctuations but later unnecessarily tax nursing personnel. By the time of the patient's transfer from the emergency department to the hospital floor, two or more measurements should be available and provide an estimate of blood pressure variability. In a stroke unit setting, we measure blood pressure hourly for the initial 4 hours, every 2 hours for the next 8 hours, and every 4 hours thereafter during the 24-48 hours the patient remains in the unit.

The clinical utility of more invasive assessment has not yet been established. Intracranial pressure (ICP) monitoring allows detection (51) and treatment (52) of changes in ICP before they become apparent clinically. ICP monitoring could also allow detection of changes in ICP potentially related to antihypertensive therapy. Invasive hemodynamic measurement of pulmonary wedge pressure and cardiac output are currently used to guide hypervolemic-hemodilation therapy (24); these measurements may become useful to guide antihypertensive and other hemodynamic therapies in the future.

Laboratory evaluation should include urinalysis and baseline electrolyte and renal function studies to determine the presence and degree of renal impairment. A chest x-ray examination and electrocardiogram should also be performed to assess the degree of cardiac involvement and the presence or absence of congestive heart failure or aortic disease. A complete blood count may also show evidence of microangiopathic hemolytic anemia, which can complicate severe or malignant hypertension. With severe hypertension (e.g., systolic BP > 200 mmHg or diastolic BP > 120 mmHg), emergency computerized tomography (CT) of the brain should be performed so as to promptly distinguish acute cerebral infarction from intracerebral hemorrhage. With the exception of acute aortic dissection, extensive investigations to detect secondary causes of hypertension should usually be deferred until the patient's blood pressure and neurological condition hav been stabilized. Indeed, measurements of plasma and urinary catecholamines and various catecholamine metabolites are frequently increased in the setting of acute stroke (22,23) and may lead to an erroneous diagnosis of pheochromocytoma.

VI. ANTIHYPERTENSIVE AGENTS

A prime consideration in the management of hypertension in the patient with an acute stroke is the selection of an antihypertensive agent that is least likely to adversely influence cerebral blood flow. The acute administration of an antihypertensive drug may influence cerebral blood flow in two ways. First, as blood pressure falls in response to the drug, cerebral blood flow will remain constant until the patient's lower limit of autoregulation is reached. When this lower limit is passed, cerebral blood flow will fall in accordance with the downslope of the autoregulation curve. Second, any direct pharmacological effect of the antihypertensive drug on the cerebral vasculature will be superimposed on the first response.

The effect of various antihypertensive drugs on cerebral blood flow have been reported in a number of recent reviews (2,53-55). However, few studies have looked at the effect of drugs on cerebral blood flow in humans because techniques of measuring cerebral blood flow have been either invasive or inaccurate. The antihypertensive agents that are currently available for clinical use in the United States are outlined in Table 2.

A. Diuretics

There is currently no information available on the acute effects of diuretics on cerebral blood flow in humans. Traub and colleagues (56) reported on the chronic effects of hydrochlorothiazide on cerebral blood flow in elderly patients with systolic hypertension. No change in cerebral blood flow was seen

Table 2 Currently Available Hypertensive Drugs

A. Diuretics
   1. Thiazides and related drugs: hydrochlorothiazide, chlorthalidone, indapamide, metolazone, etc.
   2. Loop diuretics: bumetanide, ethacrynic acid, furosemide
   3. Potassium-conserving diuretics: amiloride, spironolactone, triamterene
B. Sympatholytics
   1. Beta blockers: acebutolol, atenolol, metoprolol, nadolol, pindolol, propranolol, timolol
   2. Alpha blockers: phenoxybenzamine, phentolamine, prazosin
   3. Combined alpha and beta blockers: labetalol
   4. Central: clonidine, methyldopa, guanabenz
   5. Peripheral: reserpine, trimethaphan, guanethidine, guanadrel
C. Calcium channel antagonists: diltiazem, nifedipine, verapamil
D. Angiotensin-converting enzyme inhibitors: captopril, enalapril
E. Vasodilators: diazoxide, hydralazine, minoxidil, nitroprusside, nitroglycerin

with chronic administration of this agent. Until prospective studies are conducted to demonstrate the lack of a deleterious effect of acute diuretic administration on the cerebral circulation, it is preferable to avoid these agents in the initial management of the acute stroke patient with hypertension because of potential adverse rheological and volume contraction effects of such therapy. Indeed, a recent report from Jansen and associates (57) cautions against the use of loop diuretics such as furosemide in the setting of a recent stroke. An exception to this recommendation would be the coexistence of pulmonary edema, congestive heart failure, or other conditions that are characterized by volume expansion.

B. Sympatholytics

Sympatholytic antihypertensive drugs may be classified into a number of different categories as outlined in Table 2.

1. Beta-Adrenoceptor Blockers

Beta-adrenoceptor antagonist drugs reduce cerebral blood flow when administered acutely to either animals (58) or humans (59). However, chronic administration of these agents does not appear to lower cerebral blood flow in hypertensive subjects (60). Since the acute administration of most beta-blockers does not produce a significant reduction in blood pressure (61), these agents do not have a major role in the acute management of hypertension in the stroke patient.

2. Alpha-Adrenoceptor Blockers

The nonselective alpha-adrenoceptor blocking drugs phenoxybenzamine and phentolamine prevent the sympathetic vasoconstriction of larger inflow tract arteries of the brain that accompanies hypotension in the presence of an intact sympathetic nervous system (62). Thus, they may influence the lower limit for autoregulation of cerebral blood flow. The alpha-adrenoceptor antagonist drug prazosin apparently does change cerebral blood flow in hypertensive patients following acute or chronic administration (63,64). However, it would seem prudent to avoid the use of prazosin in the acute management of the hypertensive stroke victim because of reported excessive hypotension and syncope after the initial dose of this drug (65,66).

3. Combined Alpha-Beta Adrenoceptor Blockers

In contrast to conventional beta-blockers such as propranolol, the combined alpha-beta adrenoceptor antagonist drug labetalol has been reported to be useful in the acute management of hypertension whether administered intravenously or orally (67). Labetalol lowers blood pressure by decreasing total peripheral resistance without significantly depressing cardiac output or resting heart rate. Chronic oral therapy with labetalol has been shown not to reduce cerebral blood flow in patients with hypertension (60).

4. Centrally Acting Drugs

The centrally acting alpha-2-adrenoceptor agonist clonidine has been reported to decrease cerebral blood flow when administered intravenously to normotensives (68) or to patients with severe hypertension (69). Two published reports concerning the effects of oral methyldopa on cerebral blood flow were inconclusive (70,71). The effects of guanabenz on the cerebral circulation have not been studied in any detail. All three of these centrally acting antihypertensive agents have the potential to cause sedation, and this may lead to difficulty in the clinical assessment of the acute stroke patient. They also may cause orthostatic hypotension, and for these reasons they are best avoided in the management of the hypertensive patient with acute stroke.

5. Peripherally Acting Drugs

Reserpine, trimethaphan. and guanethidine are largely obsolete for the acute control of hypertension and have several practical disadvantages in the setting of acute stroke. All three drugs cause orthostatic hypotension and may decrease cerebral blood flow excessively. In addition, reserpine may cause sedation and interfere with the neurological assessment of the patient. The onset of action of both reserpine and guanethidine is too slow and erratic for either drug to be safe and effective for acute blood pressure reduction. Although trimethaphan may be of value in the management of aortic dissection, it may cause ileus, urinary retention, and respiratory depression.

C. Calcium Channel Antagonists

The calcium channel antagonists diltiazem, nifedipine, and verapamil have been shown to have a beneficial role in the management of a number of cardiovascular disorders including hypertension. Contractions of cerebral vessels have been shown to be highly sensitive to the effect of some calcium channel antagonists (72-74). The investigational agents nicardipine and nimodipine increase cerebral blood flow in dogs at dosages that have little effect on blood flow in peripheral vessels and on the systemic blood pressure (75). Nifedipine has been shown to lower blood pressure acutely in hypertensive crises without causing a reducton in cerebral blood flow (69). Some calcium antagonists have also been found to be effective in the prevention of postischemic impaired cerebral perfusion in animals (76) and in patients (77). These agents have also been shown to possibly reduce the severity of neurological deficits from arterial spasm in patients with subarachnoid hemorrhage (78). In contrast to the majority of sympatholytic agents, the calcium blockers do not cause significant orthostatic hypotension, which is an advantage for the stroke patient (79).

D. Angiotensin-Converting Enzyme Inhibitors

The angiotensin-converting enzyme inhibitors captopril and enalapril have been shown to have a unique effect on cerebral blood flow autoregulation (2,80,81). The agents shift both the lower and upper limits of autoregulation to a lower pressure, and the autoregulatory plateau is shortened. These effects may be mediated by a drug-induced dilatation of the larger inflow tract vessels of the brain, which is compensated for by autoregulatory constriction of the smaller resistance vessels such that cerebral blood flow remains constant. Indeed, a recent study by Safar and colleagues (82) showed that captopril dilated both the large and small arteries within the carotid circulation of patients with essential hypertension.

Thus, the risk of inducing irreversible neurological sequelae during the treatment of hypertension in the setting of acute stroke would appear to be less with drugs that belong to this class. However, since both captopril and enalapril may cause profound hypotension in patients with high plasma renin activity when administered in conventional doses (e.g., captopril 25 mg or enalapril 5 mg orally), reduced doses of these drugs are recommended for initial therapy in the acute stroke patient.

E. Vasodilators

The effect of sodium nitroprusside, which is commonly used for the management of hypertensive emergencies, on cerebral autoregulation, is rather controversial. In animal preparations, sodium nitroprusside has been shown to dilate the cerebral vasculature and to increase intracranial pressure (83). In humans, the effect on intracranial pressure is similar (84) but the effect on cerebral blood flow remains controversial (85-87). At low doses, sodium nitroprusside increases cerebral blood flow, but at higher doses a significant fall in global cerebral flow has been observed (83). The potential for sodium nitroprusside to adversely affect intracranial pressure and cerebral blood flow should be considered before using this agent in the management of severe hypertension in the stroke victim.

The direct-acting arteriolar vasodilator diazoxide has no direct pharmacological action on cerebrovascular smooth muscle in vivo, and when it lowers blood pressure, cerebral blood flow is determined only by the autoregulatory response, which remains unaltered (88). The clinically used dose of 5 mg/kg IV of diazoxide often results in an abrupt and profound fall in blood pressure, which may exceed the lower autoregulatory limit of cerebral blood flow. This results in brain hypoperfusion and occasionally may result in neurological dysfunction, cerebral infarction, blindness, or even death (89-91). This diazoxide should not be used in these doses for the acute stroke patient with hypertension. Recently, a regimen using small, repeated doses has been reported to allow gradual, safe blood pressure reduction (92), and this regimen has been used safely in the setting of acute stroke (31).

When hydralazine lowers blood pressure, a cerebral vasodilatation is superimposed on the cerebral blood flow autoregulatory response (93). Thus, when the drug reduces blood pressure below the autoregulatory limit of cerebral blood flow, its direct cerebral vasodilating effect may maintain cerebral blood flow at a stable level even at blood pressures where a marked fall in cerebral blood flow would be anticipated. However, the drug still has the potential to disturb cerebral blood flow autoregulation. Accordingly, although hydralazine may be suitable for inducing small blood pressure reductions in the stroke patient with hypertension, acute lowering of blood pressure with very large parenteral doses of the drug is not recommended.

In summary, the commonly used antihypertensive drugs have different effects on the cerebral circulation as outlined above. However, all agents have the potential to cause irreversible neurological damage if blood pressure is reduced rapidly and in an uncontrolled manner to a level that is below the lower limit of cerebral autoregulation.

VII. PRINCIPLES OF MANAGEMENT

A. Determine Target Blood Pressure

Malignant hypertension and hypertensive encephalopathy are not analogous to acute hypertension and stroke (26). Yatsu and Zivin have proposed that until controlled investigational facts regarding blood pressure management are developed, physicians should leave acute hypertension untreated (26). An alternative approach would be to treat only at a high threshold. The target systolic pressure of 160 mmHg and target diastolic pressure of 95-100 mmHg seem reasonable for the patient without preexisting hypertension (i.e., mean arterial pressure of 120 mmHg). For patients with prior hypertension, a conservative target systolic pressure would be 180 mmHg, and a conservative target diastolic pressure would be 105-110 mmHg (i.e., mean arterial pressure of 130-140 mmHg). These target pressures are considerably higher than the pressures that frequently result from current practice of emergency blood pressure management.

After the first 48-72 hours following stroke onset, long-term target blood pressures should be considered, and these will vary from patient to patient. Whatever the targets selected, they should be approached gradually, with special attention to the standing blood pressure.

B. Determine Rapidity of Blood Pressure Lowering

In the stroke patient, the core of irreversibly damaged brain is adjacent to tissue that is ischemic but still viable. Metabolically, this area of misery perfusion is characterized by a decrease in regional blood flow, a proportionately smaller decrease in oxygen metabolism, and an increase in oxygen extraction. Rapid changes in blood pressure may compromise this tissue. Positron emission tomography (PET) studies have found evidence for misery perfusion for up to 4 days after stroke onset (94), so rapid changes in blood pressure should be particularly avoided for the first week after stroke.

The target blood pressures should be achieved over the initial 12-24 hours. We would recommend that the initial rate of reduction be no more than 5-10 mm/hr for the first 4 hours. Thereafter, a rate of no more than 5-10 mmHg/4 hr should be sufficient without posing added risk. Before beginning drug therapy, the physician should recognize that a spontaneous fall in blood pressure may occur and at a rate that eliminates the need for drug therapy (18,20).

C. Choose Antihypertensive Agent

A variety of antihypertensive agents are available for the acute management of hypertension. Preferred drugs for parenteral administration are the vasodilators nitroprusside, nitroglycerine, and hydralazine and the sympatholytic agent labetalol. Preferred drugs for oral administration are the calcium channel antagonist nifedipine, the sympatholytic agent labetalol, and the angiotensin-converting enzyme inhibitor captopril. Factors to be considered in selecting the most appropriate drug for the management of hypertension in the acute stroke patient include:

1. Severity and lability of the hypertension
2. Route of drug administration

Specific therapy suggestions are detailed in Secs. VIII.A-C. For a blood pressure of >210/>120 mmHg on two readings 5 minutes apart, we would treat with intravenous sodium nitroprusside (Sec. VIII.A). For blood pressure of >180-210/>105-120 mmHg, treatment could begin with intravenous labetalol (Sec. VIII.B) (Walter). For lower initial blood pressures, oral therapy may be used (Sec. VIII.C). Diuretic agents should once again be avoided (125) if volume overload is not present. Caution should be exercised with patients suspected of having severely elevated intracranial pressure because acute systemic hypertension may be compensatory and necessary for adequate cerebral perfusion pressure (17).

REFERENCES

1. Frackowiak RSJ. The pathophysiology of human cerebral ischemia: a new perspective obtained with positron tomography. *Quart J Med New Ser* 57: 713-727, 1985.
2. Barry DI, Lassen NA. Special lecture: cerebral blood flow autoregulation in hypertension and effects of antihypertensive drugs. *J Hypertension* 53:519-526, 1984.
3. Strandgaard S. Autoregulation of cerebral blood flow in hypertensive patients. The modifying influence of prolonged antihypertensive treatment on the tolerance to acute, drug-induced hypotension. *Circulation* 53:720-727, 1976.
4. Strandgaard S, MacKenzie FT, Sengupta D, Rowan JO, Lassen NA, Harper AM. Upper limit for autoregulation of cerebral blood flow in the baboon. *Circ Res 34:435-440, 1974.*
5. McHenry LC Jr, West JW, Cooper FS, Goldberg HI, Jaffe ME. Cerebral autoregulation in man. *Stroke* 5:695-705, 1974.
6. Strandgaard S, Paulson OB. Cerebral autoregulation. *Stroke* 15:413-416, 1984.
7. Rogers RL, Meyer JS, Mortel KE, Mahurin RK, Thornby J. Age-related reductions in cerebral vasomotor reactivity and the law of initial value: a 4-year prospective longitudinal study. *J Cereb Blood Flow Metabol* 5:79-85, 1985.
8. Wolner L, McCarthy ST, Soper NDW, Macy DJ. Failure of cerebral autoregulation as a cause of brain dysfunction in the elderly. *Br Med J* 28:1117-1118, 1979.
9. White NJ. Heart-rate changes on standing in elderly patients with orthostatic hypotension. *Clin Sci* 58:411-413, 1980.
10. Minateer KL, Rowe JW, Sparrow D. Impaired cardiovascular adaptation to vasocilation in the elderly. *Gerontologist* Part 2:163, 1980.
11. Lipsitz LA, Nyquist RP Jr, Jeanne BA, Wei JY, Rowe JW. Postprandial reduction in blood pressure in the elderly. *N Engl J Med* 309:81-83, 1983.

12. Naritomi H, Meyer JS, Sakai F, Yamaguchi F, Shaw T. Effects of advancing age on regional cerebral blood flow. *Arch Neurol* 36:410-416, 1979.
13. Bentsen N, Larsen BO, Lassen NA. Chronically impaired autoregulation of cerebral blood flow in long-term diabetics. *Stroke* 6:497-502, 1975.
14. Olsen TS. Should induced hypotension ever be used in the treatment of stroke? *Acta Med Scand* (Suppl)678:113-120, 1982.
15. Meyer JS, Snimazo K, Fukuuchi Y, et al. Impaired neurogenic cerebrovascular control and dysautoregulation after stroke. *Stroke* 4:169-186, 1973.
16. Zwetnow NN. Effects of increased cerebrospinal fluid pressure on the blood flow and on the energy metabolism of the brain. An experimental study. *Acta Physiol Scand* (Suppl)339:1-31, 1970.
17. Heilbrun MP, Jorgensen PB, Boysen G. Relationships between cerebral perfusion pressure and regional cerebral blood flow in patients with severe neurological disease. *Stroke* 3:181-195, 1972.
18. Wallace JD, Levy LL. Blood pressure after stroke. *JAMA* 246:2177-2180, 1981.
19. Mohr JP, Caplan LR, Melski JW, et al. The Harvard cooperative stroke registry: a prospective registry. *Neurology* 28:754-762, 1978.
20. Britton M, Carlsson A, De Faire U. Blood pressure course with acute stroke and matched controls. *Stroke* 17:861-864, 1986.
21. Brott T, Thalinger K. Hypertension as a risk factor for spontaneous intracerebral hemorrhage. *Stroke* 17:1078-1083, 1986.
22. Myers MG, Norris JW, Hachinski VC, Sole MJ. Plasma norepinephrine in stroke. *Stroke* 2:200-203, 1981.
23. Meyer JS, Stoica E, Pascu I, Shimazu K, Hartman A. Catecholamine concentrations in CSF and plasma of patients with cerebral infarction and haemorrhage. *Brain* 96:277-288, 1973.
24. Grotta JC, Pettigrew LC, Allen S, et al. Baseline hemodynamic state and response to hemodilution in patients with acute cerebral ischemia. *Stroke* 16:790-795, 1985.
25. Wood DH. Managing the hypertensive patient with cerebrovascular disease. *J Natl Med Assoc* 76:16-23, 1984.
26. Yatsu FM, Zivin J. Hypertension in acute ischemic stroke. Not to treat. *Arch Neurol* 42:999-1000, 1985.
27. Johansson B, Strandgaard S, Lassen NA. On the pathogenesis of hypertensive "breakthrough" of autoregulation of cerebral blood flow with forced vasodilation, flow increase and blood-brain barrier damage. *Cinc Res* 34: 167-174, 1974.
28. Matashita S, Hoff JT, Ishii S. Focal brain edema associated with acute arterial hypertension. *J Neurosurg* 64:643-649, 1986.
29. Wise G, Butler R. Burkholder J. The treatment of brain ischemia with vasopressor drugs. *Stroke* 3:135-140, 1972.
30. Durward QJ, Del Maestro RF, Amacher AL, et al. The influence of systemic arterial pressure and intracaranial pressure on the development of cerebral vasogenic edema. *J Neurosurg* 59:803-809, 1983.

31. Spence JD, Maestro RF. Hypertension in acute ischemic strokes. *Arch Neurol* 42:1000-1002, 1985.
32. Spetzler RF, Zabramski JM, Kaufman B, Yeung H. NMR imaging: preliminary laboratory and clinical evaluation of focal cerebral ischemia. *J Cereb Blood Flow Metab* 3:S87-S88, 1983.
33. Bories J, Derhy S, Chiras J. CT in hemispheric ischaemic attacks. *Neuroradiology* 27:458-483, 1985.
34. Graham DI. Ischemic brain damage following emergency blood pressure lowering in hypertensive patients. *Acta Med Scand* (Suppl)678:61-69, 1982.
35. Britton M, de Faire U. Helmers C. Hazards of therapy for excessive hypertension in acute stroke. *Acta Med Scand* 207:253-257, 1980.
36. Graham DI. Ischemic brain damage of cerebral perfusion failure type after treatment of severe hypertension. *Br Med J* 4:739, 1975.
37. Ledingham JGG, Rajopalan B. Cerebral complications in the treatment of accelerated hypertension. *Quart J Med* 48:25-41, 1979.
38. Jackson G, Mahon W, Pierscianowski TA, Gordon J. Inappropriate antihypertensive therapy in the elderly. *Lancet 2:1317-1318, 1976.*
39. Jansen PAF, Schulte BPM, Meybook RHB, Gribnau, FWJ. Antihypertensive treatment as a possible cause of stroke in the elderly. *Age Ageing* 15:129-138, 1986.
40. Ruff RL, Talman WT, Petito F. Transient ischemic attacks associated with hypotension in hypertensive patients with carotid artery stenosis. *Stroke* 12:353-355, 1981.
41. Kanada SA, Kanada DJ, Hutchingons RA, et al. Angina-like syndrome with diazoxide therapy for hypertensive crisis. *Ann Intern Med* 84:696-699, 1976.
42. Robertson CR, Deen WM, Troy JL et al. Dynamics of glomerular ultrafiltration: III. Hemodynamics and autoregulation. *Am J Physiol* 223:1191–1200, 1972.
43. Huke JA, Taylor DSI, Dillon MJ. Blindness and paraplegia in severe childhood hypertension. *Lancet* 2:553, 1979.
44. Cove DH, Seddon M, Fletcher RF, et al. Blindness after treatment for malignant hypertension. *Br Med J* 2:245-246, 1979.
45. Hricik DE, Browning PJ, Kopelman R, Goorno WE, Madias NE, Dzau VJ. Captopril-induced functional renal insufficiency in patients with bilateral renal-artery stenoses or renal-artery stenosis in a solitary kidney. *N Engl J Med* 308:373-376, 1983.
46. Fallis RJ, Fisher M. Cerebral vasculitis and hemorrhage associated with phenylpropanolamine. *Neurology* 35:405-407, 1985.
47. Gerber O, Heyer EJ, Vieux U. Painless dissections of the aorta presenting as acute neurologic syndromes. *Stroke* 17:644–647, 1986.
48. Kirkendall WM, Feinleib M, Freis ED, Mark AL. Recommendations for human blood pressure determination by sphygmomanometers. *Hypertension* 3:511A-519A, 1981.

49. Yagi S, Ichikawa S, Sakamaki T, Takayama Y, Murata K. Blood pressure in the paretic arms of patients with stroke. *N Engl J Med* 315:836, 1986.
50. Messerli FH, Ventura HO, Amodeo C. Osler's maneuver and pseudohypertension. *N Engl J Med* 312:1548-1551, 1985.
51. Ropper AH, Shafran B. Brain edema after stroke; clinical syndrome and intracranial pressure. *Arch Neurol* 41:26-29, 1984.
52. Ropper AH, King RK. Intracranial pressure monitoring in comatose patients with cerebral hemorrhage. *Arch Neurol* 41:725-728, 1984.
53. Reed WG, Anderson RJ. Effects of rapid blood pressure reduction on cerebral blood flow. *Am Heart J* 111:226-228, 1986.
54. Gifford RW Jr. Effect of reducing elevated blood pressure on cerebral circulation. *Hypertension* 5(Suppl)111:17-20, 1983.
55. Graham DI, Lee WR, Cumming AMM, Robertson IS, Jones JV. Hypertension and the intracranial and ocular circulations: effects of antihypertensive treatment. In: Robertson JIS (Ed.), *Handbook of Hypertension*. Elsevier, New York, 1983, pp. 174-201.
56. Traub YM, Shapiro AP, Dujoyny M, Nelson D. Cerebral blood flow changes with diuretic therapy in elderly subjects with systolic hypertension. *Clin Exp Hypertens* A4:1193-1201, 1982.
57. Jansen PAF, Gribnau FWJ, Schulte BPM, Poels EFJ. Contribution of inappropirate treatment for hypertension to pathogenesis of stroke in the elderly. *Br Med J* 293:914-917, 1986.
58. Aogagi M, Deshmukh VD, Meyer JS, Kawamura Y, Tagashira Y. Effect of beta-adrenergic blockade with propranolol on cerebral blood flow, autoregulation and CO_2 responsiveness. *Stroke* 7:291-295, 1976.
59. Hares P, Griffith J. The effect of acebutolol on the cerebral circulation of man. *Br J Clin Pharmacol* 4:373-375, 1977.
60. Griffith DNW, Newbury JPA, Woollard ML. The effect of β-adrenergic receptor blocking drugs on cerebral blood flow. *Br J Clin Pharmacol* 7:491-494, 1979.
61. van Baak MA, Boudier HS, Smits JF. Antihypertensive mechanisms of beta-adrenoceptor blockade: a review. *Clin Exper Hypertension* A7(1):1-72, 1985.
62. Barry DI. Cerebral blood flow in hypertension. *J Cardiovasc Pharmacol* 7: S94-S98, 1985.
63. Rutland MD, Lee TY, Nimmon CC, Britton KE. Measurement of the effects of a single dose of prazosin on the cerebral blood flow in hypertensive patients. *Postgrad Med J* 56:818-822, 1980.
64. Ram CVS, Meese R, Kaplan NM, Devous MD, Bonte FJ. Cerebral blood flow and blood pressure response to prazosin therapy in the elderly hypertensive patient. *Clin Pharmacol Ther* 39:221, 1986.
65. Gabriel R, Meek D, Ghosh BC. Collapse after prazosin hydrochloride. *Lancet* 1:1095, 1975.
66. Graham RH, Thornell IR, Gain JM, Bagnoli C, Oats HF, Stokes GS. Side effects of drugs: prazosin: the first-dose phenomenon. *Br Med J* 1:1293-1294, 1976.

67. MacCarthy EP, Bloomfield SS. Labetalol: a review of its pharmacology, pharmacokinetics, clinical use and adverse effects. *Pharmacotherapy* 3:193-219, 1983.
68. James IM, Larbi E, Zaimis E. The effect of the acute intravenous administration of clonidine (St 155) on cerebral blood flow in man. *Br J Pharmacol* 39:198P-199P, 1970.
69. Bertel O, Conen D, Radu EW. Nifedipine in hypertensive emergencies. *Br Med J* 286:19-21, 1983.
70. Meyer JS, Sawada T, Kitamura A, Toyoda M. Cerebral blood flow after control of hypertension in stroke. *Neurology* 18:772-781, 1968.
71. Epina EV, Tlyina LI, Burdov AA, et al. Alteration of the functional state of the central nervous system and cerebral circulation in patients suffering from hypertensive vascular disease treated with alpha-methyldopa. *Kardiologia* 10:127, 1971.
72. Allen GS, Ranghardt SB. Cerebral arterial spasm: Part 9. In vitro effects of nifedipine on serotonin-, phenylephrine-, and potassium-induced contractions of canine basilar and femoral arteries. *Neurosurgery* 4:37-41, 1979.
73. Edvinsson L, Brandt I, Anderson KE, Bengtsson B. Effect of a calcium antagonist on experimental constriction of human brain vessels: possible efficacy in cerebrovascular spasm. *Surg Neurol* 11:327-330, 1979.
74. Van Nueten JM, Vanhoutte PM. Calcium entry blockers and vascular smooth muscle heterogeneity. *Fed Proc* 40:2862-2865, 1981.
75. Kazda S, Knorr A, Towart R. Common properties and differences between various calcium antagonists. *Prog Pharmacol* 5/2:83-116, 1983.
76. Mohamed AA, Gotoh O, Graham DI, et al. Effect of pretreatment with the calcium antagonist nimodipine on local cerebral blood flow and histopathology after middle cerebral artery occlusion. *Ann Neurol* 18:705-711, 1985.
77. Gelmers HJ. Calcium-channel blockers: effects on cerebral blood flow and potential uses for acute stroke. *Am J Cardiol* 55:144B-148B, 1985.
78. Allen GS, Ahn HS, Preziosi TJ, et al. Cerebral arterial spasm—a controlled trial of nimodipine in patients with subarachnoid hemorrhage. *N Engl J Med* 308:619-624, 1983.
79. Cubeddu LX, Aranda J, Singh B, et al. A comparison of verapamil and propranolol for the initial treatment of hypertension. Racial differences in response. *JAMA* 256:2214-2221, 1986.
80. Frei A, Muller-Brand J. Cerebral blood flow and antihypertensive treatment with enalapril. *J Hypertension* 4:365-367, 1986.
81. Paulson OB, Vorstrum S, Anderson AR, Smith J, Godtfredsen J. Converting enzyme inhibition resets cerebral autoregulation at lower blood pressure. *J Hypertension* 3(Suppl 3):S487-S488, 1985.
82. Safar ME, Bouthier JA, Laurent SM, Simon AC. Captopril and common carotid blood flow in patients with essential hypertension—a review. *Postgrad Med J* 62:31-33, 1986.
83. Candia GJ, Heros RC, Lavyne MH, Zervas NT, Nelson CN. Effect of intra-

venous sodium nitroprusside on cerebral blood flow and intracranial pressure. *Neurosurgery* 3:50-53, 1978.
84. Turner JM, Powell D, Gibson RM, McDowell DG. Intracranial pressure changes in neurosurgical patients during hypotension induced with sodium nitroprusside or trimethaphan. *Br J Anaest* 49:419-425, 1977.
85. Brown FD, Hanlon K, Crockard HA, Mullan S. Effect of sodium nitroprusside on cerebral blood flow in conscious human beings. *Surg Neurol* 7:67-70, 1977.
86. Griffith DPG, Cummins BH, Greenbaum R, et al. Cerebral blood flow and metabolism during hypotension induced with sodium nitroprusside. *Br J Anaesth* 46:671-679, 1974.
87. Henriksen L, Paulson OB. The effects of sodium nitroprusside on cerebral blood flow and cerebral venous blood gases. *Eur J Clin Invest* 12:389-393, 1982.
88. Goldbert HI, Codario RA, Banka RS, Reivich M. Patterns of cerebral dysautoregulation in severe hypertension to blood pressure reduction with diazoxide. *Acta Neurol Scand* (Suppl 64)56:64-65, 1977.
89. Graham DI. Ischemic brain damage of cerebral perfusion failure type after treatment of severe hypertension. *Br Med J* 4:739, 1975.
90. Cove DH, Sudden M, Fletcher RF, Dukes DC. Blindness after treatment of malignant hypertension. *Br Med J* 2:245-246, 1979.
91. Ledingham JGG, Rajagopalan B. Cerebral complications in the treatment of accelerated hypertension. *Quart J Med* 48:25-41, 1979.
92. McNair A, Andreasen F, Nielsen PE. Antihypertensive effect of diazoxide given intravenously in small repeated doses. *J Clin Pharmacol* 24:151-156, 1983.
93. Overgaard J, Skinhoj E. A paradoxical cerebral hemodynamic effect of hydralazine. *Stroke* 6:402-404, 1975.
94. Baron JC. Positron tomography in cerebral ischemia. *Neuroradiology* 27: 509-516, 1985.
95. Houston M. Hypertensive emergencies and urgencies: pathophysiology and clinical aspects. *Am Heart J* 111:204-210, 1986.
96. Chobanian AV. Antihypertensive therapy in evolution. *N Engl J Med* 314: 1701-1702, 1986.
97. Five-year findings of the hypertension detection and follow-up program. III. Reduction in stroke incidence among persons with high blood pressure. *JAMA* 247:633-638, 1982.
98. Freis ED. The Veterans Administration Cooperative Study of antihypertensive agents. Implications for stroke prevention. *Stroke* 5:75-77, 1974.
99. Tuomilehto J, Nissinen A, Wolf E, Geboers J, Piha T. Puska P. Effectiveness of treatment with antihypertensive drugs and trends in mortality from stroke in the community. *Br Med J* 291:857-886, 1985.
100. Amery A. Birkenhager W, Brink P, et al. Mortality and morbidity results from the European Working Party on high blood pressure in the elderly trial. *Lancet* 1:1344-1354, 1985.

membrane potential changes that facilitate synaptic transmission (15,16). The role for L channels in this latter function, termed long-term potentiation, is controversial, since L channels in general are sensitive to organic calcium antagonists whereas neuronal long-term potentiation appears to be insensitive (18,19). The seeming complexity reflected by a diversity of channels may be simplified somewhat by recent observations such as those of Jahr and Stevens that suggest that there may be only a single glutamate-operated channel, that functions differently depending upon which class of "receptor" linked to the channel is stimulated (20).

Calcium channels are effectively blocked by a number of divalent metal cations. Magnesium may be the most important of these in nature, but several others, including cobalt, cadmium, manganese, and nickel, are more effective and have gained considerable application in the laboratory. Our interest is focused on the organic calcium channel blockers, of which only three are in widespread use clinically within the United States although several others are available in Europe or under active development. There are at least four classes of organic calcium channel blockers available for research or clinical applications; representative drugs of each class are shown in Figure 2. The pharmacology of these agents has been reviewed (21,22), and we wish to make only a few important points about them here. As a group the dihydropyridines (DHP) are most important, since they comprise the largest number of drugs currently under study for their CNS effects and have a high specificity either as antagonists, agonists, or modulators of calcium channels.

As opposed to the inorganic calcium antagonists, the calcium channel blocking drugs exert their principal action by binding to membrane sites that are functionally linked to the calcium channel. These binding sites may be on either the outside or inside of the plasma membrane, and whether or not they are invariably functional receptors remains open to question. For example, Gould and colleagues examined the binding of the dihydropyridine nitrendipine in the rat (23). They found the highest density of binding sites in the brain, particularly the dentate gyrus of the hippocampus and the superficial and medial layers of the cortex, although layer 4 in cortex had relatively low density. They speculated that these binding sites may be located in regions of synaptic activity, but they found no specific binding on blood vessels. This aspect is in stark contrast to the findings reported by Towart, who found that several of the drugs in the dihydropyridine class including nitrendipine demonstrated a selective action on the cerebrovascular smooth muscle of the rabbit (24). These conflicting results suggest that selective drug binding may not correlate closely with the presence of increased numbers of functional calcium channels. Additional insight into this problem will be gained by investigating the regional distribution of subtypes of calcium channels. For example, DHP receptors may be associated

1. **Papavarine Derivatives**
   Verapamil

2. **Dihydropyridine Derivatives**
   Nifedipine
   Nimodipine
   Felodipine

3. **Benzothiazepine Derivatives**
   Diltiazem

4. **Piperazine Derivatives**
   Flunarizine

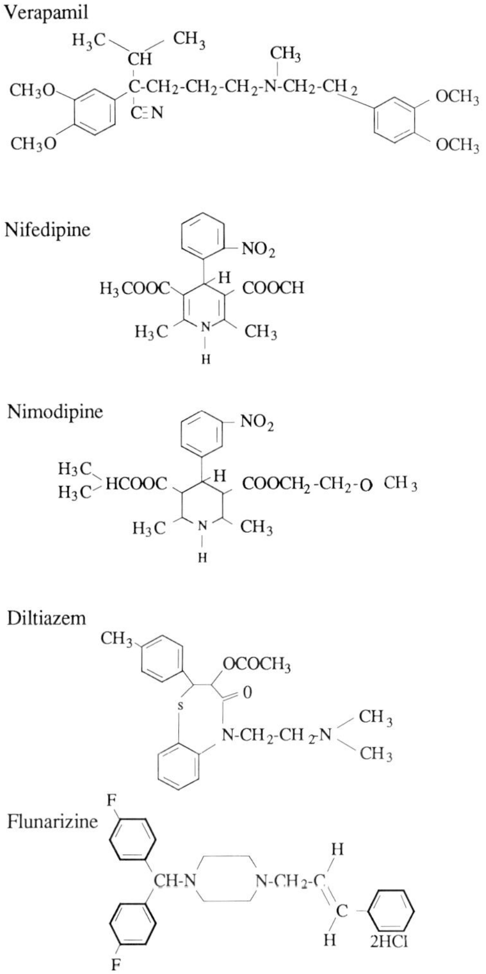

Figure 2 Organic calcium antagonists.

with L-type channels in the nervous system (15). Clearly, more investigation into this dilemma is indicated.

In summary, calcium antagonists, or the so-called calcium channel blockers, presumably act by preventing or slowing the influx of calcium from the extracellular space into the intracellular fluid, thus blocking the increase in intracellular free calcium that occurs during ischemia. Although there are some reports about direct effects of calcium blockers on mitochondrial membrane functions, this mechanism of action needs to be confirmed (25-27). Several reports have indicated that calcium antagonists are not beneficial in brain ischemia. There are others, however, that show encouraging results. Before reviewing these data we will briefly review the hypothesis of ischemic neuronal injury.

III. HYPOTHESIS OF ISCHEMIC NEURONAL INJURY

Siesjo and his collaborators have put forth two main hypotheses about the mechanisms of irreversible injury to cellular metabolic activity after incomplete ischemia. The first hypothesis states that irreversible ischemic injury in the brain is related to increased intracellular calcium levels occurring during ischemia (7). Increase in intracellular free Ca^{2+} during ischemia is caused by lack of cellular ATP and phosphocreatine resulting in an inability of energy-dependent processes such as the cation pumps—the Na-K pump as well as the Ca pump—to operate. Continuous activity of these pumps is required for removal of excess intracellular Ca^{2+} and Na^{+} to the extracellular compartment against a large concentration gradient. Intracellular free calcium also increases because of the inability of the intracellular Ca^{2+} storage sites in the brain, particularly the mitochondria and to some extent the endoplasmic reticulum, to remove the increased free cytoplasmic Ca^{2+} in the absence of an adequate energy supply. Thus, the primary insult after the mitochondrial shutdown, brought about by lack of oxygen first and lack of glucose later, is an increase in intracellular free Ca^{2+} and Na^{+}. This cation dyshomeostasis results in a cascade of detrimental enzyme-catalyzed reactions, which secondarily cause permanent damage to cellular and subcellular membranes.

The second hypothesis is based on the determination of tissue lactate and energy metabolites in the two types of ischemia, complete and incomplete, and in food-deprived and glucose-infused animals after incomplete ischemia and recirculation (7,28). This hypothesis suggests that the increased vulnerability of brain tissue in incomplete ischemia is due to the much higher lactate production during that condition and the resulting much lower pH level in incomplete ischemia as compared to complete. Currently there is not enough evidence to support either one of these hypotheses firmly.

The hypothesis on the deleterious effects of increased lactate and decreased cellular pH has received substantial attention. Effects of lowered pH on the function of normal mitochondria were studied. It has been known for a long time that heart, liver, and kidney mitochondria cease to synthesize ATP and respire maximally (in the presence of ADP) with NADH-linked substrates when pH falls to approximately 6.0 (29,30). This is particularly so when some cation shifts across the plasma membrane occur simultaneously with the falling pH, which is the case in ischemia (31). Direct measurements of intra- and extracellular brain pH during ischemia have indicated that pH can fall below 6 during ischemia and to 6.1 after 4 hours of ischemia (32,33). Rehncrona et al. (28) showed that brain lactate concentration in severe incomplete ischemia followed by recirculation reached levels as high as 42 μmol/g in glucose-supplemented animals. This is much in excess of the level reached after complete ischemia or after incomplete ischemia induced in food-deprived animals. Hillered et al. (34) compared brain mitochondrial function after 15 minutes of incomplete ischemia in fasted animals (tissue lactate 14 μmol/g tissue) and 30 minutes of incomplete ischemia in fed animals (tissue lactate 30 μmol/g tissue). The estimated intracellular pH values corresponding to these two lactate levels are 6.5 and 5.8. Hillered et al. (34) found that the high tissue lactate accumulation with a low intracellular pH resulted in irreversible mitochondrial injury; the lower level of accumulated lactate and higher intracellular pH resulted in a transient decline of mitochondrial ATP synthesis function that recovered fully during 30 minutes of recirculation. In a parallel in vitro study, incubation of brain mitochondria in a medium containing 17-20 mM lactate at pH 6.1-5.3 induced an inhibition of mitochondrial state 3 respiration and ATP synthesis, and these functions were only partially restored by further incubation at neutral pH without lactate present. It has thus been demonstrated that cellular acidosis can cause irreversible inhibition of mitochondrial function. The effects of these low pH and high lactate conditions on cellular Ca^{2+} and Mg^{2+} homeostasis, however, have not been investigated.

Recent reports on the efficacy of calcium antagonists in preventing ischemic injury in the myocardium and in the kidney make the calcium hypothesis attractive (35-37). As discussed below, controversy exists about the efficacy of calcium antagonists in preventing ischemic injury to the brain, (38-42). Theoretically, a calcium channel blocker with an ability to slow entry of extracellular calcium into the cytoplasmic compartment via voltage-sensitive channels should be efficacious in excitable cells such as neurons. Only those therapeutic agents that can gain access to the brain tissue, however, should prove beneficial. All other agents could protect the brain tissue only by indirect mechanisms such as an improved recovery of blood flow to the ischemic regions.

IV. ANIMAL MODELS OF BRAIN ISCHEMIA

Many experimental animal studies have attempted to discern whether calcium entry blockers lessen the effects of cerebral ischemia, but no consistent pattern of effect has emerged. The disparate results may reflect wide variation in the animal models used; the timing, dose, and route of administration of the experimental drug; and the lack of consistent scoring and endpoint measurement determinations. These difficulties are compounded further by the considerable molecular variation, the diverse modes of action and selectivity for the various types of calcium channels, and potential nonchannel antagonistic effects that may exist between the various types of calcium entry blockers. Finally, it is most unfortunate that in some published investigations insufficient numbers of experimental animals were used to assure a statistically valid study.

Brandt et al. studied the effects of nifedipine on the pial microvasculature of cat cerebral cortex in normal and focal ischemic conditions (43). Topical application of nifedipine (0.02-40 μg/ml) caused a marked, concentration-dependent arteriolar dilatation that was most significant within the smallest arterioles. Arterioles that constricted after middle cerebral artery occlusion invariably dilated following nifedipine application. These dilation responses were transient but recurred with repeated application. The authors concluded that nifedipine is able to dilate cerebral vessels both under normal conditions and when contracted during focal ischemia.

Phillis et al. monitored cerebral blood flow (CBF) in the rat by a venous outflow technique (44). They found that nifedipine and felodipine (administered either before or after anoxia) did not affect basal cerebral blood flow rate and, surprisingly, antagonized the increase in CBF induced by anoxia to the rats.

The effects of verapamil (VPL) on cerebral ischemia in two experiments were disappointing. Reedy et al. examined the effect of VPL on focal cerebral ischemia in cats after right MCA occlusion (45). A continuous infusion of VPL (0.2 mg/kg/hr) into the carotid artery was begun 1 hour before MCA occlusion and continued throughout the occlusion period. An additional bolus of VPL (0.5 mg/kg) was given immediately before MCA occlusion. Given this way, VPL did not improve rCBF and did not protect ischemic brain.

Roy et al. investigated the effect of verapamil and diltiazem (DTZ) in cats that underwent MCA occlusion (46). The cats received a continous intravenous infusion of either VPL (0.1 μg/kg/min) or DTZ (0.1 μg/kg/min) beginning 2 hours before MCA occlusion and continuing throughout the experiment. VPL inappropriately increased blood flow in the nonischemic hemisphere and thereby potentially worsened the focal ischemic insult. DTZ had little effect on nonischemic tissue but markedly increased perfusion of ischemic vascular beds. These results suggest that VPL may exacerbate the sequelae of acute stroke, whereas DTZ may be beneficial. Unfortunately, the beneficial effects of DTZ were limited because DTZ also caused an apparent increase in intracranial pressure and brain herniation. The investigators concluded that different calcium entry blockers probably affected several different classes of calcium channels at different brain sites during cerebral ischemia.

Particularly dramatic improvement in nervous system function was found when flunarizine (FLU) was used in dogs during resuscitation from a cardiac arrest lasting 15-20 minutes (40,47). However, these encouraging results were not supported by other studies. The effects of postischemic administration of FLU on cerebral blood flow (CBF) and metabolism ($CMRO_2$) was tested by Newberg et al. (42). They produced 10 minutes of complete cerebral ischemia in dogs by temporary ligation of both venae cavae and the ascending aorta. After reperfusion, either placebo or FLU (6 μg/kg) was infused over a 10-minute period. Flunarizine, in this model, failed to improve either CBF, $CMRO_2$, or neurological outcome. Unfortunately, only a single dose of FLU, which might be too low to afford benefit, was used. Furthermore, four of the dogs treated with FLU died of severe pulmonary edema of uncertain etiology. In a similar model in cats, Hossman et al. (48) found that FLU failed to prevent the large postischemic accumulation of Ca^{2+} within the brain and likewise did not improve the metabolic recovery in ischemic brain during reperfusions.

Deshpande and Wieloch (49) evaluated the effects of FLU in a long-term survival model of ischemia in three groups of rats. One group received FLU (40 mg/kg per dose) orally at 24 and 4 hours prior to the insult. Another group was given the drug following the insult, IV at 5 minutes (0.1 mg/kg) and orally at 8 and 24 hours (40 mg/kg per dose). The third group received only the solvent on the same schedule as the pretreated group. They found that FLU reduced ischemic cerebral damage when given postischemia. Their results did not correlate with the early recovery of either cortical energy or free fatty acid metabolism or with the improvement of postischemic delayed hypoperfusion. The mechanism, then, of this postischemic improvement in function remains speculative.

The influence of FLU on perinatal hypoxic-ischemic encephalopathy in 7-day-old rats was studied by Silverstein et al. (50), who induced hypoxic-ischemic brain injury by unilateral carotid artery ligation and subsequent exposure for 2 hours at 8% oxygen tension. Pretreatment with FLU (30 mg/kg) either parenterally or orally afforded protection against morphological brain injury.

The protective properties of PY 108-068, a potent calcium antagonist of the dihydropyridine type, against brain ischemia in vitro and in vivo was studied by Wiernsperger et al. (51). The competitive inhibiton of the effect of calcium by PY 108-068 was demonstrated in isolated calcium-loaded arterial rings of cat cerebral arteries. The results in vivo showed that PY 108-068 improved oxygen supply in the cortex of cats subjected to epicerebral arterial occlusion, reversed the spastic state of cortical microvessels in a model of cerebral vasospasm, and

58. Barnett GH, Bose B, Little JR, Jones SC, Friel HT. Effects of nimodipine on acute focal cerebral ischemia. *Stroke 17*:884-890, 1986.
59. Mohamed AA, Gotoh O, Graham DI, Osborne KA, McCulloch J, Mendelow AD, Teasdale GM, Harper AM. Effect of pretreatment with the calcium antagonist nimodipine on local cerebral blood flow and histopathology after middle cerebral artery occlusion. *Ann Neurol 18*:705-711, 1985.
60. Steen PA, Newberg LA, Milde JH, Michenfelder JD. Cerebral blood flow and neurologic outcome when nimodipine is given after complete cerebral ischemia in the dog. *J Cereb Blood Flow Metab 4*:82-87, 1984.
61. Steen PA, Gisvold SE, Milde JH, Newberg LA, Scheithauer BW, Lanier WL, Michenfelder JD. Nimodipine improves outcome when given after complete cerebral ischemia in primates. *Anesthesiology 62*:406-414, 1985.
62. Hakim AM. Nimodipine moderates the cerebral acidosis in MCA occluded rats (abstract). *Stroke 17*:22, 1986.
63. Hakim AM. Cerebral acidosis in focal ischemia: II. Nimodipine and verapamil normalize cerebral pH following middle cerebral artery occlusion in the rat. *J Cereb Blood Flow Metab 6*:676-683, 1986.
64. Meyer FB, Anderson BE, Sundt TM, Sharbrough FW. Selective central nervous system calcium channel blockers—a new class of anticonvulsant agents. *Mayo Clinic Proc 61*:239-247, 1986.
65. Germano I, Bartkowski H, Nishimura M, Cassel B, Pitts L. The effects of nimodipine in acute experimental cerebral ischemia in the rat (abstract). *Stroke 17*:22, 1986.
66. Heffez DS, Passonneau JV. Effect of nimodipine on cerebral metabolism during ischemia and recirculation in the mongolian gerbil. *J Cereb Blood Flow Metab 5*:523-528, 1985.
67. Mabe H, Nagai H, Takagi T, Umemura S, Ohno M. Effect of nimodipine on cerebral functional and metabolic recovery following ischemia in the rat brain. *Stroke 17*:501-505, 1986.
68. Arrigo A, et al. Flunarizine in the therapy of chronic cerebrovascular insufficiency. Multicentric controlled study. *Clin Ter 30*:110(6):541-548(Ita), 1984.
69. Deshpande JK, et al. Amelioration of ischemic brain damage by postischemic treatment with flunarizine. *Neurol Res 71*:27-29, 1985.
70. Allen GS, Ahn HS, Preziosi TJ, Battye R, Boone SC, Chou SN, Kelly DL, Weir BK, Crabbe RA, Lavik PJ, Rosenbloom SB, Dorsey FC, Ingram CR, Mellits DE, Bertsch LA, Boisvert DPJ, Hundley MB, Johnson RK, Strom JA, Transou CR. Cerebral arterial spasm—a controlled trial of nimodipine in patients with subarachnoid hemorrhage. *N Engl J Med 308*:619-624, 1983.
71. Gelmers HJ. The effects of nimodipine on the clinical course of patients with acute ischemic stroke. *Acta Neurol Scand 69*:232-239, 1984.
72. Mathew NT, Meyer JS, Rivera VH. Double blind evaluation of glycerol treatment in acute cerebral infarction. *Lancet 2*:1327-1333, 1972.
73. Gelmers HJ, Gorter K, de Weerdt CJ, Wiezer JHA. A controlled trial of nimopidine in acute ischemic stroke. *N Engl J Med 318*:203-207, 1988.

74. Sherman DG, Easton JD, Hart RG, Sherman CP, Battye R. Nimodipine in acute cerebral infarction. A double blind study of safety and efficacy. In: Battistini N, Fiorani P, Courbier R, Plum F, Fieschi C (Eds.), *Acute Brain Ischemia Medical and Surgical Therapy*. Raven Press, New York, 1986, pp. 257-262.
75. Denny-Brown D. The treatment of recurrent cerebrovascular symptoms and the question of "vasospasm." *Med Clin N Am 35*:1457-1475, 1951.
76. The Prostacyclin Study Group. Intravenous prostacyclin in acute non-hemorrhagic stroke: a placebo controlled double blind trial. *Stroke* 1987.
77. Meldrum B. Excitatory amino acids and anoxic/ischaemic brain damage. *Trends Neurosci 8*:47-48, 1985.
78. Mayer ML, Westbrook GL. Cellular mechanisms underlying excitotoxicity. *Trends Neurosci 10*:59-61, 1987.
79. Scott CK, Persico FJ, Carpenter K, Chasin M. The effects of flunarizine, a new calcium antagonist, on human red blood cells in vitro. *Angiology 31*: 320-330, 1986.
80. DeClerck F, Beerens M, Thone F, Borgers M. Effect of flunarazine on the human red cell shape changes and calcium deposition induced by A23187. *Thromb Res 24*:1-24, 1981.

10

Neuropeptides and Cerebral Ischemia

Robert J. Fallis*

Brigham and Women's Hospital, Harvard Medical School, Boston, Massachusetts

I. INTRODUCTION

Since the initial discovery of an endogenous opiate receptor within the central nervous system (CNS) (1), there has been rapid progress in defining families of

**Present affiliation*: Neuroimmunology Branch, National Institutes of Health, Bethesda, Maryland

Table 1 Major Categories of Neuropeptides in the Central Nervous System

Precursor	Derived peptides
A. Endogenous Opioids	
1. Pro-opiomelanocortin	ACTH
	β-lipotropin
	β-endorphin
	α-MSH, β-MSH, γ-MSH
2. Proenkephalin	Met-enkephalin
	Leu-enkephalin
	Met-enkephalin-arg-gly-leu
	Met-enkephalin-gly-phe
	Peptides B, E, F, I
	Amidorphin
	Metorphamide
3. Prodynorphin (proenkephalin B)	α-neoendorphin
	β-neoendorphin
	Dynorphin A
	Dynorphin B
	Rimorphin
	Leu-enkephalin
B. Brain-gut neuropeptides	
1. Provasoactive intestinal polypeptide	Vasoactive intestinal polypeptide
	PHM-27
2. Procholecystokinin	Cholecystokinin
3. Preprotachykinin (α and β forms)	Substance P
	Substance K
4. Preprogastrin	Gastrin
5. Proproglucagon	Glucagon
6. Others	Neurotensin
	Insulin
	Motilin
C. Hypothalamic releasing hormones	
1. Preprosomatostatin	Somatostatin
2. Others	Thyrotropin-releasing hormone
	Gonadotropin-releasing hormone
D. Neurohypophyseal neuropeptides	
1. Preprovasopressin	Vasopressin
	Neurophysin II
	Glycoprotein
2. Prepro-oxytocin	Neurophysin I
	Oxytocin
E. Hypophyseal neuropeptides	Prolactin
	Growth hormone
	Luteinizing hormone

Table 1 (Continued)

Precursor	Derived peptides
F. Others	
1. Preproangiotensin	Angiotensin
2. Preprobradykinin	Bradykinin
3. Other	Atrial natriuretic factor

Source: Modified from Refs. 7, 15, and 27.

opiate and nonopiate receptors, as well as families of endogenous neuropeptide ligands for these receptors. The neuropeptides have been proposed to function in various cases either as putative neurotransmitters or as hormones. The functions of the various neuropeptides have proven to be diverse, ranging from the mediation of pain to the modulation of cardiovascular, autonomic, and behavioral functions. Following reports suggesting that the opiate antagonist naloxone may be efficacious in the clinical management of cerebral ischemia (2), there has been additional interest in the role that neuropeptides may play in the pathogenesis of stroke. This chapter reviews the neuropeptides as they relate to cerebrovascular disease and discusses the therapeutic potential of these peptides and their analogs in the management of stroke.

II. NEUROPEPTIDES: BASIC CONCEPTS

More than 50 biologically active neuropeptides have been characterized (Table 1). They may be classified into a number of families on the basis of their biochemical and pharmacological characteristics. Functionally, the neuropeptides have all been proposed to mediate their actions through neurotransmitter mechanisms. Some of them, such as ACTH, are also known to function through classical hormonal pathways. Although the functions of many of the peptides have yet to be fully elucidated, their known functions are diverse. Of particular interest is the fact that vasoactive properties have been demonstrated in experimental systems for a number of the neuropeptides. A complete review of all of the neuropeptides and their functions is outside the scope of this chapter (see Ref. 3 for a review). Here emphasis is on those peptides that are known or suspected to have vasoactive properties.

A. The Endogenous Opioids

The discovery of the endogenous opiate receptor was made in 1973 (1). In 1975, the endogenous opiate receptor ligands methionine-enkephalin (met-enkephalin) and leucine-enkephalin (leu-enkephalin) were described (4). Since then, advances in the field have been rapid. As a result of this work, families of neuropeptides have been described that are related on a biochemical and pharmacological level. As a rule, members of each family are derived from high molecular weight precursor peptides termed polyproteins. The derivation of biologically active lower molecular weight daughter peptides from a high molecular weight precursor through a variety of processing events has emerged as a general concept in the study of neuropeptide families. For example, the enkephalins are now known to be derived from a common high molecular weight precursor peptide called proenkephalin. Computer analysis of the nucleotide sequences of precursor genes have directly substantiated this relationship (5).

There are three families of opioid peptides in vertebrates, each characterized by a unique precursor peptide: proenkephalin A (PE), pro-opiomelanocortin (POMC), and prodynorphin (PD), which is also known as proenkephalin B (Fig. 1). POMC was the first precursor peptide to be well characterized in relation to its daughter peptides and the various processing events that generate these peptides. When fully processed, POMC gives rise to ACTH, β-lipotropin (β-LPH), β-endorphin (which is a low molecular weight product derived from β-LPH), and three forms of melanocyte-stimulating hormone (α-MSH, β-MSH, and γ-MSH). Each of these peptides is biologically active. In addition, POMC contains a sequence sufficient to code for met-enkephalin. Biologically active met-enkephalin is probably not derived from this sequence, however, due to the lack of a proteolytic processing site in the sequence. The biologically active form of met-enkephalin derives from a different polyprotein, proenkephalin A. Genetic analyses of the nucleotide sequence coding for the POMC polyprotein through recombinant DNA techniques have been instrumental in verifying these relationships. These techniques also predicted the existence of a POMC derivative product, γ-MSH, prior to its isolation (6). POMC processing may give rise to different daughter peptides depending on the tissue in which the polyprotein is found. Tissue-specific POMC processing events are best understood in the rat pituitary gland system (reviewed in Ref. 7). In the intermediate lobe of the rat pituitary, which is absent in humans, POMC is processed to produce lower molecular weight products, such as α-MSH and β-endorphin. In the anterior lobe, higher molecular weight derivatives are produced, including ACTH and β-LPH. Anatomically, POMC is found in restricted locations. It is found primarily in the pituitary gland, the nucleus of the tractus solitarius, and the medial basal hypothalamus. POMC-rich fibers project from the hypothalamus to the limbic system and the brainstem (8). Outside of the CNS, POMC is found along with PE and PD in the adrenal medulla and is widely distributed throughout the autonomic nervous system.

The daughter peptides derived from POMC have a variety of known functions. Some of the derivative products of POMC and the other pro-opioids func-

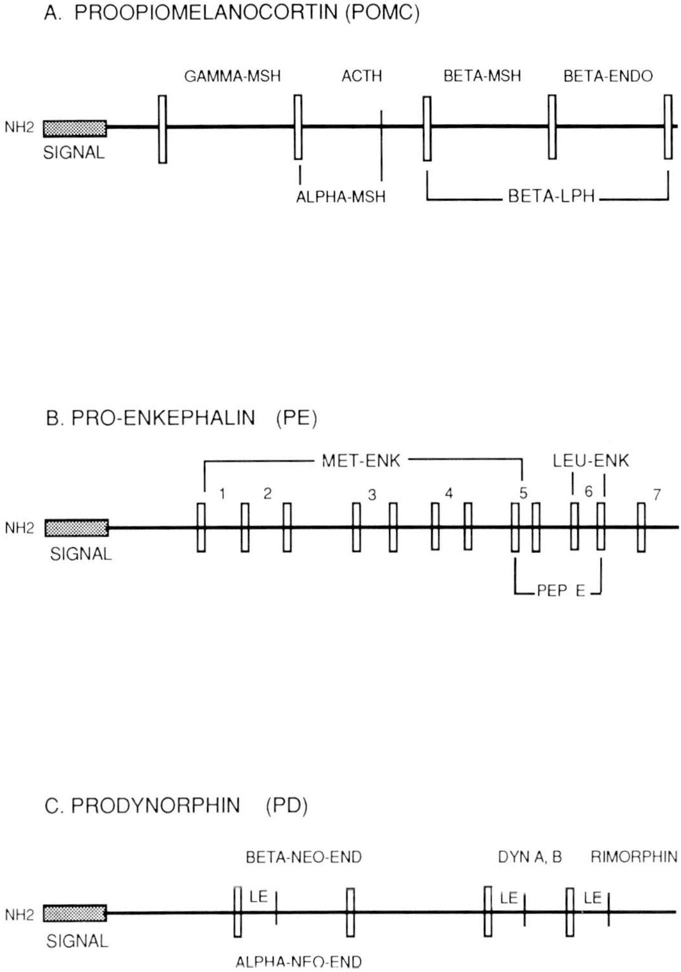

Figure 1 Schematic representation of the structures of the three opioid precursor polyproteins. (Modified from Refs. 8 and 27.) The precursor protein is indicated in each case, along with the major derived functional peptides. Enzymatic processing cleavage sites (occuring at dibasic amino acid sites) are denoted by vertical bars. The precursor peptides are not drawn to scale. (*A*) POMC is processed to ACTH, β-endorphin (beta-endo), β-lipotropin (beta-LPH), and MSH. (*B*) Proenkephalin contains four copies of met-enkephalin (met-enk) distributed between sites 1, 2, 3, and 5. Two peptides modified around the met-enk sequence are also present, one at site 4 and one at site 7. One copy of leu-enkephalin (leu-enk) is found at site 6. Peptide E (pep E) is also shown. (*C*) Prodynorphin is processed to α and β-neo-endorphin (neo-end) dynorphin A and B (dyn A and B), rimorphin, and three copies of leu-enkephalin (LE).

tion in blood pressure homeostasis. Of interest in this regard is the known physiological relationship between the vagal-solitary complex in the brainstem, a rich source of POMC, and its function in blood pressure homeostasis through baroreceptor and chemoreceptor reflex arcs. POMC is found in the nucleus of the solitary tract along with the two other known precursor polypeptides in the opioid family. This site is the only location in the nervous system, other than the hypothalamus, known to contain the POMC, PE, and PD families of opioids, suggesting a complex interrelationship between these peptides and blood pressure control (9).

The POMC daughter peptide β-endorphin is known to have a number of important effects on cardiovascular function. Modulation of cardiovascular homeostasis has been studied in several systems including the anesthetized rat, where β-endorphin was found to induce hypotension following intracisternal administration. Treatment with the opiate antagonist naloxone effectively inhibited this hypotensive effect (10). Intravenous or intrathecal administration of β-endorphin has produced hypotension and bradycardia in conscious rats and monkeys and anesthetized dogs (9). The peptide has not been reported to selectively modulate cerebral blood flow. It is reported that β-endorphin is secreted during periods of experimental stress (11) and may also be involved in reducing behavioral responses to the pain of repetitive foot shock, thus leading to stress-induced analgesia (12). In humans, β-endorphin levels in the plasma are elevated during pregnancy and labor (13), suggesting a role for the peptide in the modulation of this physiological stress.

The other major POMC products, ACTH and MSH, also function in blood pressure control. These functions are mediated through hormonal mechanisms. ACTH is known to modulate pressor responses by directly regulating adrenal cortical function, thus leading to the regulation of salt and water balance through secondary mechanisms. By potentiating steroidogenesis, γ-MSH may influence these responses (14). MSH also has a well-described role in the regulation of melanocyte function. ACTH may have additional central effects within the brain and may function in certain behavioral responses, such as analgesia and memory (15).

The second precursor peptide in the opioid family is proenkephalin (PE). The pentapeptides met-enkaphalin and leu-enkephalin are both derived from this polyprotein. Met-enkephalin is distinguished by a methionine residue at its carboxyl terminus, whereas leu-enkephalin contains a leucine at that position. The remaining four amino acids in the sequences (tyr-gly-gly-phe) are common to both met-enkephalin and leu-enkephalin. Four copies of met-enkephalin and one copy of leu-enkephalin are found within the PE polyprotein. An additional eight peptides modified around the met-enkephalin nuclear pentapeptide sequences are also derived from PE. Proenkephalin is distributed widely. It is found throughout the CNS and also in locations outside of the CNS, such as the gastrointestinal tract and the adrenal medulla (16). As is the case with POMC, PE processing is carried to different stages according to the anatomical localization of this polyprotein. All of the products derived from PE have opioid properties and are therefore involved in the mediation of analgesic responses. The enkephalins also affect cardiovascular homeostasis and exert a pressor effect in a number of experimental systems, although this varies according to the system under study. The pressor effect mediated by centrally administered enkephalins is relatively naloxone-resistant (10), whereas the pressor responses generated by intravenously injected enkephalins are not (17). In addition to increasing blood pressure following their administration, the enkephalins are capable of increasing both heart rate and respiratory rate (18).

The last precursor peptide in the opioid system is prodynorphin (PD). Prodynorphin gives rise to five known peptides, each a modification of the basic leu-enkephalin sequence. These are α-neoendorphin, β-neoendorphin, dynorphin A, dynorphin B, and rimorphin. With full processing of this precursor peptide, three copies of leu-enkephalin are produced. Prodynorphin is distributed primarily in the gastrointestinal tract, in the pituitary, and in the brain, where it is found in the hypothalamus and within the brain stem (19). Dynorphin and alpha-neoendorphin are high-affinity ligands of the κ opioid receptor and, in experimental models, generate hypotension through a diuretic mechanism mediated by this receptor (20). These opioids may also regulate blood pressure by direct modulation of the sympathetic nervous system (21). The magnitude of these cardiovascular effects, however, is variable and depends on the experimental paradigm under study (8,9).

1. *Opiate Receptors*

The biological effects of the endogenous opiates are mediated by specific, high-affinity receptors for these peptides. As the number of identified endogenous opioids has grown, so have the number of opioid receptors. Five unique classes of endogenous opioid receptors have been described: μ, δ, κ, σ, and ϵ (22,23). Evidence suggests that subclasses, or isotypes, of some receptor types exist as well (24). These various receptor types differ in their neuropharmacology, in their anatomical distribution within the CNS, and in their putative functional properties. Autoradiography of CNS tissue using radiolabeled ligands has permitted the localization of the various receptor types within the nervous system. The μ receptors are found in the hippocampus, hypothalamus, thalamus, and the periaqueductal grey (25). The κ receptors are found deep in the cortex and in the cerebellum (26). The δ receptor is distributed in the amygdala and in the nucleus accumbens as well as in the substantia gelatinosa, which also contains μ receptors (25).

The restricted anatomical locations of different receptor types within the CNS has suggested that the endogenous opiates exert their effects in an anatomically constrained fashion through their respective receptors. As a result, the endogenous opiates may function on a number of levels depending on the specific neuronal pathways with which the peptides and their receptors are associated. Each receptor types has various functions associated with it. The mu receptor is concerned with traditional analgesic responses. This receptor binds morphine with high affinity. The κ or ketocyclazocine receptor is distinguished pharmacologically from the μ receptor by the inability of κ-specific ligands to induce bradycardia or precipitate a morphine withdrawal crisis when given in vivo. The sedative effects of some opiate drugs are mediated through this receptor. Although it is unclear if the dynorphins represent the endogenous ligands for the κ receptor, they are able to ligate this receptor with high affinity (27). The delta or enkephalin receptor may be involved in limbic seizures and some behavioral responses (28). Met-enkephalin and leu-enkephalin bind to the delta receptor and to the μ receptor with high affinity. It is known that β-endorphin binds preferentially to the μ receptor but will also bind to δ receptors (23). It has also been postulated that β-endorphin binds to an ε receptor (29). The σ receptor is known to bind the drug SKF-10047 in a nonstereospecific manner. When the drug is administered, general CNS activation, such as tachycardia, pupillary dilatation, and mania result. The characteristics of this opiate receptor are controversial. The receptor does not display the stereospecificity characteristic of the μ, δ, and κ receptors. In addition, some evidence suggests that it may be the receptor for the nonopiate drug phencyclidine (8,22).

The identification of unique receptor types has largely been dependent on the development of highly specific drugs that are able to bind to these receptors with very high affinities. A number of pharmacological agents are available that may be characterized as opiate antagonists or agonists at the receptor level. These drugs have proven to be useful in the characterization of the opiate receptors, but most are not purely selective and bind with differential affinities to various receptor classes when used at different concentrations. By using highly selective pharmacological probes, workers have begun to identify specific receptors responsible for a biological effect. Holaday and his coworkers, for example, were able to show with the aid of a specific delta receptor antagonist that the production of experimental hypotension could be inhibited. This inhibition did not occur when an irreversible μ-selective antagonist was added to the preparation. This was in contrast to the inhibition seen following the administration of naloxone, which is a μ receptor antagonist with much less restricted specificity. Through the use of these receptor-specific agents, these workers were able to postulate that the generation of hypotension in this system, and its reversal by naloxone, was not mediated through μ-receptor-specific mechanisms (30).

Naloxone is probably the opiate antagonist most widely used in clinical practice today. It preferentially binds to the μ receptor and thus is widely used as a morphine antagonist. At higher doses, however, it is clear that naloxone is not a pure μ antagonist, and the drug in fact can show opiate agonist activities (31, 32). This dose-dependent change in the neuropharmacological properties of naloxone underscores the need for careful interpretation of studies using drugs, such as naloxone, that are mixed in their ability to bind opiate receptors.

B. Nonopiate Vasoactive Neuropeptides

1. Vasoactive Intestinal Polypeptide

The brain-gut peptides, found in both the gastrointestinal tract and the CNS, comprise one of the nonopioid families of neuropeptides (Table 1). Vasoactive intestinal polypeptide (VIP) is an important member of this family. This peptide exists as a high molecular weight precursor peptide, provasoactive intestinal polypeptide. This polyprotein is then processed into VIP and a second, lower molecular weight protein, PHM-27 (33). Vasoactive intestinal polypeptide and VIP-specific receptors are distributed both within the CNS and peripherally. In the nervous system, VIP is found in the neocortex, hippocampus, hypothalamus, amygdala, stria terminalis, and periaqueductal grey. In the periphery, VIP is found in association with autonomic nerve terminals in the gastrointestinal tract (where this peptide was first discovered) and in the genitourinary and respiratory tracts (34,35). The peptide has also been detected in nerve endings supplying blood vessels in both the intestine (36) and the brain. In the cerebrovascular system, VIP is especially rich in distribution in nerves supplying the anterior cerebral, posterior communicating, and proximal middle cerebral arteries. It appears to be less widely distributed through the vertebral-basilar system (37). VIP has been shown to exert a vasodilatory effect on cerebral arteries (37) and in cerebral arterioles, where the degree of vasodilation is directly dose-dependent (38). Infusions of VIP have been shown to increase cerebral blood flow in several experimental animal models, including the dog (39), goat (40), and baboon (41). Although these studies provide a number of insights into the modulation of cerebral blood flow by VIP, this peptide has not been implicated in the pathogenesis of stroke or cerebral ischemia despite its known distribution and vasoactive properties. Further investigation will be essential in defining the role that VIP may play in the modulation of cerebral blood flow.

2. Other Vasoactive Neuropeptides

A number of nonopioid neuropeptides have been reported to influence blood pressure regulation and salt and water balance, although none have been implicated in the pathogenesis of cerebral ischemia or stroke. These include substance P, bradykinin, angiotensin, vasopressin, neurotensin, and atrial natriuretic factor. These peptides are found within the CNS as well as peripherally. Some have been detected in nerve terminals closely associated with the cerebral vasculature (15). Substance P, neurotensin, and atrial natriuretic factor have all been found to be capable of producing hypotension in experimental systems (27). Atrial natriuretic factor may do so through both central and peripheral effects. Angiotensin is a potent pressor agent that acts through vasoconstrictor mechanisms (9,27). Vasopressin is able to regulate blood pressure through its regulator effects on water retention and excretion by the kidneys. Bradykinin has been demonstrated to generate both hypotension and hypertension according to how it is administered in the experimental system (42). In addition to these cardiovascular effects of the neuropeptides, it has been suggested that the vasoactive neuropeptides may play a role in the pathognesis of migraine and vasospasm (43). This hypothesis has not been supported by firm experimental evidence.

The nonopioid tripeptide thyrotropin-releasing hormone (TRH) has been found to affect cardiorespiratory functions (9). It does not bind to opiate receptors, but has been found to antagonize many opiate effects without antagonizing analgesic effects (44). The therapeutic effects of this peptide in the treatment of experimental models of spinal cord trauma (45) and shock (46) and cerebral ischemia (47) have been studied.

C. Excitatory Neuropeptides

The major excitatory neurotransmitters of the central nervous system are the excitatory amino acids, particularly L-glutamate and L-aspartate. There appear to be four distinct receptor systems for these excitatory amino acids: The *N*-methyl-*D*-aspartate (NMDA), kainate (K), and quisqualate (Q) receptors have been described on the basis of the actions of selective agonists; a fourth receptor has been defined by specific antagonist effects of L-2-aminophosphobutyric acid (48). These four receptor types each have characteristic electrophysiological, anatomical, and biochemical profiles. The NMDA receptors form a system complementary to the K and Q receptors. Glutamatergic synapses often function by utilizing the K and/or Q receptors to generate a fast depolarizing response; if an appropriate membrane potential is reached, the NMDA receptors become activated. Current derived from NMDA receptors is longer lasting than K- or Q-derived current; it also allows entry of calcium in addition to sodium ions. Magnesium ions serve as noncompetitive antagonists of NMDA-receptor activation by gating voltage-dependent cation channels normally opened by NMDA. The activity of both NMDA and non-NMDA receptors at glutamatergic synapses help provide synaptic plasticity for the CNS (48).

The distribution of NMDA receptors is of particular interest as a potential explanation of the phenomenon of selective vulnerability of the CNS to hypoxic-ischemic injury. In the adult, hypoxic-ischemic insult preferentially affects cerebral cortical layers III, V, and VI; Sommer's sector or CA1 of hippocampus;

amygdala; and cerebellar neurons, particularly Purkinje cells. Spinal cord and thalamic neurons are more resistant to hypoxic-ischemic injury. Autoradiographical studies localizing NMDA sites have demonstrated substantial similarity of distribution (with the exception of Purkinje cells) between regions of high density of NMDA receptors and the known regions selectively vulnerable to hypoxic-ischemic injury (49).

D. Summary: Neuropeptides and Their Functions

A number of neuropeptides, both opioid and nonopioid, are known to effect cardiovascular homeostasis in experimental models. Some have been suggested, based on indirect evidence, to modulate cerebral blood flow. It is evident that the functional heterogeneity of the neuropeptides and their known receptors is complex. Functional diversity is generated as a result of this complexity in a number of ways. A given polypeptide, for example, may generate multiple daughter peptides with diverse functions as it is subjected to various degrees of processing, and some polyproteins, such as POMC, may be processed differentially according to the tissue in which the peptide is found. As predicted by DNA sequence data, additional biologically active daughter peptides derived from precursor polyproteins may exist, although they remain undiscovered. There is controversy surrounding the classes and characteristics of the neuropeptide receptors, but the field is advancing rapidly as pharmacological probes with more highly defined specificities are developed. Many available receptor ligands, such as naloxone, have mixed receptor specificities, and this has confused the interpretation of experimental and clinical studies that utilize these relatively nonspecific drugs.

Despite the fact that none of the neuropeptides have been firmly established as cerebrovascular regulatory peptides, the existing evidence has generated interest in exploring the therapeutic potential of the neuropeptides and their exogenous analogues in the treatment of cerebral ischemia. The analogue that has been most commonly used is the morphine antagonist naloxone.

III. EXPERIMENTAL STUDIES

A. Naloxone

In 1978, Holaday and Faden demonstrated that the opiate antagonist naloxone could significantly improve the hypotension associated with experimentally induced endotoxemia (50,51). Later, the same workers extended their observations to show that naloxone was also effective in modulating the hypotension associated with hypovolemic shock (52), transection of the cervical spinal cord (53), and cervical spinal cord trauma (54,55). Naloxone was shown to generate these effects in a stereospecific manner (56). Others have confirmed and extended these findings to show that naloxone not only improves neurological outcome following spinal cord injury but also improves spinal cord blood flow and preserves somatosensory evoked potential responses (57). In these systems, levels of β-endorphin were found to be increased in the blood following experimental manipulation, suggesting that spinal cord injury or shock caused activation of the endorphin system. Holaday and Faden hypothesized (58) that β-endorphin release led to irreversible cord injury by generating local hypoperfusion, ischemia, and infarction around the region of injury. Naloxone was postulated to antagonize this endorphin effect through specific receptor mechanisms (53), thus reversing local hypoperfusion and minimizing spinal cord ischemia in the region of trauma. Since local perfusion was improved, areas of infarction were minimized following the injury. This hypothesis has provided a foundation for additional studies of experimentally induced cerebral ischemia.

The beneficial effects of naloxone in experimental models of hypotension and spinal cord injury promoted interest in applying opiate antagonists to the treatment of experimental models of cerebral ischemia. Hosobuchi et al. (59) reported that naloxone, given in an intraperitoneal dose of 1 mg/kg, was effective in reversing the ischemic neurological deficits induced in gerbils after permanent unilateral carotid artery ligation. Unfortunately, this promising observation was not confirmed by others who attempted to repeat the work using similar methodology (60-62). Holaday and D'Amato (63) were able to show that temporary bilateral carotid artery occlusion in gerbils was associated with hypotension that could be reversed with intravenous naloxone at a dose of 5 mg/kg, although no effect on neurological function was seen with this dose. Using an air embolism model of cerebral ischemia in dogs, Faden et al. (47) demonstrated improvements both in cerebral blood flow, as measured by ^{14}C-iodoantipyrine autoradiography, and in the cortical somatosensory evoked responses after 1 hour of ischemic injury. Naloxone was given as an initial 2 mg/kg bolus, followed by an infusion at 2 mg/kg/hr. Although neurological outcome was not reported, these investigators suggested that naloxone may have acted in a protective role to help limit the extent of cerebral ischemia. A number of other studies have reported that naloxone is effective in improving neurological recovery after experimental cerebral ischemia. These experimental models have involved studies of permanent middle cerebral artery occlusion in the cat (64), spontaneous stroke-prone rats fed a high salt diet (65), middle cerebral artery occlusion in the baboon (66,67), and ischemic spinal injury in the rabbit (68). The dosages of naloxone used in these studies ranged between 1 mg/kg in the rat model to 7 mg/kg in the baboon. Improved functional recovery was reported in all instances and was correlated in one study with a reduction in pathology in the responding animals (66). Only one study (69), involving both permanent and temporary middle cerebral artery occlusion in the baboon, failed to show any improvement in neurological function following treatment with a naloxone bolus of 10 mg/kg followed by a 10 mg/kg/hr infusion. Cerebral blood flow and infarct size were also measured in this study and found to be unchanged after naloxone treatment. Faden (68) has suggested that the optimal dose of naloxone for the treatment of experimental ischemia is between 2 and 5 mg/kg. Therefore, the failure of this last study to demonstrate improvement may have been due to the use of an excessively high dosage of the drug.

The experimental evidence to date suggests that the experimentally induced hypotension associated with a number of experimental models can be effectively modulated by the opiate antagonist naloxone in a stereospecific manner. A dose of 2-5 mg/kg, much higher than the 0.006 mg/kg dose required for antagonism of the pharmacological effects of morphine, is needed for this effect. The mechanisms through which naloxone exerts its effects on neurological function and outcome following cerebral ischemia or infarction have remained controversial. It has not been possible to identify a unique neuropeptide pathway in this system, partially because naloxone has been utilized at dosages at which its functions are complex and not limited to morphine receptor antagonism. Additional effects, other than antagonism at the mu receptor, may be critically important in the modulation of hypotension by naloxone in experimental models. Although generally viewed as a pure opiate antagonist, naloxone has long been known to exert opiate agonist properties when used at high dosages (31). The drug is known to have a number of effects at these dosages, some of which are not directly mediated through the opiate system. For example, naloxone may exert a number of inhibitory effects on a variety of nonopiate compounds, including substance P (32). The dosages required are in general much higher than those needed to antagonize the effects of narcotic drugs such as morphine. When given to human volunteers in high doses (up to 4 mg/kg), naloxone has been shown to produce dose-dependent increases in the systolic blood pressure and in the respiratory rate (70). Other studies have shown naloxone to have a number of other functional properties unrelated to neuropeptide antagonism, such as antagonism of the GABA system (71). The effects of this compound are, therefore, complex and dose-dependent.

B. Excitatory Neurotransmitters

Much of the interest in excitatory neurotransmitters in stroke stems from work done on cultures of rat hippocampus. Rothman (72) observed that mature neurons (at least 2 weeks in vitro) with spontaneous synaptic activity were more sensitive to anoxia than were younger neurons. Additionally, mature neurons tolerated prolonged anoxia without morphological changes when in the presence of a high concentration of magnesium (73).

The initial studies of hypoxic neuronal injury have been followed by a series of experiments that generally support the concept that NMDA receptor blockade can reduce ischemic neuronal injury. Intrahippocampal injections of the competitive inhibitor 2-amino-7-phosphonoheptanoic acid reduce the early ischemic neuronal changes associated with carotid occlusion and hypotension in the rat (74). Later studies have used MK-801, a noncompetitive NMDA-receptor antagonist with putative action at an ion channel site. Ozyurt et al. (75) reported reduced volume of ischemic damage at 6 hours following focal cerebral ischemia in pretreated cats. Kochlar et al. (76) reported protective effects of MK-801 pretreatment in rabbit models of cerebral embolism and spinal cord ischemia.

There are several explanations for the apparent efficacy of NMDA-receptor blockade in cerebral ischemia. The most widely held view is that a synaptically released excitatory neurotransmitter, probably glutamate, accumulates to neurotoxic concentrations under ischemic or anoxic conditions. Glutamate accumulation during ischemia or hypoxia is probably due to both excessive release and reduced neuronal and glial reuptake. The consequences of toxic (greater than 100 μM in vitro) glutamate concentration appear to be (1) immediate neuronal swelling and lysis due to influx of sodium, calcium, and chloride ions and (2) calcium-mediated destruction of neuronal membranes and neurofilaments (77).

There are many important questions regarding the role of excitatory neurotransmitters in stroke. These include:

1. What is the effectiveness of NMDA-receptor blockade in cerebral ischemia in primates?
2. Is the effect of excitatory neurotransmitter blockade in stroke a manifestation of antiepileptic properties of these agents? If so, they are less likely to be effective in human stroke.
3. Does the reduction of ischemic change with NMDA blockade result in reduction in size of the ultimate infarct, or is infarct development simply delayed? That is, does ischemic change become similar to the delayed neuronal death seen 3 days following four-vessel occlusion in the rat, a process that is probably not a typical feature of human cerebral ischemia (75,78)?
4. What is the effect of delay of treatment after the onset of cerebral ischemia?
5. What are the roles of other neurotransmitters with excitatory activity, especially dopaminergic transmitters? Initial studies have implicated the excitatory D2 receptor as having significance in ischemic neuronal injury (79).

These and other questions will be of great importance as the role of excitatory neurotransmitters in stroke is fully elucidated.

IV. CLINICAL STUDIES

A. Naloxone

Brandt and colleagues (80) reported a case of subacute necrotizing encephalomyelopathy characterized by increased levels of CSF beta-endorphin and clinical symptoms mimicking those of morphine poisoning. Naloxone was able to transiently reverse these symptoms when given in dosages ranging from 0.2 to 1.8 mg. Following this initial report, Baskin and Hosobuchi (2) treated two selected postoperative patients with cerebral ischemia and depressed states of consciousness with intravenous naloxone at a dose of 0.4 mg (approximately 0.006 mg/kg) and described transient improvement in neurological function following treatment of these patients, but not in a third patient with CT evidence of cerebral infarction. Four subsequent studies have demonstrated either no benefit or only minimal benefit from naloxone when the drug was used in dosages ranging up to 4 mg per patient (approximately 0.06 mg/kg) (81-84). These studies have in general involved the treatment of patients with radiological evidence of cerebral infarction, and in each of these studies patients were treated with naloxone hours to days following the onset of neurological symptoms using dosages much lower than those that have been shown to provide benefit in experimental models. Jabaily and Davis (81) utilized naloxone in doses ranging between 0.8 and 1.2 mg (approximately 0.016-0.018 mg/kg) in the treatment of cerebral infarction and ischemia. Patients were treated between 4 and 36 hours following the onset of stroke. In three of seven patients, transient improvement in neurological function lasting up to 1 hour was noted. Bredesen and colleagues (82) were unable to demonstrate an improvement in neurological function in a group of 10 patients who had suffered stroke from a variety of causes, including ischemic infarction, hemorrhage, and subarachnoid hemorrhage. Patients were treated with 0.4-0.8 mg (0.006-0.012 mg/kg) with naloxone. The treatment with naloxone was delayed up to 14 days following the stroke onset. These workers later extended their study to include 19 patients: 14 with stroke, four with brain hemorrhage, and one with subarachnoid hemorrhage (83). All patients were treated within 72 hours following the onset of symptoms using 0.8-2.0 mg of naloxone. No improvement was seen in neurological function in any patient treated. Fallis et al. (84), in a double-blind trial comparing naloxone in dosages of 0.4-4.0 mg (0.006-0.060 mg/kg) to normal saline found no improvement in neurological function following naloxone treatment in a group of 15 patients who had suffered either cerebral infarction or hemorrhage. Patients were treated between 8 and 60 hours following the onset of symptoms. No significant alterations in mean blood pressure and no significant elevations of plasma β-endorphin levels in the treated population were detected during the study.

The results of the clinical studies involving the use of naloxone in stroke have remained controversial, although most studies have found naloxone to be ineffective in improving neurological outcome following stroke. These results have been disappointing when compared to the beneficial effect of naloxone in the treatment of experimental hypotension. These results in the clinical use of naloxone for treatment of human stroke may be due to a number of discrepancies between experimental and clinical studies. First, although the doses used in these clinical trials were up to 10 times the amount initially reported to be of benefit in the treatment of human cerebral ischemia (2), these doses of naloxone were nevertheless up to a thousandfold less than the 2-5 mg/kg doses shown to be effective in experimental models of spinal cord injury and hypotension. In an effort to address the question of proper dosage, later studies focused on the safety of giving high doses of naloxone to stroke patients. Adams et al. (85) studied the effects of escalating doses of naloxone in the treatment of stroke. Total naloxone doses of up to 4978 mg, divided between an initial bolus and a subsquent 24-hour infusion, were administered per patients to a group of 15 stroke victims. This total dose was approximately 1000 times the highest total dose used in previous clinical trials of naloxone in stroke and is within the range shown to be efficacious in experimental models of spinal cord trauma and shock. Neurological improvement was reported in nine patients treated with the larger dosages of naloxone used in this study. No toxic effects of such large naloxone doses were reported, with the exception of modest hypotension in one patient.

A second discrepancy in the available clinical studies concerns the interval between the onset of stroke and treatment with naloxone. The treatment of stroke victims with naloxone has generally been delayed for hours to days following stroke onset in the reported clinical series. This is in contrast to experimental studies describing a beneficial effect of naloxone in the treatment of hypotension. In the latter studies, naloxone was generally administered immediately after the experimental manipulation. Although a delay following the onset of stroke may prove to be unavoidable in clinical practice, delaying treatment with naloxone may allow irreversible damage to occur following the stroke. An unanswered question is whether or not treatment with naloxone immediately following the event would be of benefit. Finally, it is not clear from studies performed using experimental models of cerebral infarction that treatment with naloxone will lead to improved neurological outcome following stroke (63,69). On the basis of these experimental studies, therefore, patients suffering from cerebral infarction may not be expected to benefit from treatment with naloxone. It is possible that naloxone may act to protect ischemic brain parenchyma surrounding the area of infarction. This has been postulated as a potential mechanism for naloxone in an experimental canine model of cerebral ischemia (47).

The evidence suggests that in high doses (2-5 mg/kg) naloxone may be of benefit in the treatment of experimental models of spinal cord injury, endotoxemia, hypovolemic shock, and even cerebral ischemia. The mechanisms through which naloxone acts to produce improvement in these models have not been fully defined but may involve both opiate and nonopiate pathways. Additional study will be required to define the precise mode of action that naloxone has in these experimental systems. The clinical results implicating a beneficial effect of naloxone in the treatment of human cerebral ischemia have remained controversial. The successful completion of future clinical trials utilizing dosages of naloxone comparable to those used in the experimental systems may prove decisive in defining a possible role for naloxone in the treatment of human cerebrovascular disease.

B. Nonopiate Neuropeptides

Although unproven, a number of vasoactive nonopiate neuropeptides, including VIP, substance P, neurotensin, angiotensin, oxytocin, vasotocin, and vasopressin, may be involved in the regulation of cerebral blood flow. All are known to have vasoactive properties in experimental systems (35,86). None of these peptides has been implicated in the pathogenesis of cerebrovascular disease, however, and no systematic studies of any of them have been carried out in experimental models of cerebral ischemia. Only one other neuropeptide, thyrotropin-releasing hormone (TRH) has been used as a therapeutic agent in experimental models of cerebral ischemia, shock, and spinal cord injury. Unlike naloxone, TRH did not improve cerebral blood flow or cortical somatosensory evoked responses in a canine model of air embolism induced cerebral ischemia (47). The peptide may be of benefit, however, in the treatment of cord injury and shock (45,46).

V. CONCLUSIONS

The known neuropeptides comprise a complex group of compounds with diverse functions. Of these many functions, the regulation of cardiovascular system and autonomic nervous system homeostasis by the neuropeptides is of particular interest in the study of cerebral ischemia and stroke. Many opiate and nonopiate neuropeptides are known to have vasoactive properties. Compelling evidence suggests that treatment with naloxone has a beneficial effect in experimental models of hypotension. It is possible that this effect may be mediated through both opiate and nonopiate mechanisms. It is not clear whether naloxone provides a clear improvement in neurological function following stroke. Therefore, the suggestion that the endogenous opiates are involved in the pathogenesis of stroke or cerebral ischemia remains controversial, and the use of naloxone in the routine clinical management of cerebral ischemia cannot be recommended.

Despite the complexity of the neuropeptides and their receptors, rapid progress has been made in defining these various molecules since their initial discovery. In addition to the enormous importance of excitatory neurotransmitters in neuronal function, current evidence suggests a major role for a number of neuropeptides in the control of cardiovascular function. Indirect evidence suggests roles for several peptides in the control of cerebral blood flow. As the neuropharmacology of the neuropeptides is developed, their effects on cerebrovascular function will become clarified. Improved therapeutic strategies for the treatment of human cerebral ischemia and stroke may thus become available.

REFERENCES

1. Pert CS, Snyder SH. Opiate receptor: demonstration in nervous tissue. *Science* 179:1011-1014, 1973.
2. Baskin DS, Hosobuchi Y.Naloxone reversal of ischemic neurological deficits in man. *Lancet* 2:272-275, 1981.
3. Krieger DT, Brownstein MJ, Martin JB (Eds.). *Brain Peptides*. Wiley, New York, 1983.
4. Hughes J, Smith TW, Kosterlitz HW, Fothergil L, Morgan BA, Morris HR. Identification of two related pentapeptides from the brain with potent opiate agonist activity. *Nature* 258:577-579, 1975.
5. Schwartz JP, Costa E. Hybridization approaches to the study of neuropeptides. *Ann Rev Neurosci* 9:277-304, 1986.
6. Nakanishi S, Inone A, Kita T, Nakamura M, Chang ACY, Cohen SN, Numa S. Nucleotide sequence of cloned cDNA for bovine corticotropin-β-lipotropin precursor. *Nature* 278:423-427, 1979.
7. Douglass J, Civelli O, Herbert E. Polyprotein gene expression: generation of diversity of neuroendocrine peptides. *Ann Rev Biochem* 53:665-715, 1984.
8. Akil H, Watson SJ, Young E, Lewis ME, Khachaturian H, Walker JM. Endogenous opioids: biology and function. *Ann Rev Neurosci* 7:223-255, 1984.
9. Holaday JW. Cardiovascular effects of endogenous opiate systems. *Ann Rev Pharmacol Toxicol* 23:541-594, 1983.
10. Bolme P, Fuxe K, Agnati LF, Bradley R, Smythies J. Cardiovascular effects of morphine and opioid peptides following intracisternal administration in chloralose anesthetized rats. *Eur J Pharmacol* 48:319-324, 1978.
11. Guillemin R, Vargo TM, Rossier J, Minick S, Ling N, Rivier C, Vale W, Bloom, F. Beta-endorphin and adrenocorticotropin are secreted concomitantly by the pituitary gland. *Science* 197:1367-1369, 1977.
12. Madden J, Akil H, Patrick RL, Barchas JD. Stress-induced parallel changes in central opioid levels and pain responsiveness in the rat. *Nature* 265:358-360, 1977.
13. Thomas TA, Fletcher JE, Hill RG. Influence of medication, pain and progress in labour on plasma β-endorphin-like immunoreactivity. *Br J Anaesthesiol* 54:401-408, 1982.

14. Pederson RC, Brownie AC, Ling N. Pro-adrenocorticotropin/endorphin-derived peptides: coordinate action on adrenal steroidogenesis. *Science* 208: 1044-1046, 1980.
15. Cooper PE, Martin JB. Neuroendocrinology and brain peptides. *Ann Neurol* 8:551-557, 1980.
16. Watson SJ, Akil H, Sullivan SO, Barchas JD. Immunocytochemical localization of methionine-enkephalin: preliminary observations. *Life Sci* 21:733-738, 1977.
17. Schaz K, Stock G, Simon W, Schlor K-H, Unger T, Rockhold R, Ganten D. Enkephalin effects on blood pressure, heart rate, and baroreceptor reflex. *Hypertension* 2:395-407, 1980.
18. Sander GE, Giles TD, Kastin AJ, Quiroz AC, Kaneish A, Coy DH. Cardiopulmonary pharmacology of enkephalins in the conscious dog. *Peptides* 2: 403-407, 1981.
19. Khachaturian H, Watson SJ, Lewis ME, Coy D, Goldstein A. Dynorphin immunocytochemistry in the rat central nervous system. *Peptides* 3:941-954, 1982.
20. Leander JD. A kappa opioid effects increased urination in the rat. *J Pharmacol Exp Ther* 224:89-94, 1982.
21. Schultzberg M, Hokfelt T, Lundberg J, Terenius L, Elfvin L-G, Elde R. Enkephalin-like immunoreactivity in nerve terminals in sympathetic ganglia and adrenal medulla and in adrenal medullary cells. *Acta Physiol Scand* 103:475-477, 1978.
22. Zukin RS, Zukin SR. Multiple opiate receptors: emerging concepts. *Life Sci* 29:2681-2690, 1981.
23. Lord JAH, Waterfield AA, Hughes J, Kosterlitz HW. Endogenous opioid peptides: multiple agonists and receptors. *Nature* 267:495-499, 1977.
24. Wuster M, Schulz R, Herz A. Multiple opiate receptors in peripheral tissue preparations. *Biochem Pharmacol* 30:1883-1887, 1981.
25. Goodman RR, Snyder SH, Kuhar MJ, Young WS. Differentiation of delta and mu receptor localizations by light microscopic autoradiography. *Proc Natl Acad Sci USA* 77:6239-6243, 1980.
26. Robson LE, Foote RW, Maurer R, Kosterlitz HW. Opioid binding sites of the κ type in guinea-pig cerebellum. *Neuroscience* 12:621-627, 1984.
27. Lynch DR, Snyder SH. Neuropeptides: multiple molecular forms, metabolic pathways, and receptors. *Ann Rev Biochem* 55:773-799, 1986.
28. Urca G, Frenk H, Liebeskind JC, Taylor AN. Morphine and enkephalin: analgesic and epileptic properties. *Science* 197:83-86, 1977.
29. Akil H, Hewlett WA, Barchas JD, Li CH. Binding of $[^3H]\beta$-endorphin to rat brain membranes: characterization of opiate properties and interaction with ACTH. *Eur J Pharmacol* 64:1-8, 1980.
30. Holaday JW, Ruvio BA, Robles LE, Johnson DE, D'Amato RJ. M154,129, a putative delta antagonist, reverses endotoxic shock without altering morphine analgesia. *Life Sci* 31:2209-2212, 1982.
31. McMillan DE, Wolf PS, Carchman RA. Antagonism of the behavioral effects of morphine and methadone by narcotic antagonists in the pigeon. *J Pharmacol Exp Ther* 175:443-458, 1970.

32. Sawynok J, Pinsky C, LaBella FA. Minireview on the specificity of naloxone as an opiate antagonist. *Life Sci* 25:1621-1632, 1979.
33. Itoh N, Obata K, Yanaihara N, Okamoto H. Human preprovasoactive intestinal polypeptide contains a novel PHI-27-like peptide, PHM-27. *Nature* 304:547-549, 1983.
34. Fahrenkrug J. Vasoactive intestinal polypeptide: measurement, distribution, and putative neurotransmitter function. *Digestion* 19:149-169, 1979.
35. Iverson LL. Nonopioid neuropeptides in mammalian CNS. *Ann Rev Pharmacol Toxicol* 23:1-27, 1983.
36. Itoh T, Sasaguri T, Makita Y, Kanmura Y,Kuriyama H. Mechanisms of vasodilation induced by vasoactive intestinal polypeptide in rabbit mesenteric artery. *Am J Physiol* 249:H231-H240, 1985.
37. Larrson L-I, Edvinsson L, Fahrenkrug J, Hakanson R, Owman C, Schaffalitzky de Muckadell O, Sundler F. Immunohistochemical localization of a vasodilatory polypeptide (VIP) in cerebrovascular nerves. *Brain Res* 113: 400-404, 1976.
38. Wei EP, Kontos HA, Said SI. Mechanism of action of vasoactive intestinal polypeptide on cerebral arterioles. *Amer J Physiol* 239:H765-H768, 1980.
39. Wilson DA, O'Neill JT, Said SI, Traystman RJ. Vasoactive intestinal polypeptide and the canine cerebral circulation. *Circ Res* 48:138-148, 1981.
40. Larson JJ, Boeck V, Otteson B. Effect of vasoactive intestinal polypeptide on cerebral blood flow in the goat. *Actu Physiol Scand* 111:471-474, 1981.
41. Edvinsson L, McCulloch J, Cerebral circulation and metabolic effects of vasoactive intestinal polypeptide. *J Physiol* (*Lond*) 291:42P-43P, 1979.
42. Unger T, Ganten D, Lang RE, Rascher W. Brain peptides and blood pressure control. *Trends Pharm Sci* 2:289-292, 1981.
43. Moskowitz MD, Reinhard JF Jr, Romero J, Melamed E, Pettibone DJ. Neurotransmitters and the fifth cranial nerve: is there a relation to the headache phase of migraine? *Lancet* 2:883-884, 1979.
44. Tache Y, Lis M, Collu R. Effects of thyrotropin-releasing hormone on behavioral and hormonal changes induced by beta-endorphin. *Life Sci* 21: 841-846, 1977.
45. Faden AI, Jacobs TP, Holaday JW. Thyrotropin-releasing hormone improves neurologic recovery after spinal trauma in cats. *N Engl J Med* 305: 1063-1067, 1981.
46. Holaday JW, D'Amato R, Faden AI. Thyrotropin-releasing hormone improves cardiovascular function in experimental endotoxic and hemorrhagic shock. *Science* 213:216-218, 1981.
47. Faden AI, Hallenbeck JM, Brown CQ. Treatment of experimental stroke: comparison of naloxone and thyrotropin-releasing hormone. *Neurology* (*NY*) 32:1083-1087, 1982.
48. Cotman C, Iversen L. Excitatory amino acids in the brain—focus on NMDA receptors. *Trends Neurosci* 10:263-265, 1987.
49. Greenamyre JT,Olson JMM, Penney JB. Autoradiographic characterization

of *N*-methyl-*D*-aspartate-, quisqualate- and kainate-sensitive glutamate binding sites. *J Pharmacol Exp Ther* 233:254-263, 1985.
50. Holaday JW, Faden AI. Naloxone reversal of endotoxin hypotension suggests role of endorphins in shock. *Nature* 275:450-451, 1978.
51. Faden AI, Holaday JW. Experimental endotoxin shock: the pathophysiologic function of endorphins and treatment with opiate antagonists. *J Infect Dis* 142:229-238, 1980.
52. Faden AI, Holaday JW. Opiate antagonists: a role in the treatment of hypovolemic shock. *Science* 205:317-318, 1979.
53. Holaday JW, Faden AI. Naloxone acts at central opiate receptors to reverse hypotension, hypothermia, and hypoventilation in spinal shock. *Brain Res* 189:295-299, 1980.
54. Faden AI, Jacobs TP, Mougey E, Holaday JW. Endorphins in experimental spinal injury: therapeutic effect of naloxone. *Ann Neurol* 10:326-332, 1981.
55. Faden AI, Jacobs TP, Holaday JW. Neuropeptides and spinal cord injury. In: Costa E, Trabucchi M (Eds.), *Regulatory Peptides: From Molecular Biology to Function*. Raven Press, New York, 1982, pp. 131-138.
56. Faden AI, Jacobs TP. Opiate antagonist WIN 44,441-3 stereospecifically improves neurologic recovery after ischemic spinal injury. *Neurology* 35:1311-1315, 1985.
57. Young W, Flamm ES, Demopoulos HB, Tomasula JJ, DeCrescito V. Effect of naloxone on posttraumatic ischemia in experimental spinal contusion. *J Neurosurg* 55:209-219, 1981.
58. Holaday JW, Faden AI. Naloxone reverses the pathophysiology of shock through an antagonism of endorphin systems. In: Martin JB, Reichlin S, Bick KL (Eds.), *Neurosecretion and Brain Peptides*. Raven Press, New York, 1981, pp. 421-434.
59. Hosobuchi Y, Baskin DS, Woo SK. Reversal of induced ischemic neurologic deficit in gerbils by the opiate antagonist naloxone. *Science* 215:69-71, 1982.
60. Holaday JW, D'Amato RJ. Naloxone or TRH fails to improve neurologic deficits in gerbil models of "stroke." *Life Sci* 31:385-392, 1982.
61. Kastin AJ, Nissen C, Olsen RD. Failure of MIF-1 or naloxone to reverse ischemic-induced neurologic deficits in gerbils. *Pharmacol Biochem Behavior* 17:1083-1085, 1982.
62. Levy DE, Pike CL, Rawlinson DG. Failure of naloxone to limit clinical or morphological brain damage in gerbils with unilateral carotid artery occlusion. *Soc Neurosci Abstr* 8:248, 1982.
63. Holaday JW, D'Amoto RJ. Naloxone and ischemic neurologic deficits in the gerbil: is there an effect? *Science* 218:592-593, 1982.
64. Levy R, Feustel P, Severinghaus J, Hosobuchi Y. Effect of naloxone on neurologic deficit and blood flow during focal cerebral ischemia in cats. *Life Sci* 31:2205-2208, 1982.
65. Dullien VK, Giardina WJ, Wiese J. Naloxone's effect on reversing hyperir-

ritability in the early stages of stroke in the spontaneously hypertensive stroke-prone rat. *Soc Neurosci Abstr* 8:2481, 1982.

66. Zabramski JM, Spetzler RF, Selman WR, Hershey LA, Roessman U. Naloxone improves neurologic function during and outcome after temporary focal cerebral ischemia. *Stroke* 14:123, 1983.
67. Baskin DS, Kieck CF, Hosobuchi Y. Naloxone reversal of ischemic neurologic deficits in baboons is not mediated by systemic effects. *Life Sci* 31: 2201-2204, 1982.
68. Faden AI. Opiate antagonists in the treatment of stroke. *Stroke* 15:575-578, 1984.
69. Nehls DG, Gaines C, Crowell RM. Effects of naloxone in the treatment of experimental stroke in awake monkeys. *Stroke* 14:123, 1983.
70. Cohen MR, Cohen RM, Pickar D, Murphy DL, Bunney WE Jr. Physiological effects of high dose naloxone administration to normal adults. *Life Sci* 30: 2025-2031, 1982.
71. Dingledine R, Iverson LL, Breuker E. Naloxone as a GABA antagonist: evidence from iontophoretic, receptor binding and convulsant studies. *Eur J Pharmacol* 47:19-27, 1978.
72. Rothman SM, Samaie M. Synaptic activity mediates death of hypoxic neurons. *Science* 220:536-537, 1983.
73. Rothman S. Physiology of excitatory synaptic transmission in cultures of dissociated rat hippocampus. *J Neurophysiol* 54:701-713, 1985.
74. Simon R, Swan J, Griffiths T, Meldrum B. Blockade of *N*-methyl-*D*-aspartate receptors may protect against ischemic damage in the brain. *Science* 226:850-852, 1984.
75. Ozyurt E, Graham D, Wordruff G, McCulloch J. Protective effect of the glutamate antagonist, MK-801 in focal cerebral ischemia in the cat. *J Cerebral Blood Flow Metab* 8:138-143, 1988.
76. Kochhar A, Zivin J, Lyden P, Mazzarella V. Glutamate antagonist therapy reduces neurologic deficits produced by focal central nervous system ischemia. *Arch Neurol* 45:148-153, 1988.
77. Rothman S, Olney J. Glutamate and the pathophysiology of hypoxic-ischemic brain damage. *Ann Neurol* 19:105-111, 1986.
78. Pulsinelli W, Brierly J, Plum F. Temporal profile of neuronal damage in a model of transient forebrain ischemia. *Ann Neurol* 11:491-498, 1982.
79. Globus M, Ginsberg M, Harik S, Busto R, Dietrich W. Role of dopamine in ischemic striatal injury: metabolic evidence. *Neurology* 37:1712-1719, 1987.
80. Brandt NJ, Terenius L, Jacobsen BB, Klinken L., Nordius A, Brandt S, Blegvad K, Yssing M. Hyper-endorphin syndrome in a child with necrotizing encephalomyelopathy. *N Engl J Med* 303:914-916, 1980.
81. Jabaily J, Davis JN. Naloxone partially reverses neurologic deficits in some but not all stroke patients. *Neurology* (*Minneap*) 32:A197, 1982.
82. Bredesen DE, Cutler JR, Simon RP. Failure of naloxone to reverse vascular neurologic deficit. *Neurology* (*Minneap*) 32:A79, 1982.

83. Cutler JR, Bredesen DE, Edwards R, Simon RP. Failure of naloxone to reverse vascular neurologic deficits. *Neurology* 33:1517-1518, 1983.
84. Fallis RJ, Fisher M, Lobo R. A double-blind trial of naloxone in the treatment of acute stroke. *Stroke* 15:627-629, 1984.
85. Adams HP, Olinger CP, Butler MJ, Barson WG, Graff-Radford NR, Brott TG, Biller J, Damasio H, Tomsick T, Spilker JA. A dose-escalation study of large doses of naloxone for treatment of patients with acute cerebral ischemia. *Neurology* 35(Suppl 1):143, 1985.
86. Faden AI. Neuropeptides and stroke: current status and potential application. *Stroke* 14:169-172, 1983.

11

Steroid Therapy in Stroke

Richard A. Shubin and Mark Fisher
University of Southern California School of Medicine, Los Angeles, California

I. INTRODUCTION

Glucocorticosteroids (steroids) have been employed in the treatment of stroke for more than a generation. A 1986 survey of 70 physicians in Toronto found that 39 used steroids "sometimes," while 30 "never" used steroids in the treatment of stroke (1). The actual extent of steroid use is unknown but is probably substantial. The divergence in clinical practice reflects the frankly contradictory conclusions of a multitude of reports in the literature. This chapter will review human and animal studies of the efficacy of steroids in the treatment of cerebral infarction and intracranial and subarachnoid hemorrhage.

II. ISCHEMIC STROKE: CLINICAL TRIALS

The use of steroids for the treatment of ischemic stroke dates to the 1950s. In four uncontrolled trials, steroids appeared to markedly ameliorate deficits due to

Table 1 Uncontrolled Trials of Steroids in Cerebral Infarction

Author (Ref.)	Year	*n*	Effect of steroids on outcome
Russek et al. (2)	1954	12	9/12 marked improvement
Sheely et al. (4)	1955	5	Less spasticity
Russek et al. (3)	1955	35	21/35 improvement in 12-24 h; 27/35 improvement in 3 weeks
Roberts (5)	1958	20	9/20 marked improvement; 6/20 mild improvement
Candelise et al. (18-20)	1975	227	No benefit
Gilsanz et al. (21)	1975	61	No benefit

stroke. Russek et al. (2,3) observed dramatic improvement in strength, sensation, speech, mood, and level of consciousness in two studies (47 patients total). Sheely et al. (4) found that use of hydrocortisone decreased spasticity, increased range of motion, and improved ambulation in patients with acute and chronic deficits following a stroke. Roberts (5) reported that treatment with hydrocortisone led to rapid improvement in a variety of focal deficits in 14 of 20 patients with acute stroke (Table 1).

Cortisone was then found to be ineffective in the treatment of ischemic stroke in two controlled trials (Table 2). Dyken and White (6) studied 36 patients who presented within 48 hours of the development of a focal neurological deficit. Patients were randomized to receive placebo or hydrocortisone. There was no statistically significant difference in morbidity or mortality between the two groups; death occurred in 13 of the 19 patients who received cortisone and

Table 2 Controlled Trials of Steroids in Human Cerebral Infarction

Author (Ref.)	Year	*n*	Effect of steroids on outcome
Dyken and White (60	1956	36	No benefit
Hetzel et al. (7)	1957	12	No benefit
Rubinstein (16)	1965	40	Beneficial for large hemispheric strokes
Patten et al. (17)	1972	31	Beneficial, especially for the most severely affected
Bauer and Tellez (23)	1973	54	No benefit
Norris (24)	1976	53	No benefit, possibly deleterious
Mulley et al. (25)	1978	113	No benefit
Santambragio et al. (22)	1978	89	No benefit
Norris and Hackinski (1)	1986	113	No benefit

in 10 of the 17 patients who received placebo. Hetzel et al. (7) began a double-blind study, which they terminated upon publication of the results of Dyken and White. There was no significant difference in morbidity or mortality between the treated and untreated groups (12 enrolled patients).

Early mortality following stroke is most commonly due to transtentorial herniation (8-11), usually occurring 3-5 days poststroke in association with edema in the ischemic region (12). The demonstration that dexamethasone was effective in the treatment of vasogenic brain edema (13-15) renewed interest in steroids as a treatment of stroke. In two trials between 1965 and 1972, dexamethasone was reported to augment recovery from stroke. Rubinstein (16) studied 19 patients with severe cerebral hemisphere infarction. There were four deaths among the 13 patients who received dexamethasone, while four of six patients receiving placebo died. Five of the nine survivors in the treatment group showed marked improvement, all within 24-48 hours. Patten et al. (17) randomly assigned 31 patients to received dexamethasone (n = 14) or placebo (n = 17). Neurological status and functional ability was evaluated daily. Dexamethasone-treated patients demonstrated a greater rate (64% vs. 41%) and magnitude (+23% vs. −14%, $p < 0.02$) of improvement according to the scale designed by the authors. The mortality rate was not noted.

Dexamethasone was found to be ineffective in all subsequent series. Candelise, with Spinnler (18) and Colombo and Spinnler (19,20), found no difference in morbidity and mortality between 227 patients treated with dexamethasone alone or in combination with mannitol and historic controls. Gilsanz et al. (21) reported that treatment with dexamethasone did not improve functional recovery in 61 patients compared to historic controls. Santambragio et al. (22) found no statistically significant difference in morbidity or mortality among 89 patients randomized to receive (1) a mixture of three ergot derivatives; (2) dexamethasone, 24 mg/day in divided doses; (3) a 20% solution of mannitol, 0.8-0.9 g/kg body weight; or (4) routine care. Bauer and Tellez (23) sudied 54 patients who developed a focal deficit within 48 hours of admission. Half received dexamethasone 4 mg four times per day. Patients were rated every other day for 2 weeks according to a scale of neurological function designed by the authors. There were no statistically significant differences in morbidity or mortality between dexamethasone- and placebo-treated patients. Norris (24) studied 53 patients who presented within 24 hours of the development of a focal neurological deficit. Of these, 27 received placebo and 26 received dexamethasone; patients were followed for 4 weeks. Mortality was not statistically significantly different between the two groups. Dexamethasone-treated patients, however, did not show as much improvement as placebo-treated patients. Norris speculated that dexamethasone may be not only ineffectual but also possibly deleterious in the treatment of acute stroke. Mulley et al. (25) found that treatment with dexamethasone for 118 patients did not alter the mortality rate or functional outcome 1 year following a stroke. Norris and Hachinski (1) studied 113 patients who presented within 48 hours of the development of a focal neurological deficit and had a computerized tomography scan of the brain confirming the diagnosis. Half the patients received placebo while the others received "megadose" dexamethasone, consisting of 24 mg every 6 hours initially; this was gradually decreased over 12 days. Patients were followed for 3 weeks. Treatment with "megadose" dexamethasone did not improve mortality or morbidity as assessed by the Toronto stroke scoring system (26).

The use of steroids in ischemic stroke has not been associated with a significant rate of complications. Russek et al. (2,3), Sheely et al. (4), and Roberts (5) found no serious adverse effects in their studies during a 3-week course of hydrocortisone. Sheely et al. reported that one patient became mildly euphoric and two developed episodes of confusion and depression coincident with steroid use. Patten et al. (17) noted exacerbation of diabetes mellitus in one of 16 patients; this resolved when dexamethasone was stopped. Bauer and Bellez (23) found gastrointestinal hemorrhage more frequently among the control than among the dexamethasone-treated patients. Norris (24) noted a significant incidence of side effects during treatment of stroke with dexamethasone. Several patients suffered a serious exacerbation of diabetes mellitus, two patients died of pneumonia, one became septic, and another developed a brain abscess. Gastrointestinal hemorrhage occurred in 3 of 27 treated patients versus 1 of 26 controls. Steroid-treated patients fared no worse than those given placebo in the study by Mulley et al. (25), with the exception of one instance of reactivation of tuberculosis, which was readily controlled with appropriate antibiotics. Ottonello and Primavera (27) found a higher rate of gastrointestinal lesions at autopsy in patients treated with dexamethasone compared to untreated patients. Norris and Hachinski (1) excluded patients thought to be at risk for developing complications, such as a history of diabetes mellitus or gastrointestinal hemorrhage. Insulin-requiring hyperglycemia developed in four patients treated with dexamethasone. Serious infections occurred in four of the controls, while gastrointestinal hemorrhage developed in both groups. In summary, the use of a short course of steroids for treatment of ischemic stroke is associated with a relatively low rate of serious complications. Steroids can exacerbate diabetes mellitus and precipitate hyperglycemia but do not appear to increase the incidence of infections or fluid and electrolyte disturbances. The evidence with respect to gastrointestinal bleeding is inconclusive.

The early uncontrolled trials of steroids in stroke were provocative. However, benefits were not demonstrated in any of the later, larger trials. Spence and Donner (28) critically evaluated published trials up to 1976 and found a variety of flaws in study design. Trials designed with the above critiques in mind still have not demonstrated efficacy with either conventional or megadose dexamethasone. The overwhelming evidence indicates that steroids are ineffective in the treatment of acute ischemic stroke.

Table 3 Experimental Trials of Steroids in Ischemic Stroke

Author (Ref.)	Year	Animal	Conclusion
Plum et al. (32)	1963	Rat	No effect
Kahn et al. (33)	1972	Gerbil	No effect
Siegel et al. (34)	1972	Rat	No effect
Harrison and Ross Russell (44)	1972	Gerbil	Improved survival
Harrison et al. (45)	1973	Gerbil	Edema reduced
Donley and Sundt (39)	1973	Squirrel monkey	No effect
Bartko et al. (30)	1972	Cat	Improved survival
Hoppe et al. (41)	1974	Cat	Effective in infarcted but not ischemic tissue
Lee et al. (37)	1974	Cat	No effect
De La Torre and Surgeon (43)	1976	Rhesus monkey	Edema reduced
Yamaguchi et al. (35)	1976	Rat	No effect
Little (38)	1978	Cat	Improvement at 6-12 hours, no change at 48 hours
Fenske et al. (40)	1979	Cat	Improved level of consciousness in survivors
Ito et al. (36)	1980	Gerbil	No effect
Hartmann et al. (31)	1982	Baboon	Improved survival
Barbosa-Coutinho et al. (42)	1985	Baboon	Peri-infarct edema diminished
Sapolsky and Pulsinelli (46)	1985	Rat	Increased neuronal injury

III. ISCHEMIC STROKE: EXPERIMENTAL STUDIES

The effect of steroids on infarction has been studied in a variety of animal models. The multitude of species and models of stroke make a direct comparison between experiments problematical. Most experiments were designed to ascertain the effect of steroids on the formation of cerebral edema. Several studies investigated the effect of steroids on outcome (Table 3). Recently, attention has been directed to the effect of steroids on blood flow and neuronal function following ischemia.

Kostron and Fischer (29) established that steroids penetrate regions of infarction. Tritiated dexamethasone was administered to rats that had undergone ligation of the right common carotid artery. Dexamethasone was concentrated in the infarcted hemisphere. Neurons displayed higher levels of uptake compared to other cellular elements. Ultrastructural examinations revealed that dexamethasone was selectively present in microsomes, lysosomes, and the cytoplasm.

Treatment of experimental stroke with steroids increases cerebral blood flow to the affected hemisphere following infarction. Bartko et al. (30) measured the cerebral blood flow of cats before and after occluding one middle cerebral artery. Animals that received dexamethasone for 3 days prior to the infarction demonstrated greater blood flow to the affected hemisphere than those that received placebo over the first 4 hours following infarction. Hartmann et al. (31), measured regional cerebral blood flow in 13 baboons by the intra-arterial xenon-133 method before, and for 28 days following the production of stroke by occlusion of the left middle cerebral artery. Dexamethasone-treated animals showed improved regional and total cerebral blood flow from day 7 onwards compared to controls.

Most investigators have not found steroids to improve outcome or inhibit edema formation following experimental infarction. Plum et al. (32) randomized adult male Sprague-Dawley white rats to receive dexamethasone or placebo. Animals were placed in a hypoxic environment following ligation of the right carotid artery. Mortality was significantly higher among animals pretreated with dexamethasone (14 of 43, 43%) compared to controls (11 of 75, 15%). There was no significant difference in histological appearance, distribution or volume of edema, or electrolyte content between the treated and untreated animals. Kahn et al. (33) randomized 60 gerbils to receive saline or dexamethasone beginning 1 hour after unilateral carotid ligation and then every 8 hours for 5 days. Treatment with dexamethasone did not alter survival or the histological appearance of the brain. Siegel et al. (34) produced infarction in female rats by intra-arterial injection of microspheres into the right common carotid artery. Animals received either dexamethasone or saline. Use of dexamethasone did not alter mortality or inhibit the formation of edema. Yamaguchi et al. (35) produced a stroke in rats by bilateral carotid ligation. Treatment with hydrocortisone or dexamethasone had no effect on edema formation. Ito et al. (36) studied gerbils receiving beta-methasone or placebo following left middle cerebral artery occlusion; there was no significant difference between groups in water content, electrolyte concentration, or the integrity of the blood-brain barrier. Lee et al. (37) randomized cats to receive either placebo or dexamethasone for 2 weeks starting either 2 weeks prior to or at the time of occlusion of one middle cerebral artery. Dexamethasone treatment beginning before or at the time of the stroke did not alter morbidity, mortality, infarct size, or histological appearance compared to placebo. Little (38) found that high-dose dexamethasone with mannitol had no effect on edema formation following left middle cerebral artery occlusion in cats. Donley and Sundt (39) studied squirrel monkeys subjected to temporary occlusion of the middle cerebral artery; there was no benefit of dexamethasone in morbidity or the histological appearance of the areas of infarction. Fenske et al. (40) produced a stroke in cats by occlusion of the middle cerebral artery. Beginning at the time of occlusion, animals received either placebo or dexamethasone, 2.5 mg/kg initially, then 0.625 mg/kg body weight every 6 hours for 24 hours. Treatment did not alter mortality or reduce hemispheric swelling, although the level of consciousness was higher among treated surviving animals.

A few investigators found that treatment with steroids lessened edema formation following experimental stroke. Hoppe et al. (41) subjected 10 cats to transorbital occlusion of the middle cerebral artery. Thirty minutes after surgery, and every 12 hours for the next 2 days, half of the cats received dexamethasone; the others received placebo. All animals were sacrificed at the end of 48 hours. One hour before death, each cat received an injection of sodium pertechnetate to define regions of infarction and integrity of the blood-brain barrier. Dexamethasone treatment resulted in less edema formation and a more intact blood-brain barrier compared to placebo. Barbosa-Coutinho et al. (42) randomized baboons to receive dexamethasone 1 mg/kg or placebo starting 1 hour after occlusion of the left middle cerebral artery. Animals were sacrificed after 1 week. The volume of infarction was unchanged by treatment, but the volume of peri-infarct edema was significantly reduced compared to controls. De La Torre and Surgeon (43) randomized rhesus monkeys to receive dexamethasone or dimethyl sulfoxide (DMSO) following occlusion of one middle cerebral artery. Dexamethasone-treated animals had significantly less edema than controls. Harrison and Ross Russell (44) randomized gerbils to receive placebo or high-dose dexamethasone (5 mg/kg body weight every 8 hours for 2 days) following ligation of the right carotid artery. After 1 week, 15 of 16 treated with dexamethasone survived compared to only 9 of 26 controls ($p < 0.01$). Harrison et al. (45) found that treatment with dexamethasone inhibited the formation of edema compared to placebo.

Norris (24) noted that patients who received steroids did not show the same degree of recovery as the untreated controls. Sapolsky and Pulsinelli (46) investigated the effect of steroids on neuronal function during global ischemia. Ischemia was produced via transient four-vessel occlusion (47,48). At the time of reperfusion, animals were randomized to receive one of the following treatments: (1) sham adrenalectomy plus corticosterone, 10 mg intravenously; (2) adrenalectomy; or (3) adrenalectomy followed by infusion of cortisone. The animals were subsequently observed for 72 hours and then sacrificed. The degree of ischemic neuronal injury was assessed by light microscopy. Sapolsky and Pulsinelli found that the severity of the ischemic damage was related to the level of corticosterone; ischemic injury was potentiated by the administration of steroids and attenuated with adrenalectomy. This result could not be attributed to the effects of steroids on respiratory or cardiovascular mechanisms; there was no difference in mean arterial pressure, carbon dioxide tension, pH, body temperature, or hematocrit between the two groups. Sapolsky and Pulsinelli speculated that cortisone may modulate neuronal injury through release of excitatory neurotransmitters leading to ATP depletion and accumulation of intracellular calcium. They also suggested that inhibition of corticosteroid synthesis or treatment with glucocorticoid receptor antagonists may be appropriate to lessen ischemic neuronal injury.

Steroids have been tested in a wide variety of animal models of cerebral infarction. The weight of experimental evidence indicates that steroids do not reduce morbidity, mortality, or edema formation following cerebral infarction. Steroids may well aggravate ischemic neuronal injury. The lack of convincing, consistent favorable effects of steroids on experimental cerebral infarction suggests that further clinical studies of steroids in ischemic stroke are unwarranted.

IV. INTRACRANIAL HEMORRHAGE

The use of steroids to treat intracranial hemorrhage (ICH) has been predicated on the assumption that steroids can reduce elevated intracranial pressure from the clot or from surrounding edema. However, steroids have not been shown to improve outcome following ICH in any clinical trial (Table 4). Russek et al. (2) treated three patients who had suffered intracranial hemorrhages with hydrocortisone. All were comatose when treatment was initiated, and all subsequently died in 2-5 days. All six of Rubinstein's patients with ICH died despite treatment with dexamethasone, 4 mg intravenously followed by 4 mg intramuscularly every 6 hours for 3 days (16). Six patients with ICH were included in French's series of 433 patients treated with dexamethasone for cerebral edema (15). All had large intracerebral hematomas and increased intracranial pressure. Dexamethasone was administered for variable periods of time prior to evacuation of hematoma; none of the patients improved. Hooshmand et al. (49) found that dexamethasone was effective in lowering intracranial pressure in experimental and spontaneous intracerebral hemorrhage. Experimental hemorrhage was produced by injecting 8 cc of autologous blood into the right hemisphere of dogs. A single intravenous injection (1 mg/kg) of dexamethasone produced a

Table 4 Steroids and Human Intracerebral Hemorrhage

Author (Ref.)	Year	*n*	Effect of steroids on outcome
Russek et al. (2)	1954	3	No benefit
Rubinstein (16)	1965	6	No benefit
French (15)	1966	6	No benefit
Hooshmand et al. (50)	1972	30	No benefit
Tellez and Bauer (51)	1973	40	No benefit
Poungvarin et al. (52)	1987	93	No benefit

gradual, consistent drop in intracranial pressure that persisted for 8 hours. Hooshmand et al. (50) performed a prospective, randomized trial of dexamethasone (6 mg every 4 hours) versus dexamethasone plus a single dose of mannitol (2 mg/kg) intravenously versus placebo. Intracranial pressure was assessed by comparing shifts of the third ventricle (assessed by M-mode echoencephalography) on admission and after 24 hours of treatment. The use of dexamethasone resulted in a statistically significant ($p < 0.01$) decrease in shift of the third ventricle at 24 hours, and patients who received placebo were less responsive on days 2 through 4. However, there was no difference with respect to morbidity or mortality at 3 months.

Tellez and Bauer (51) found dexamethasone to be ineffective treatment for intracranial hemorrhage. Twenty-one patients were randomized to receive placebo and 19 received dexamethasone (12 mg intravenously on admission, followed by 4 mg intramuscularly every 6 hours for 3 days). Treatment was started within 48 hours of the onset of the ictus. The diagnosis of intracranial hemorrhage was made on the basis of a focal neurological deficit accompanied by a decrease in the level of consciousness and the presence of at least 200 red blood cells in the cerebrospinal fluid. Patients were evaluated for 14 days. Treatment did not alter morbidity or mortality; 14 deaths occurred in patients receiving dexamethasone versus 15 receiving placebo.

Poungvarin et al. (52) found dexamethasone ineffective in treating primary supratentorial intracranial hemorrhage. Their study was the first to use computerized tomography (CT) scans for making the diagnosis of ICH (53,54). Patients were grouped on the basis of their clinical state and randomized to receive placebo or dexamethasone (10 mg initially, followed by 5 mg every 6 hours for 6 days, 5 mg every 12 hours for 2 days, and 5 mg for 2 day). The study was terminated after enrollment of 93 patients because of a significantly higher rate of complications in the dexamethasone-treated group. These complications included sepsis and diabetes. There was no statistically significant difference in mortality, residual disability, need for neurosurgical intervention, length of hospitalization, or cause of death.

In summary, clinical studies have indicated that steroids provide no benefit in the treatment of ICH. There is no convincing experimental evidence supporting the use of steroids in ICH. The routine use of steroids following ICH should be abandoned.

V. SUBARACHNOID HEMORRHAGE

Many clinicians include dexamethasone as part of their routine preoperative and/or postoperative management of the patient with subarachnoid hemorrhage (15, 55-62). French (15) commented on the effect of steroids on the preoperative management of subarachnoid hemorrhage (SAH). He found "unquestionable symptomatic improvement" in four of six obtunded patients treated with dexamethasone. However, he did not note the duration of the improvement or the effect on long-term morbidity or mortality. Synckers (63) found that the use of high-dose dexamethasone at the induction of anesthesia was associated with a low rate of postoperative vasospasm. Only one patient of 37 in his series displayed vasospasm, in contrast to an expected rate of 10%.

Cerebral vasospasm is associated with the presence of extensive blood collection in the subarachnoid space. Some histological examinations of affected arteries reveal inflammatory infiltrate in the vessel wall. Chyatte et al. (64) found that chronic vasospasm could be ameliorated through treatments with anti-inflammatory drugs, methylprednisolone (30 mg/kg intravenously every 8 hours), and ibuprofen. Chronic cerebral vasospasm was produced by the use of the canine "double hemorrhage" model, in which 4 cc of autologous blood is twice injected into the cisternal magna. Treatment with either methylprednisolone or ibuprofen reduced vasospasm and hastened clinical recovery. There were no side effects in animals receiving a single agent. There was a high incidence of severe gastrointestinal hemorrhage in animals that received both agents, with no improvement in outcome. Low-dose methylprednisolone (15 mg/kg intravenously every 8 hours) was not as effective as high-dose methylprednisolone (30 mg/kg intravenously every 8 hours) (65). Chyatte et al. (66) treated 21 patients with aneurysmal SAH judged to be at high risk for developing vasospasm. Patients received high-dose methylprednisolone; their outcome was compared to matched contemporary controls. The former had a reduced incidence and severity of vasospasm and improved morbidity and mortality. Treatment was associated with a 20% incidence of insulin-requiring hyperglycemia; there was no increased risk of sepsis or gastrointestinal hemorrhage.

This is the best instance where the clinical application of steroids in stroke has a reasonable experimental foundation. There is a need for a large, randomized, controlled trial to assess the efficacy of steroids in preventing vasospasm following SAH. Subarachnoid hemorrhage appears to be the only form of stroke in which steroids may have a therapeutic role.

ACKNOWLEDGMENTS

We thank Carol Flores and Nina Morales for preparation of the manuscript. Supported in part by NIH Awards NS 884 and NS 20989.

REFERENCES

1. Norris JW, Hachinski VC. High dose steroid treatment in cerebral infarction. *Br Med J* 292:21-23, 1986.

2. Russek HI, Zohman BL, Russek AS. Cortisone in the immediate therapy of apoleptic stroke. *J Am Ger Soc* 2:216-222, 1954.
3. Russek HI, Russek AS, Zohman BL. Cortisone in the immediate therapy of apoleptic stroke. *JAMA* 159:102-105, 1955.
4. Sheely RF, Johnson CH, Baker JJ, Harbarugh R. Effect of cortisone and hydrocortisone on hemiplegia after cerebral infarction. *JAMA* 159:803-806, 1955.
5. Roberts HJ. Supportive adrenocortical steroid therapy in acute and subacute cerebrovascular accidents. *J Am Geriatr Soc* 6:686-702, 1958.
6. Dyken M, White PT. Evaluation of cortisone in the treatment of cerebral infarction. *JAMA* 162:1531-1534, 1956
7. Hetzel BS, Lander H, Robson HN. Immediate treatment of apoplexy (letter). *Br Med J* 1:1122, 1957.
8. Van Trotsenburg L, Vinken PJ. Fatal cerebral infarction simulating an acute expanding lesion. *J Neurol Neurosurg Psychiatry* 29:241-243, 1966.
9. Adams JH, Graham DI. Twelve cases of fatal cerebral infarction due to arterial occlusion in the absence of atheromatous stenosis or embolism. *J Neurol Neurosurg Psychiatry* 30:479-488, 1967.
10. Ng LKY, Nimmannitya J. Massive cerebral infarction with severe brain swelling: a clinicopathologic study. *Stroke* 1:158-163, 1970.
11. Silver FL, Norris JW, Lewis AJ, Hachinski VL. Early mortality following stroke: a prospective review. *Stroke* 15:492-496, 1984.
12. Shaw QM, Alvord EC Jr, Berry RG. Swelling of the brain following ischemic infarction with arterial occlusion. *Arch Neurol* 1:161-177, 1959.
13. Klatzo I. Neuropathological aspects of brain edema. *J Neuropathol Exp Neurol* 26:1-14, 1967.
14. Fishman R. Brain edema. *N Engl J Med* 293:708-711, 1975.
15. French LA. The use of steroids in the treatment of cerebral edema. *Bull NY Acad Med* 42:301-311, 1966.
16. Rubinstein MK. The influence of adrenocortical steroids in severe cerebrovascular accidents. *J Nerv Ment Dis* 141:291-299, 1965.
17. Patten BN, Mendell J, Bryun B, Curtin W, Carter S. Double-blind study of the effects of dexamethasone in acute stroke. *Neurology* 22:377–383, 1972.
18. Candelise L, Spinnler H. (Letter) *Med J Aust* 5:335, 1972.
19. Candelise L, Colombo A, Spinnler H. (Letter) *Lancet* 1:806, 1974.
20. Candelise L, Colombo A, Spinnler H. Therapy against brain swelling in stroke patients. *Stroke* 6:353-356, 1975.
21. Gilsanz V, Buencuerpo J, Rebollar JL, Chantres MT. Controlled trial of glycerol versus dexamethasone in the treatment of cerebral edema in acute cerebral infarction. *Lancet 1*:1049-1051, 1975.
22. Santambragio S, Martinotti R, Sardella R, Porro F, Randazzo A. Is there a real treatment for stroke? Clinical and statistical comparison of different treatments in 300 patients. *Stroke* 9:130-132, 1978.
23. Bauer RB, Tellez H. Dexamethasone as treatment in cerebrovascular disease. 2. A controlled study in acute cerebral infarction. *Stroke* 4:547-555, 1973.
24. Norris JW. Steroid therapy in acute cerebral edema. *Arch Neurol* 33:69-71, 1976.

25. Mulley G, Wilcox RG, Mitchell JRA. Dexamethasone in acute stroke. *Br Med J* 2:994-996, 1978.
26. Norris JW, Hachinski VC. Comment on "study design of stroke treatments." *Stroke* 13:527-528, 1982.
27. Ottonello GA, Primavera A. Gastrointestinal complications of high-dose corticosteroid therapy in acute cerebrovascular patients. *Stroke* 10:108-110, 1979.
28. Spence JD, Donner A. Problems in design in stroke treatment trials. *Stroke* 13:94-99, 1982.
29. Kostron H, Fischer J. Regional cellular, and subcellular distribution of [^{3}H] dexamethasone in rat brain edema. *Surg Neurol* 20:48-54, 1983.
30. Bartko D, Reulen HJ, Koeh H. Effect of dexamethasone on the early edema following occlusions of the middle cerebral artery in cats. In: Reulen HJ, Schurmann K (Eds.), *Steroids and Brain Edema*, Springer-Verlag, Berlin, 1972, pp. 127-157.
31. Hartmann A, Menzl J, Buttinger C. Effect of dexamethasone on regional cerebral blood flow in ischemic cerebral infarction. In: Hartmann A, Broeck M (Eds.), *Treatment of Cerebral Edema*. Springer-Verlag, Berlin, 1962, pp. 157-170.
32. Plum F, Alvord ED Jr, Posner JB. Effects of steroids on experimental cerebral edema. *Arch Neurol* 9:571-573, 1963.
33. Kahn K, Pranzarone GF, Newman T. Dexamethasone treatment of experimental cerebral infarction (abstract). *Neurology* 22:406-407, 1972.
34. Siegel BA, Studer RK, Potchen EJ. Steroid therapy of brain edema. *Arch Neurol* 27:209-212, 1972.
35. Yamaguchi M, Shirakata S, Yamasaki S, Matsumoto S. Ischemic brain edema and compression brain edema. *Stroke* 7:77-83, 1976.
36. Ito U, Ohno K, Sugaruma Y, Suzuki K, Inaba Y. Effect of steroid on ischemic brain edema. *Stroke* 11:166-172, 1980.
37. Lee NL, Martin AR, Waltz AG, Loewenson RE. Ineffectiveness of dexamethasone for treatment of experimental cerebral infarction. *Stroke* 5:216-218, 1974.
38. Little JR. Modification of acute focal ischemia by treatment with mannitol and high dose dexamethasone. *J Neurosurg* 49:517-524, 1978.
39. Donley RF, Sundt TM. The effect of dexamethasone on the edema of focal cerebral ischemia. *Stroke* 4:148-155, 1973.
40. Fenske A, Fisher M, Regli F, Hase U. The response of focal ischemic cerebral edema to dexamethasone. *J Neurol* 220:199-209, 1979.
41. Hoppe WH, Waltz AG, Jordan MM, Jacobson RL. Effects of dexamethasone on distributions of water and pertechnitate in brains of cats after middle cerebral artery occlusion. *Stroke* 5:617-622, 1974.
42. Barbosa-Coutinho M, Hartmann A, Hossman KA, Rommel T. Effect of dexamethasone on serum protein extravasation in experimental brain infarcts of monkey. An immuno-histochemical study. *Acta Neuropathol (Berlin)* 65:255-260, 1985.

43. De La Torre JC, Surgeon JW. Dexamethasone and DMSO in experimental transorbital cerebral infarction. *Stroke* 7:577-583, 1976.
44. Harrison MJG, Ross Russell RW. Effect of dexamethasone on experimental cerebral infarction in the gerbil. *J Neurol Neurosurg Psychiatry* 35:520-521, 1972.
45. Harrison MJG, Brownhill D, Lewis PD, Ross Russell RW. Cerebral edema following carotid artery ligation in the gerbil. *Arch Neurol* 28:389-391, 1973.
46. Sapolsky RM, Pulsinelli WA. Glucocorticords potentiates ischemic injury of neurons; therapeutic implications. *Science* 229:1397-1400, 1985.
47. Pulsinelli WA, Brierly JB. A new model of bilateral hemispheric ischemia in the unanesthesized rat. *Stroke* 10:267-276, 1979.
48. Pulsinelli WA, Duffy TE. Regional energy balance in rat brain after transient forebrain ischemia. *J Neurochem* 40:1500-1503, 1983.
49. Hooshmand H, Dove J, Houff S, Suter C. Effects of diuretics and steroids on CSF pressure. *Arch Neurol* 21:499-509, 1969.
50. Hooshmand H, Quinn JC, Houff SA. Cerebrospinal fluid pressure changes with chemotherapy for intracerebral hemorrhage. *Neurology* 22:56-61, 1972.
51. Tellez H, Bauer RB. Dexamethasone as treatment in cerebrovascular disease. 1. A controlled study in intracerebral hemorrhage. *Stroke* 4:541-546, 1973.
52. Poungvarin N, Bhoopat W, Virlyavejakul A, Rodprasart P, Buranasiri P, Sukondhabhant S, Hensley MJ, Strom BC. Effects of dexamethasone in primary supratentorial intracerebral hemorrhage. *N Engl J Med* 316:1229-1233, 1987.
53. Hier DB, Davis KB, Richardson EP, Mohr JP. Hypertensive putaminal hemorrhage. *Ann Neurol* 1:152-159, 1977.
54. Weisberg L. Computerized tomography in intracranial hemorrhage. *Arch Neurol* 36:422-426, 197.
55. Poppin JL. Operative treatment for aneurysms of the anterior communicating artery. *Clin Neurosurg* 22:8-13, 1964.
56. Ballinger DM, Solerman N, Ducker TB, Perot P. Prognosis of surgically treated intracranial aneurysm patients. *JAMA* 237:1845-1847, 1977.
57. French LA, Ortiz-Suarez HJ. Anterior communicating artery aneurysms. Technique of operation and results. *Clin Neurosurg* 22:115-119, 1974.
58. Giannotta SL, Kindt GN. Total morbidity and mortality rates of patients with surgically treated intracranial aneurysms. *Neurosurgery* 4:125-128, 1979.
59. Salazar JL. Treatment of ruptured and unruptured internal carotid artery aneurysms. *Surg Neurol* 11:451-455, 1979.
60. Hamby WB. Intracranial surgery for aneurysms. *Prog Neurol Surg* 3:1-65, 1969.
61. Hunt WE, Kosnik EG. Timing and perioperative care in intracranial aneurysm surgery. *Clin Neurosurg* 22:79-89, 1974.

62. Wallace CT. Anesthesia for intracranial aneurysms. *South Med J* 68:275-729, 1985.
63. Synckers FD. The treatment of cerebral aneurysms. *S Afr Med J* 50:835-839, 1976.
64. Chyatte D, Rusch N, Sundt TM. Prevention of chronic experimental cerebral vasospasm with ibuprofen and high-dose methylprednisolone. *J Neurosurg* 59:925-932, 1983.
65. Chyatte D, Sundt TM. Response of chronic experimental cerebral vasospasm to methylprednisolone and dexamethasone. *J Neurosurg* 60:929-926, 1984.
66. Chyatte D, Fode NC, Nichols DA, Sundt TM. Preliminary report: effects of high dose methylprednisolone on delayed cerebral ischemia in patients at high risk for vasospasm after aneurysmal subarachnoid hemorrhage. *Neurosurgery* 21:157-160, 1987.

12

Percutaneous Transluminal Angioplasty for the Treatment of Stroke

F. Y. Tsai
University of Missouri, Kansas City School of Medicine, Kansas City, Missouri

G. B. Hieshima and R. T. Higashida
University of California, San Francisco, California

I. ISCHEMIC STROKE

Percutaneous transluminal angioplasty (PTA) for vascular occlusive disease was pioneered by Dotter and Judkins in 1964 (1). Their technique was not initially appreciated by American physicians, although various European centers began to report its usefulness. In 1973, Portsman introduced the use of a caged balloon catheter, hoping to improve the PTA technique (2). However, PTA in the United States was not widely accepted until the introduction of the Grüntzig and Hopff double-lumen balloon catheter in 1974 (3).

Although the use of PTA has been extended rapidly from coronary and iliofemoral arteries to most other vascular systems in the body, the treatment of brachiocephalic artery stenosis by PTA has progressed very cautiously. Dilatation of stenotic lesions in the head and neck territory in an attempt to improve intraoperative methods for the treatment of fibromuscular hyperplasia of the carotid artery was first reported by Morris et al. in 1968 (4). Prior to PTA, surgical endarterectomy or bypass was considered the treatment of choice to relieve high-grade stenotic lesions.

Percutaneous transluminal angioplasty for brachiocephalic artery stenosis has been slow to evolve because of the high potential risk of distal cerebral embolization. Over the past few years, PTA of brachiocephalic arteries has slowly increased in frequency. A number of reports have described the successful treatment of stenotic atherosclerotic vessels by PTA as an alternative to direct surgical endarterectomy or bypass. These reports are extremely favorable and indicate that PTA may be effective in the treatment of brachiocephalic arterial occlusive disease (5-29).

The purpose of this chapter is to describe the practical aspects of PTA in the treatment of brachiocephalic arterial occlusive disease associated with stroke.

II. MATERIALS AND TECHNIQUE

We have established a research protocol and stroke committee consisting of neurologists, vascular surgeons, neurosurgeons, and neuroradiologists to evaluate patients with cereborovascular disease. All patients receive complete neurological, clinical, and radiological tests referable to the cerebral vascular circulation including aortic arch and selective carotid and vertebral angiography. Only if patients fail to respond to conventional medical therapy are they considered for PTA.

The angioplasty balloon catheter (manufactured by Medi-Tech, Inc.) is modified so that it has a short distal tip and is used in conjunction with a soft tip or a tight J guidewire. The size of the balloon is critical in avoiding complications. We prefer to use a balloon that approximates the normal luminal diameter prior to disease in order to avoid overdilatation of the vessel, which could result in rupture.

All patients are pretreated with heparin 20,000 u IV drip, and aspirin, 325-650 mg, for 5-10 days prior to treatment. For carotid and vertebral artery PTA EEG monitoring during the entire procedure is used, and fresh heparinized blood is injected during the actual dilatation. Systemic anticoagulation with heparin, 5000 units, is also administered during the procedure. Following the procedure, all patients are monitored neurologically in the hospital for 1-2 days. They receive prednisolone for 1 week and dipyridamole and/or aspirin for 3-6 months.

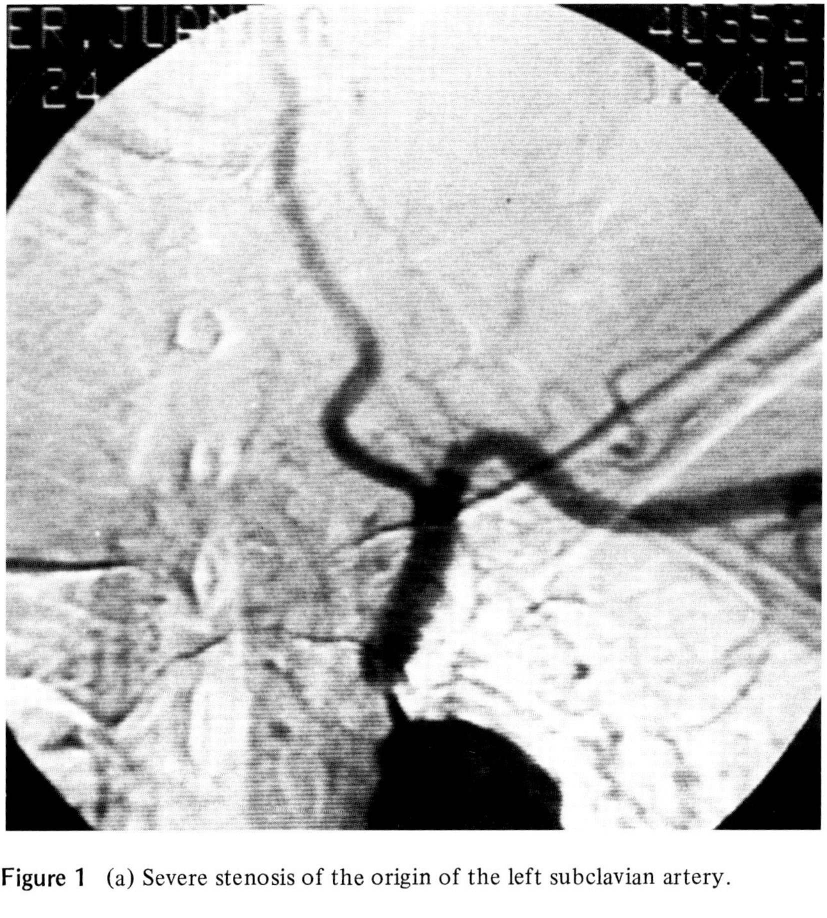

Figure 1 (a) Severe stenosis of the origin of the left subclavian artery.

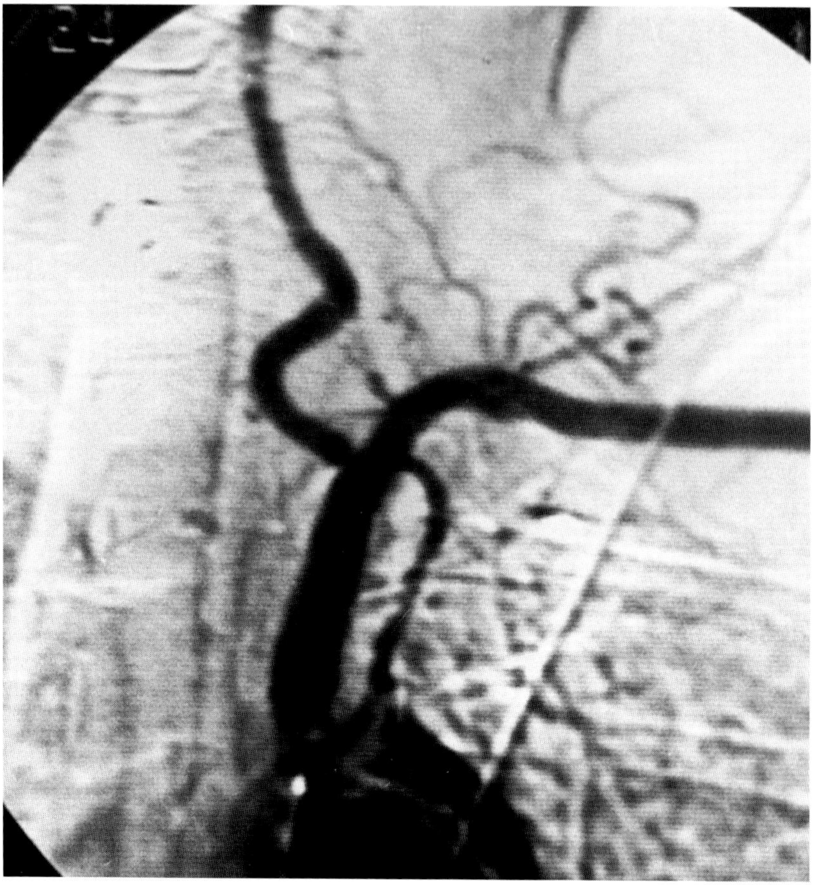

Figure 1 (b) The stenotic origin of the left subclavian artery has been reopened.

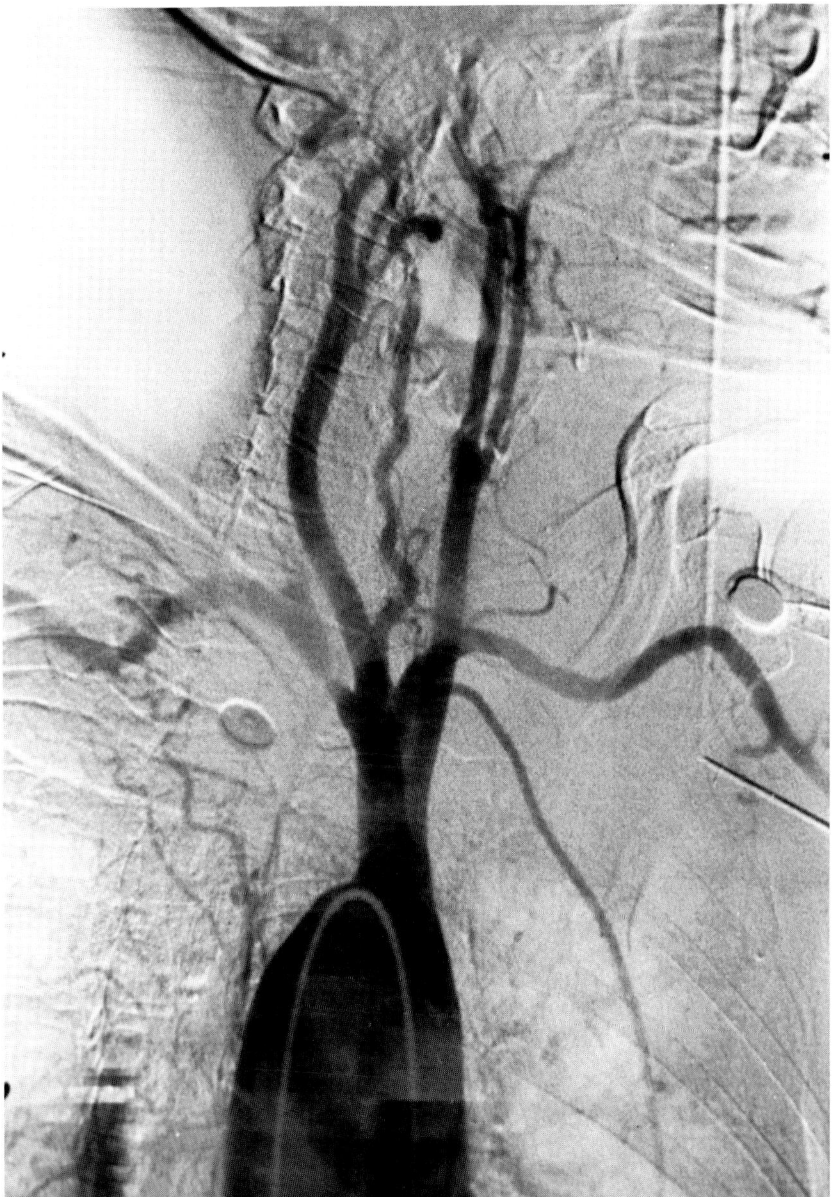

Figure 2 (a) Stenosis of the right subclavian artery is demonstrated by an arch angiogram with no antegrade filling of the right vertebral artery.

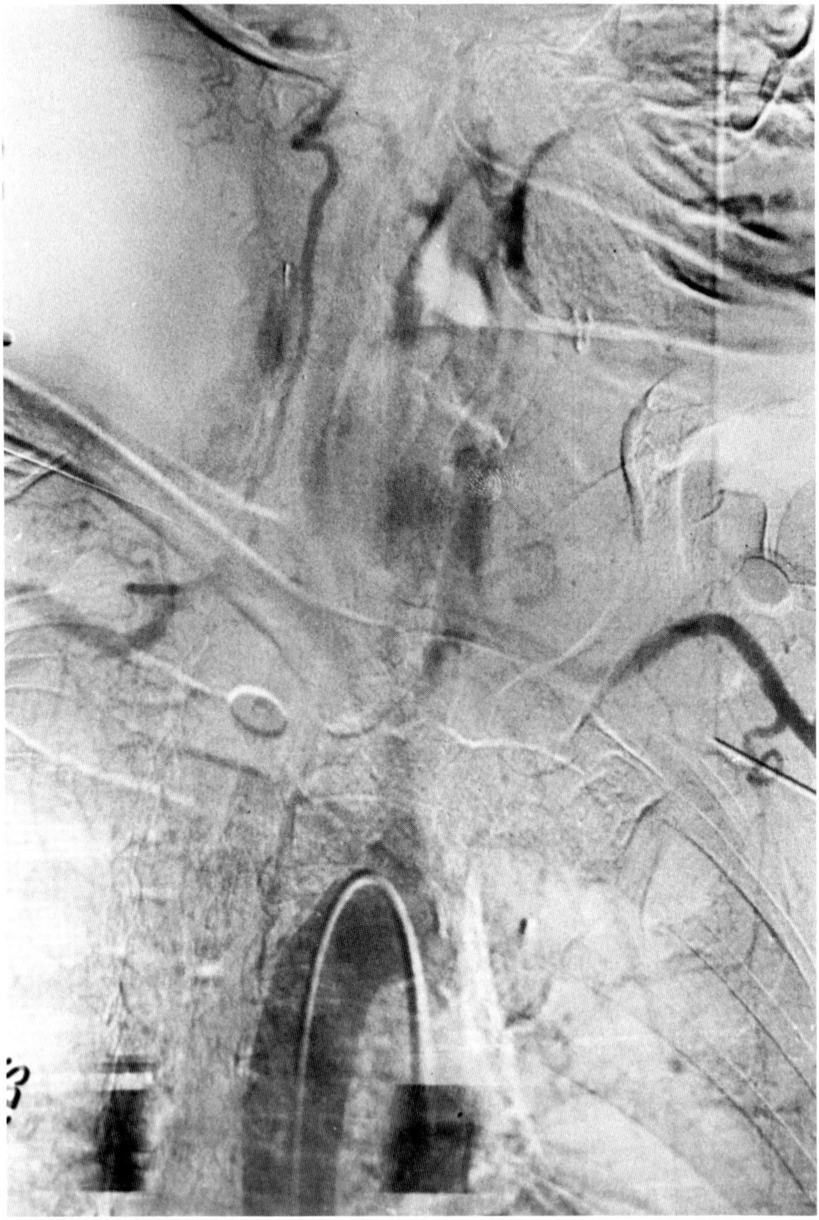

Figure 2 (b) The right vertebral artery is filled retrograde from the left vertebral artery.

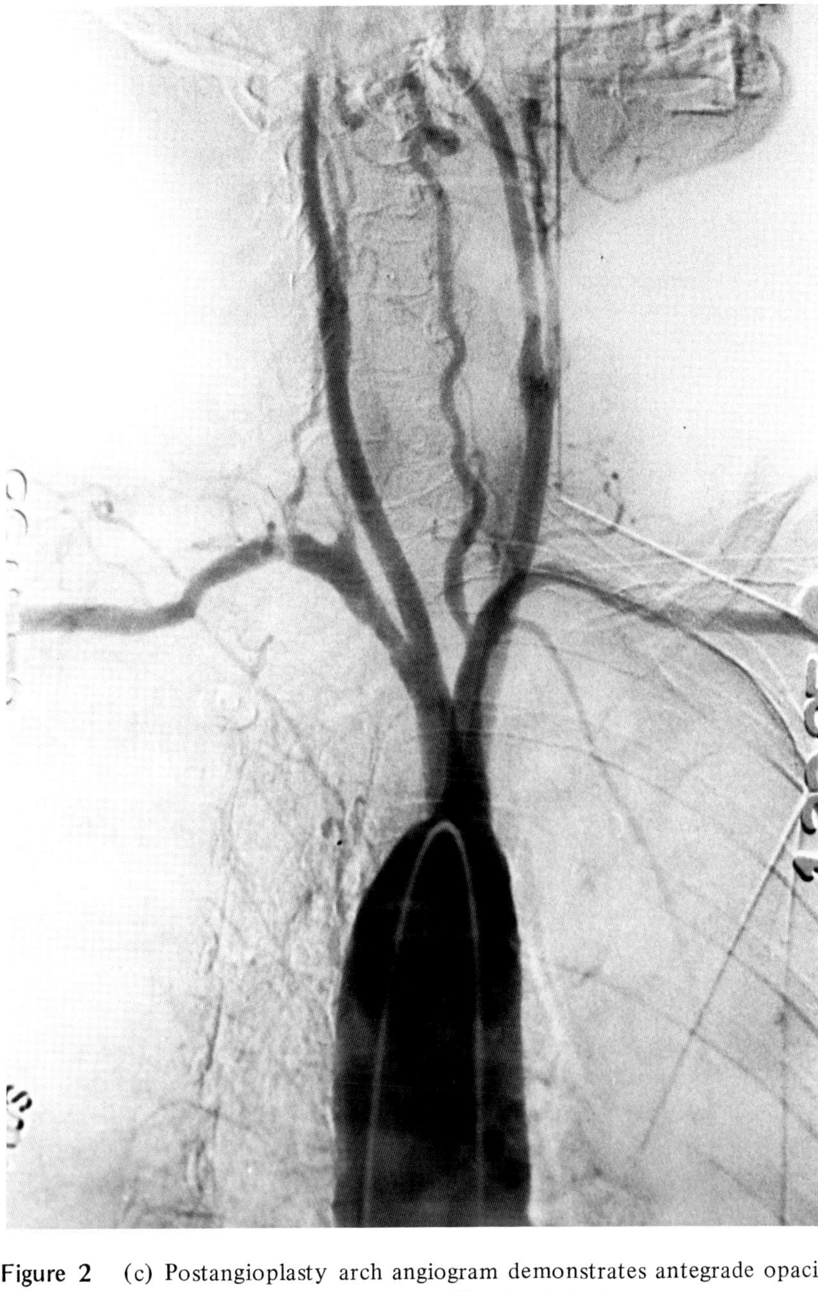

Figure 2 (c) Postangioplasty arch angiogram demonstrates antegrade opacification of the right vertebral artery via postdilated subclavian artery.

III. SUBCLAVIAN ARTERY STENOSIS

Subclavian arterial occlusive disease accounts for 17% of extracranial cerebrovascular disease. It is second in frequency to carotid bifurcation for atherosclerotic involvement. The surgical treatment of subclavian arterial occlusive disease has been simplified with the use of extrathoracic bypass to avoid the surgical risk associated with transthoracic vascular reconstruction (Figure 1). However, the surgical risks remain rather high, with complication rates reported in the range of 4-23% (24,30-32). Thus, alternative nonsurgical procedures have become important considerations in this vascular territory.

Angioplasty for subclavian artery stenosis was first reported by Zeitler and Holik in 1977 (5). Backman and Kim first described PTA for subclavian steal syndrome in 1980 (6). Since then there have been a number of reports describing PTA for subclavian arterial occlusive disease (7-29). Proximal subclavian lesions may produce simple stenosis or be associated with subclavian steal syndrome (Fig. 2). Clinically, patients with subclavian artery obstruction present with vertebral-basilar insufficiency. Only 11 of 67 of our patients had primary symptoms of arm ischemia. Twenty-four of 67 patients had angiographic evidence of subclavian steal. In treating patients with subclavian steal, reversal of ipsilateral blood flow may play a protective role during angioplasty if emboli become dislodged proximal to the lesion (6,8,24-28). Occasionally, severe eccentric stenotic lesions may be dilated at two different times by using a smaller balloon first and then a larger balloon 4-6 weeks later.

Potential complications of subclavian artery PTA include dissection and occlusion of proximal side branch vessels, which may occur if the vessel is overdistended by the balloon. Another potential complication is compression and occlusion of adjacent vessels due to balloons that are too long. This is illustrated in Figure 3. Both the proximal subclavian and proximal vertebral artery demonstrate high-grade stenotic lesions. A 2.0-cm long balloon was initially placed across the proximal subclavian lesion. However, upon inflation, it slipped downward into the aortic arch or migrated distally into the subclavian artery. A 3.0-cm balloon may have compressed the proximal vertebral artery and caused occlusion. Therefore, it was decided to place a tapered 3.0-cm balloon catheter across both the proximal subclavian and vertebral artery lesions simultaneously and perform angioplasty of both vessels at the same time.

In the past several years, we have performed PTA of the subclavian artery in 67 patients without major complications. Only one minor complication occurred, in a patient who had asymptomatic partial occlusion of the right internal mammary artery. The literature contains reports of only three complications, consisting of digital artery emboli (29).

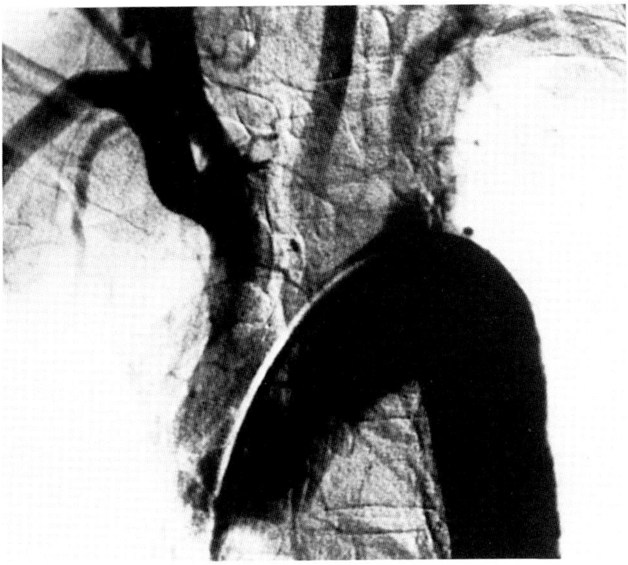

(a)

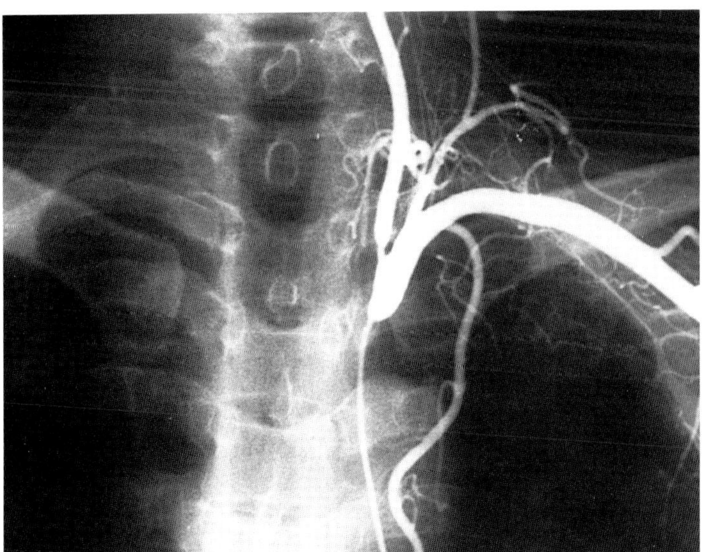

(b)

Figure 3 (a) Arch angiogram showing severe stenosis of the left subclavian artery. (b) Additional stenosis of the left vertebral artery is demonstrated by angiographic catheter passing beyond the stenotic proximal left subclavian artery.

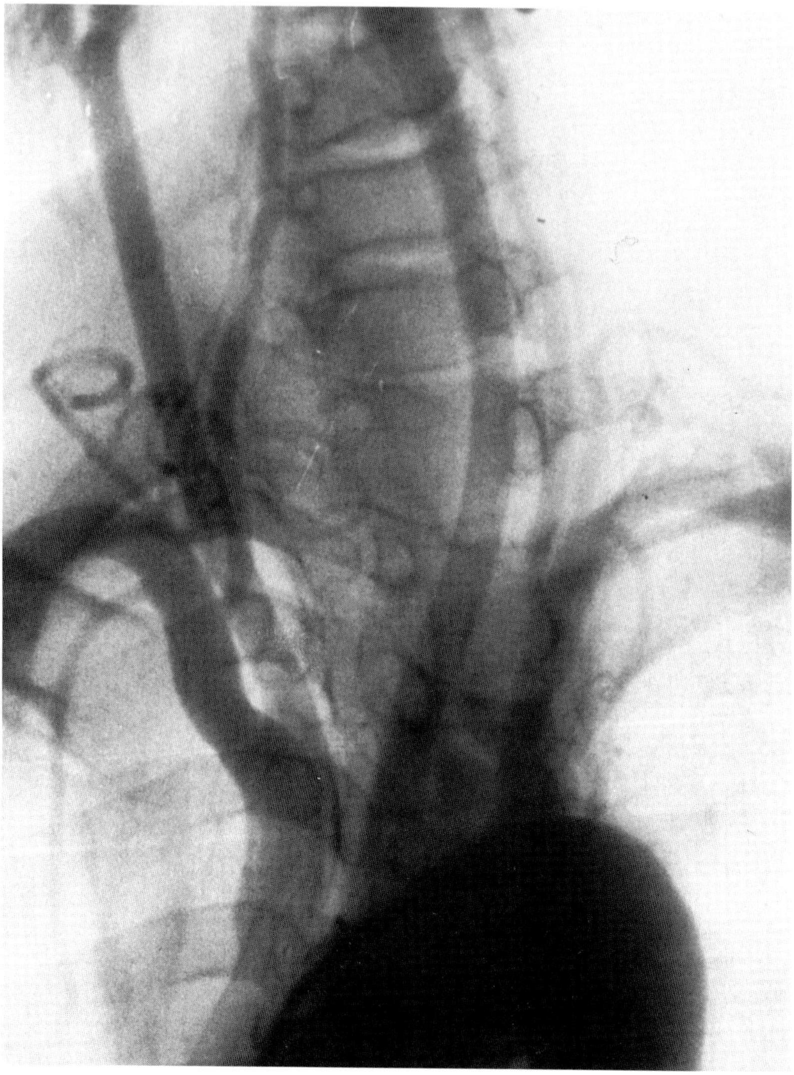

Figure 3 (c) Postangioplastic arch angiogram shows reopening of left subclavian and vertebral arteries.

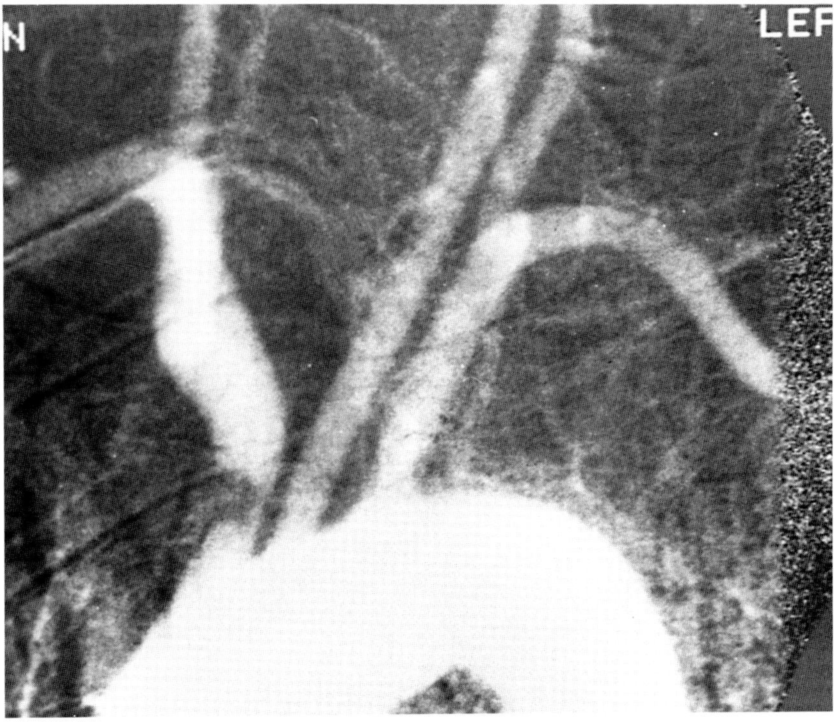

Figure 4 (a) Arch angiogram showing severe stenosis of right innominate artery origin.

IV. INNOMINATE ARTERY STENOSIS

The innominate artery has two major branches, the right common carotid artery and the subclavian artery. It accounts for less than 2% of cerebral ischemic episodes associated with extracranial arteriosclerotic disease. Although the innominate artery gives rise to the right vertebral artery, brainstem ischemia is infrequent when right vertebral stenosis occurs. This is due to the usual predominance of the right vertebral artery. The risk from surgical intervention for innominate artery stenosis is extremely high; the mortality from trans-sternal bypass or direct endarterectomy is reported to be as high as 6% (33). Extrathoracic bypass has become an alternative surgical procedure. However, surgical reconstruction for stenotic innominate artery lesions still remains quite complicated. Thus, alternatives for treatment of patients with stenosis of the innominate artery should be considered. In 1981, Lowman et al. (33) reported intraoperative

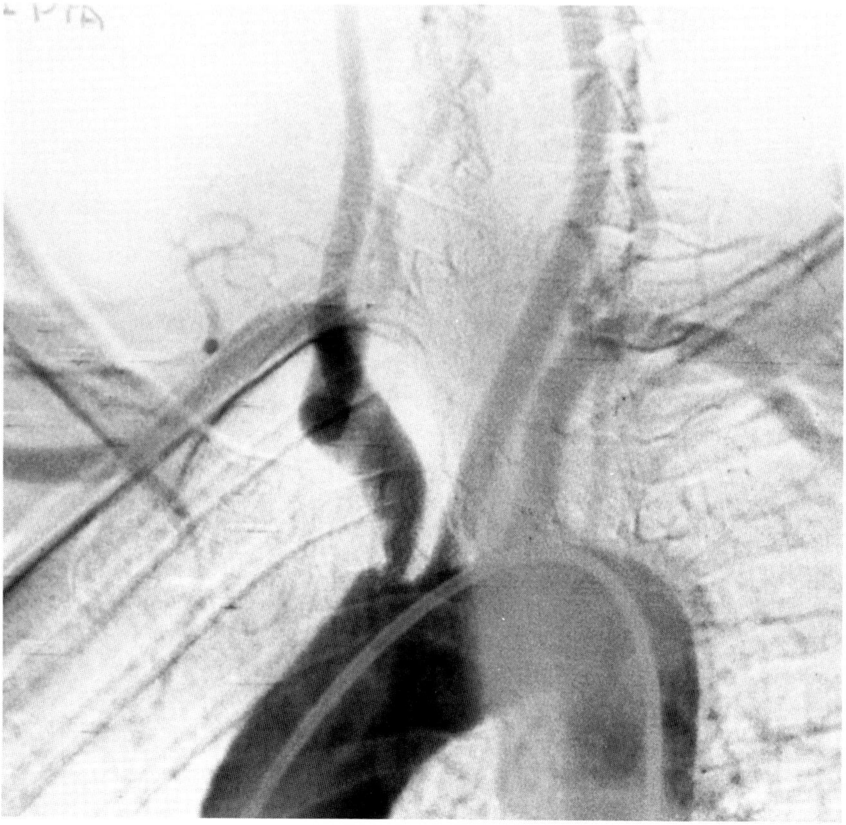

Figure 4 (b) Postangioplasty angiogram demonstrated partial dilatation of the stenotic origin, but the clinical symptoms were eliminated without further intervention.

retrograde transluminal angioplasty of the innominate artery through a right common carotid arteriotomy. Although intraoperative angioplasty may prevent the possibility of cerebral emboli, it does carry the same risk as carotid surgery (34). In 1983, Garrido and Garofola (34) reported a single case of successful PTA for innominate artery stenosis. Angioplasty may be better than intraoperative dilatation if patients have high surgical risk or coexistent vascular disease. Preliminary results from PTA of the innominate artery have been excellent (33-35). We have performed PTA in seven patients with stenosis of the innominate artery and there have been no complications (Fig. 4).

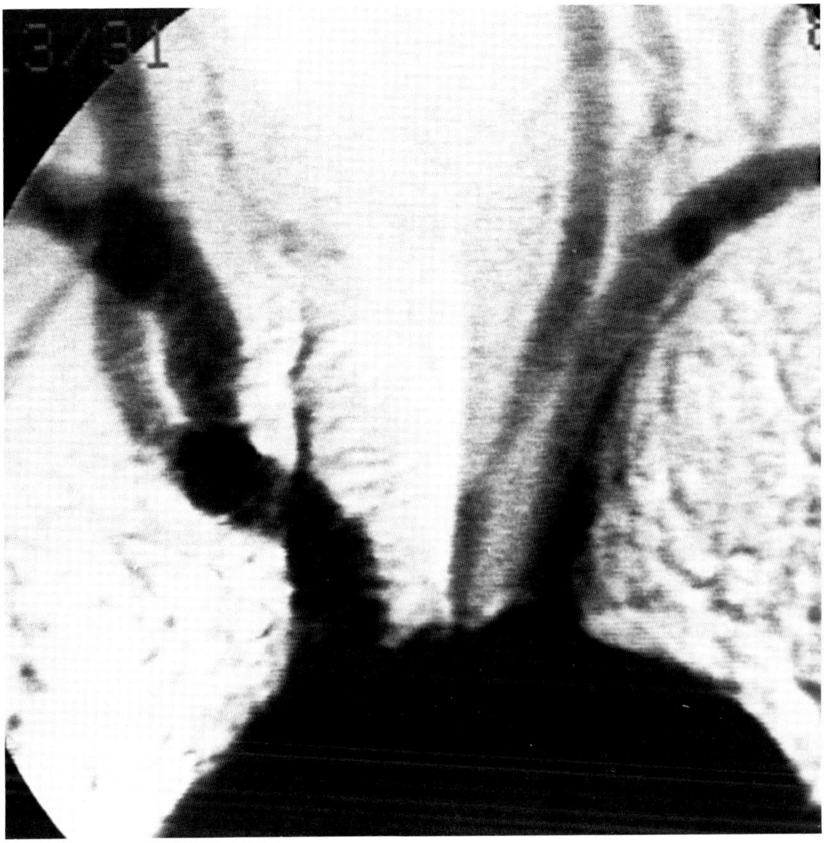

Figure 5 (a) Arch and (b) left carotid DSA demonstrated severe stenosis of left proximal common carotid artery.

V. CAROTID ARTERY STENOSIS

The treatment of choice for carotid artery bifurcation disease is usually surgical endarterectomy. Endarterectomy for carotid bifurcation lesions has been relatively effective and safe. However, surgical endarterectomy of the proximal common carotid artery, as it arises from the aortic arch carries a much higher risk and is also a more complex procedure; cervical carotid bypass is preferred to direct endarterectomy, even though complications may still be quite extensive (30,31,37-41). A review of the published complications following surgical endarterectomy for carotid bifurcation disease varies from 0.8% to 19.0% morbidity and from 1.9% to 19% mortality. The disparity in results is related in part to

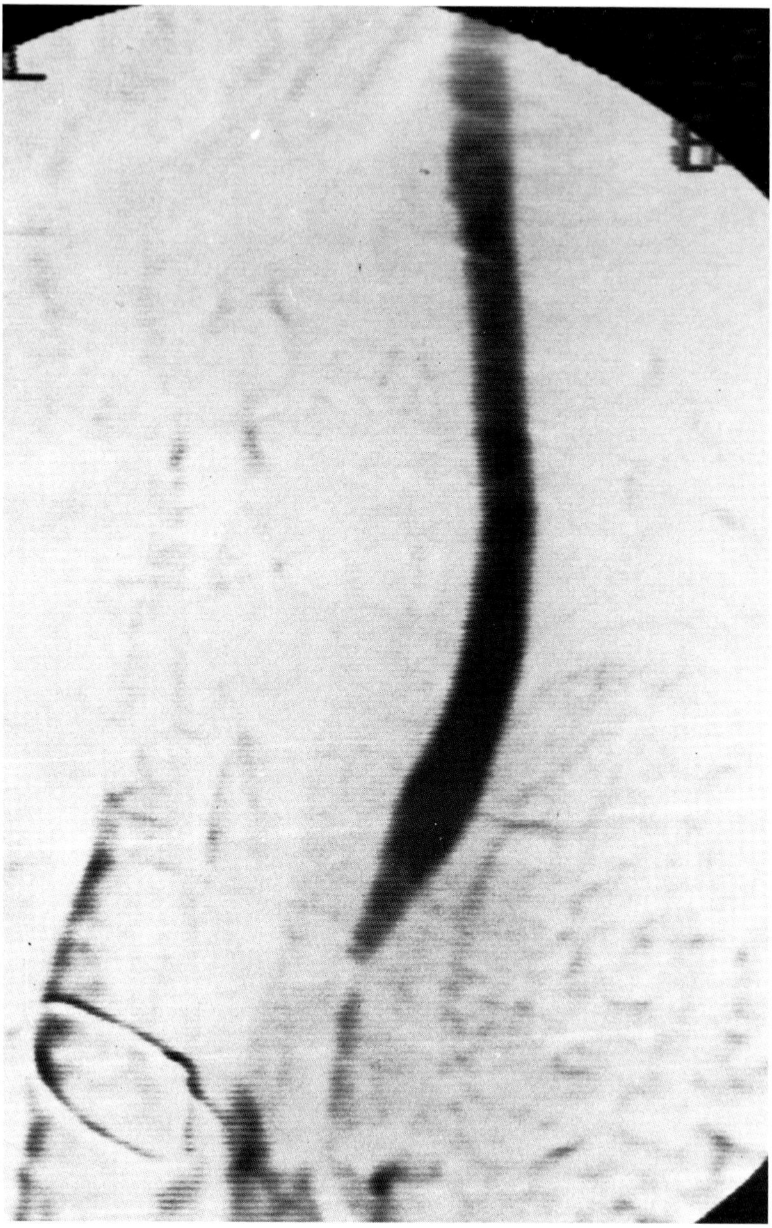

Figure 5 (b)

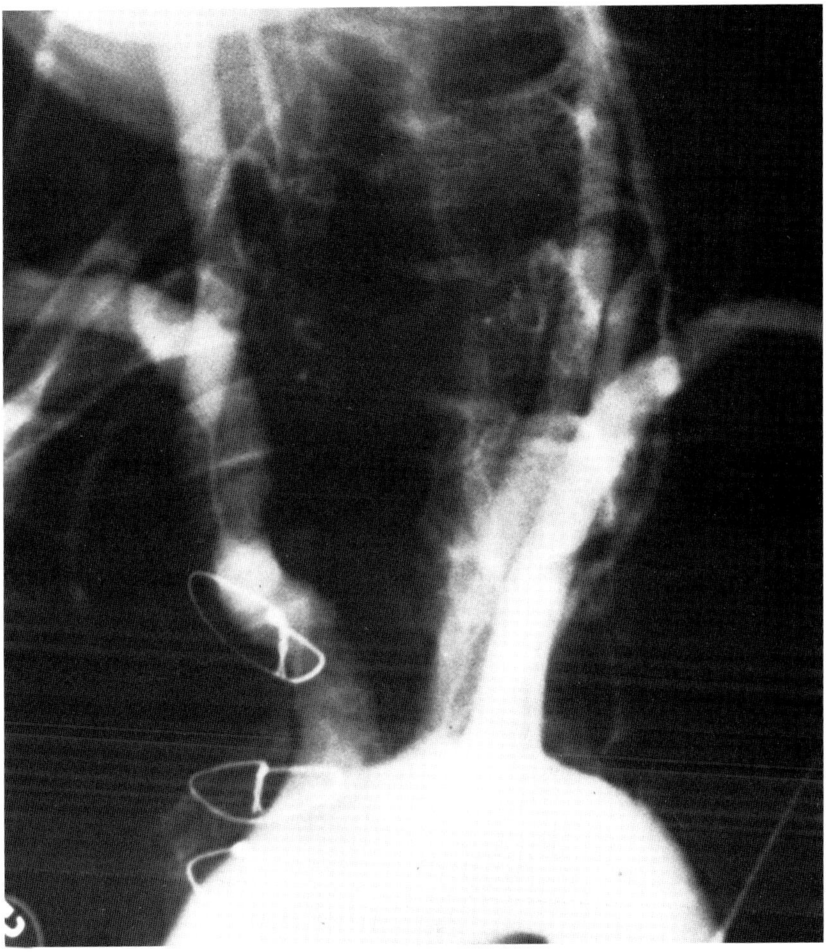

Figure 5 (c) Postangioplasty angiography showed restoration of left proximal common carotid artery. Note: This patient had previous cardiac bypass surgery.

variation in the population, patient selection, surgical technique, and preoperative status of the patients (38). Therefore those patients with high surgical risk may be candidates for PTA to relieve carotid stenosis (Fig. 5).

In 1968, Morris et al. (4) described the successful dilatation of a patient with fibromuscular dysplasia using a bile duct dilator intraoperatively. In 1980, Kerber et al. (42) reported successful intraoperative balloon angioplasty of a carotid artery. Later that year, Mathias (43) reported successful angioplasty from a percutaneous route. Since then numerous other authors have reported successful PTA for carotid atherosclerotic disease (44-56).

At our institution, all patients undergoing PTA for high-grade, hemodynamically significant carotid artery lesions are monitored by EEG. We have had seven patients with EEG changes (slow waves and spikes) immediately after the balloon catheter was passed through the stenotic segment. The angioplasty procedure of those patients was abandoned without complication. The EEG changes were probably due to ischemia from total cessation of blood flow. Therefore, we feel that injecting fresh heparinized arterial blood is important in order to avoid cerebral ischemia during balloon inflation. We have had two two patients in whom ischemic symptoms developed during inflation; symptoms subsided immediately after deflation of the balloon. Since we began injecting fresh arterial blood into the carotid artery, we have not experienced this problem (33, 54,55).

Subtotal occlusion of the internal carotid artery may appear as total occlusion on a standard angiogram. Therefore digital subtraction angiography should be routinely obtained to avoid this mistake. The nearly occluded internal carotid artery may be reopened by PTA with balloon dilatation techniques (54) (Fig. 9).

The external carotid artery may have an extremely important role for collateral supply to the intracranial circulation in those patients with total occlusion of the internal carotid artery. Stenosis may also occur at the proximal external carotid artery. Although an external carotid to internal carotid (EC-IC) bypass may increase flow to the cerebral circulation, stenosis of the proximal external carotid artery may prevent improvement of collateral circulation. In these cases, PTA of the external carotid artery will improve the collaterals and increase the cerebral circulation (33,50-56). It will also aid in keeping open the EC-IC anastomosis.

In performing PTA for external carotid artery lesions, one must be catious because the external carotid artery is inclined to spasm. Unnecessary manipulation must be avoided. Once spasm occurs, the artery must be kept open wth anticoagulants to prevent thrombosis. Hypotension is another complication that may occur during proximal external or carotid bifurcation PTA. This is due to compression on the carotid body. Atropine should be given prior to PTA to avoid this problem. We have successfully performed PTA on 41 patients with common, internal, or external carotid arterial occlusive lesions without complication (33,54,55) (Figs. 5-10).

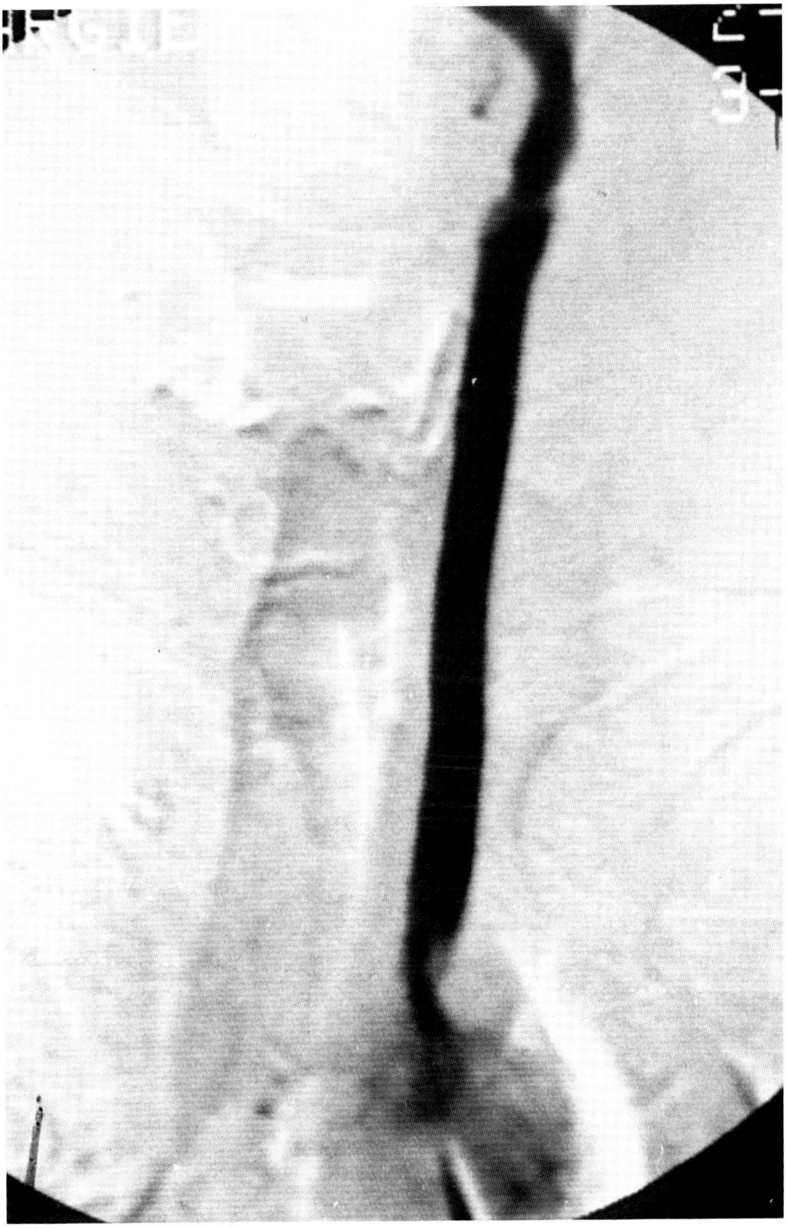

Figure 6 (a) Stenosis of proximal left common carotid artery was noted as a tandem lesion with the stenosis of carotid bifurcation.

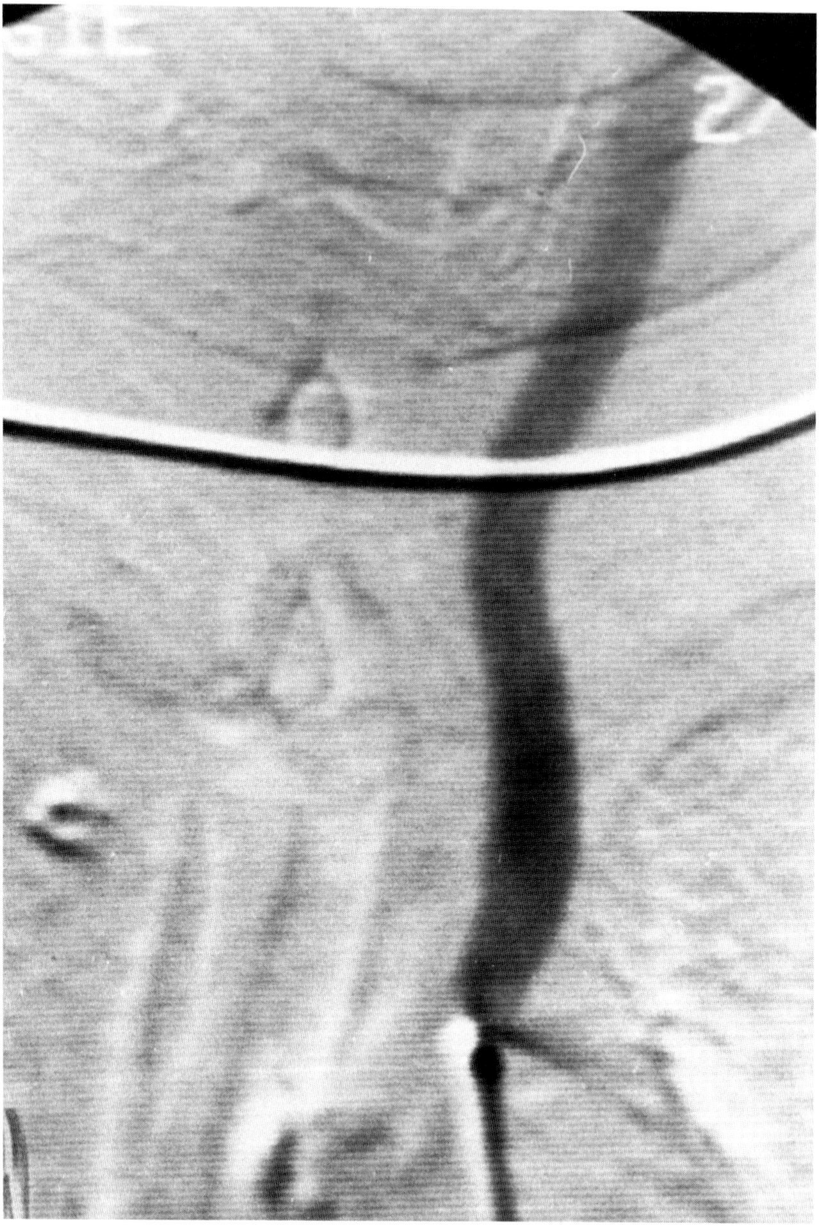

Figure 6 (b) After angioplasty, the stenotic common carotid artery was reopened.

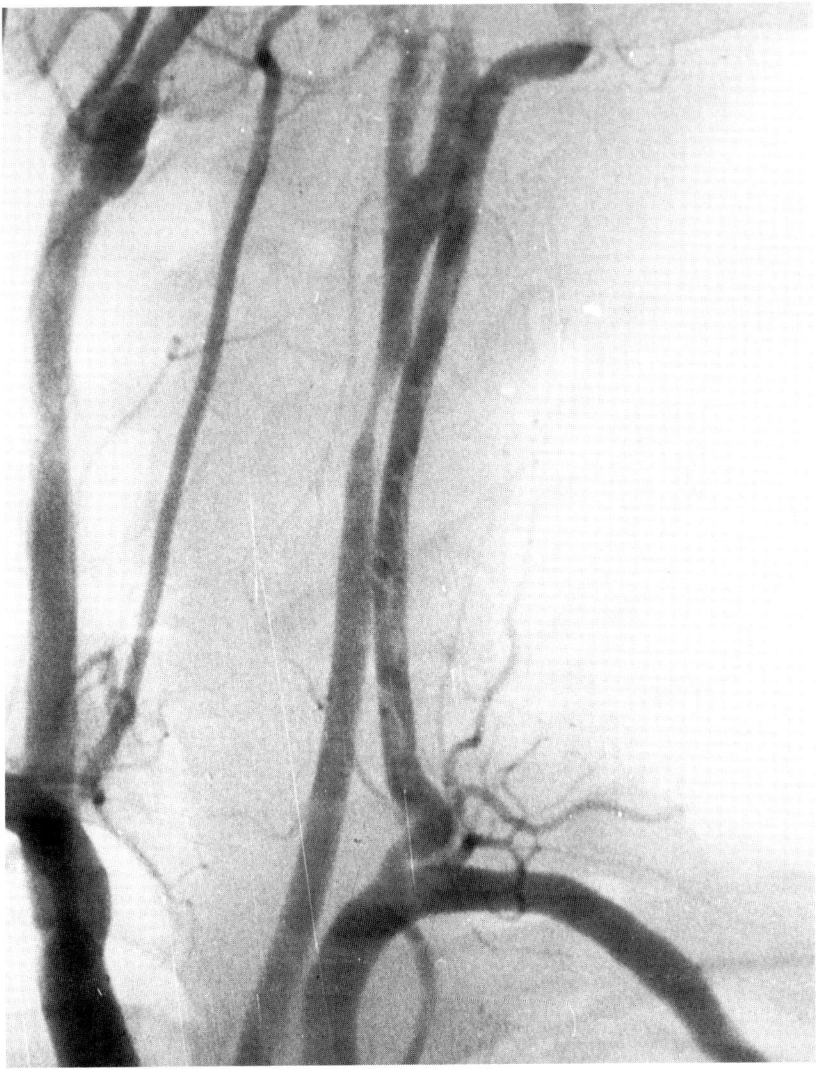

Figure 7 (a) Arch angiography showed a smooth luminal stenosis of the distal left common carotid artery, thought to be Takayasu's arteritis in this patient, who was in his thirties.

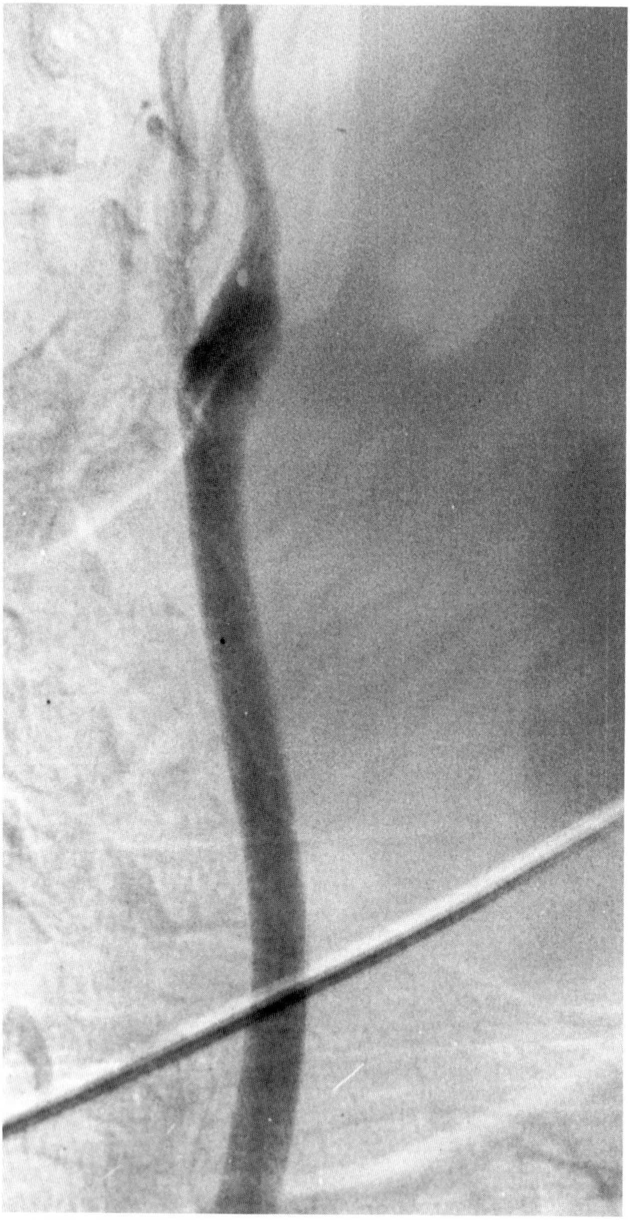

Figure 7 (b) Postangioplasty disclosed restoration of the left common carotid artery.

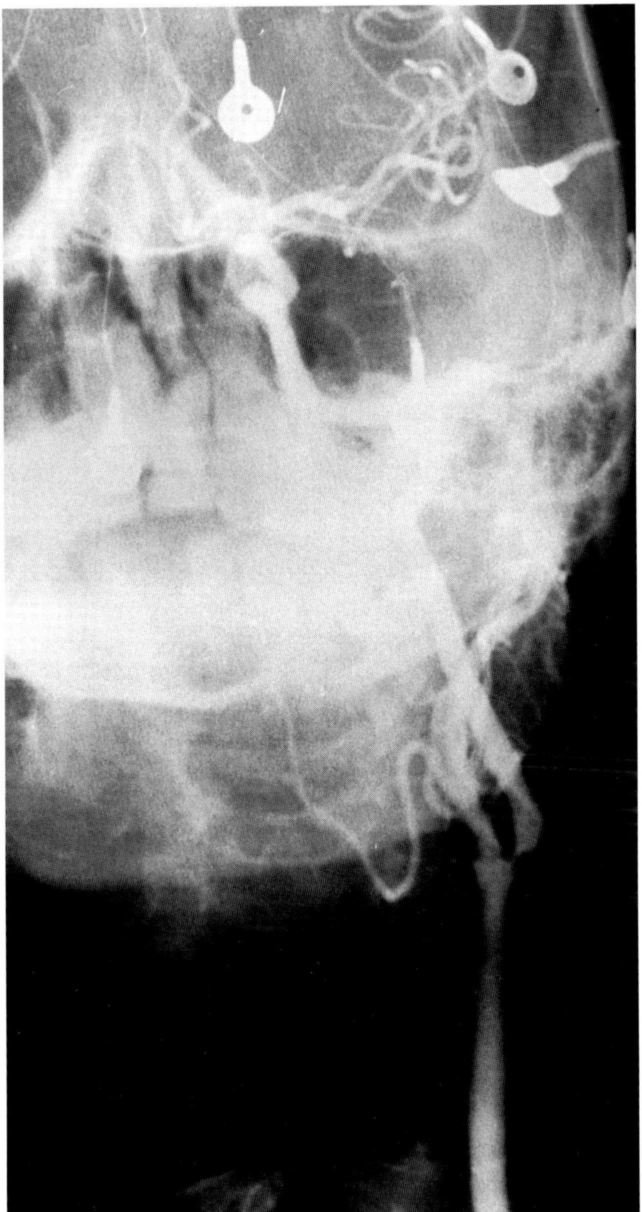

Figure 8 (a) Common carotid angiography demonstrated severe stenosis of the left internal carotid artery origin, just at the carotid bifurcation.

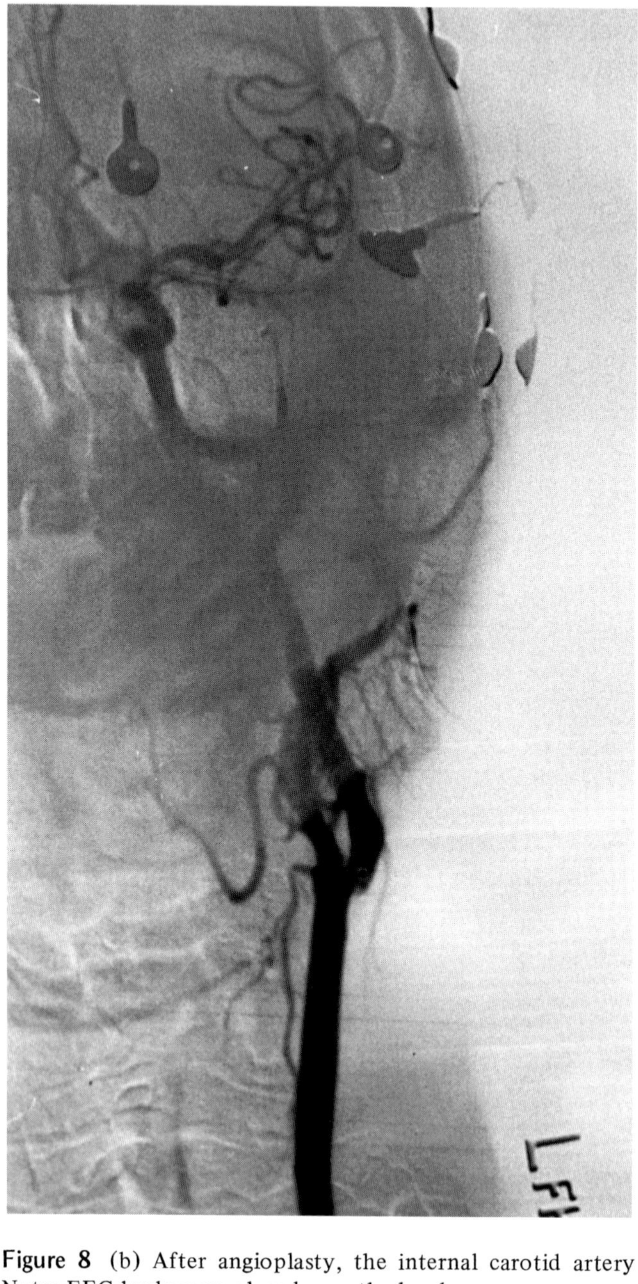

Figure 8 (b) After angioplasty, the internal carotid artery was well restored. Note: EEG leads were placed over the head.

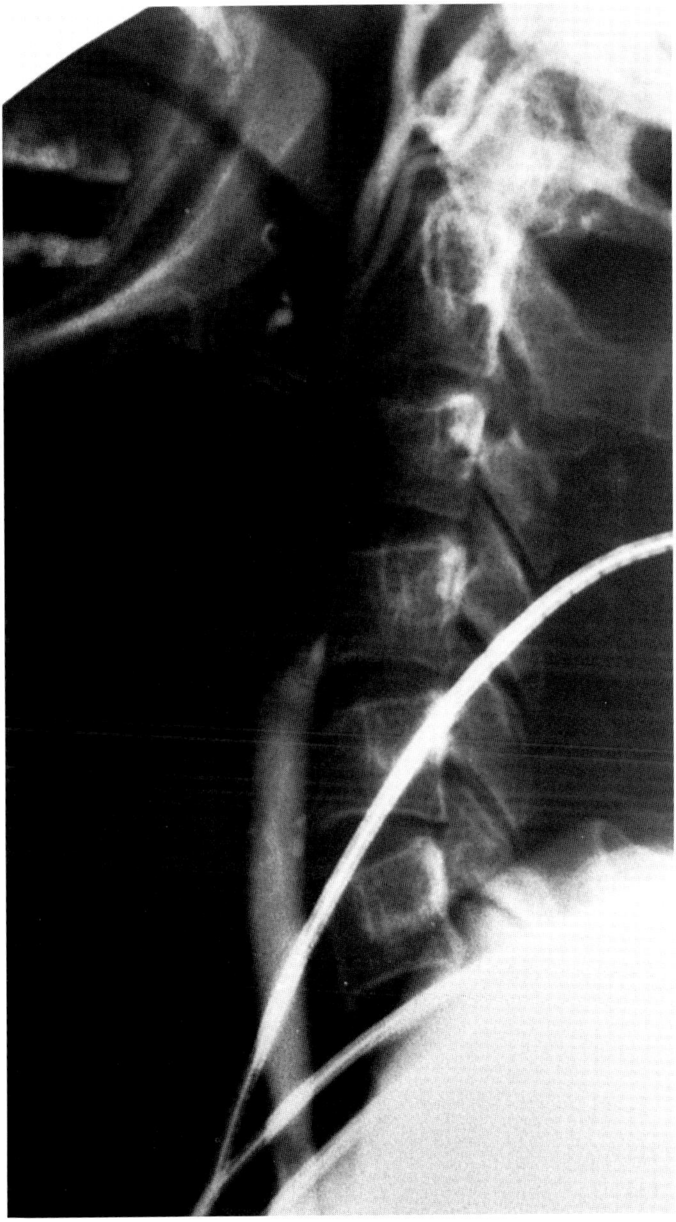

Figure 9 (a) Right common carotid angiogram showed a total occlusion of the internal carotid artery.

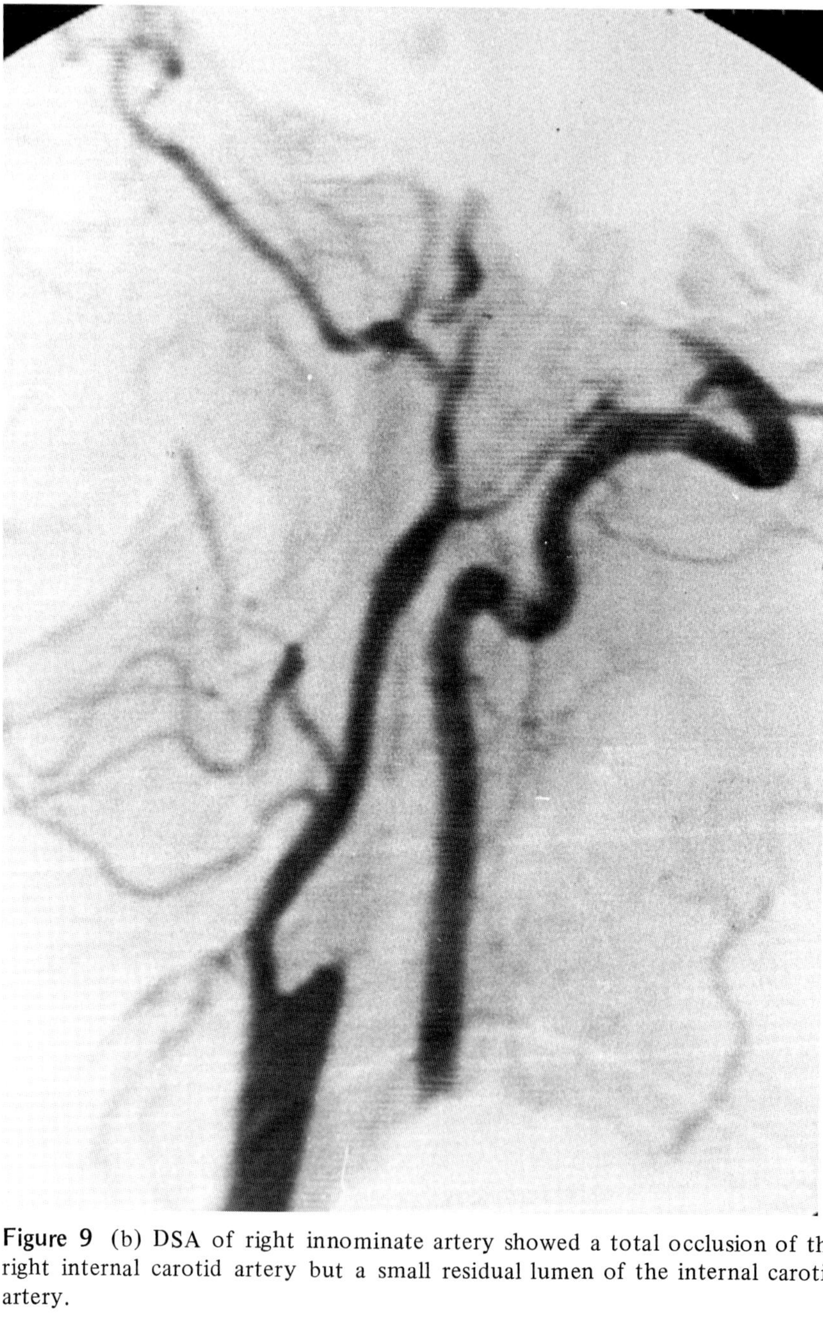

Figure 9 (b) DSA of right innominate artery showed a total occlusion of the right internal carotid artery but a small residual lumen of the internal carotid artery.

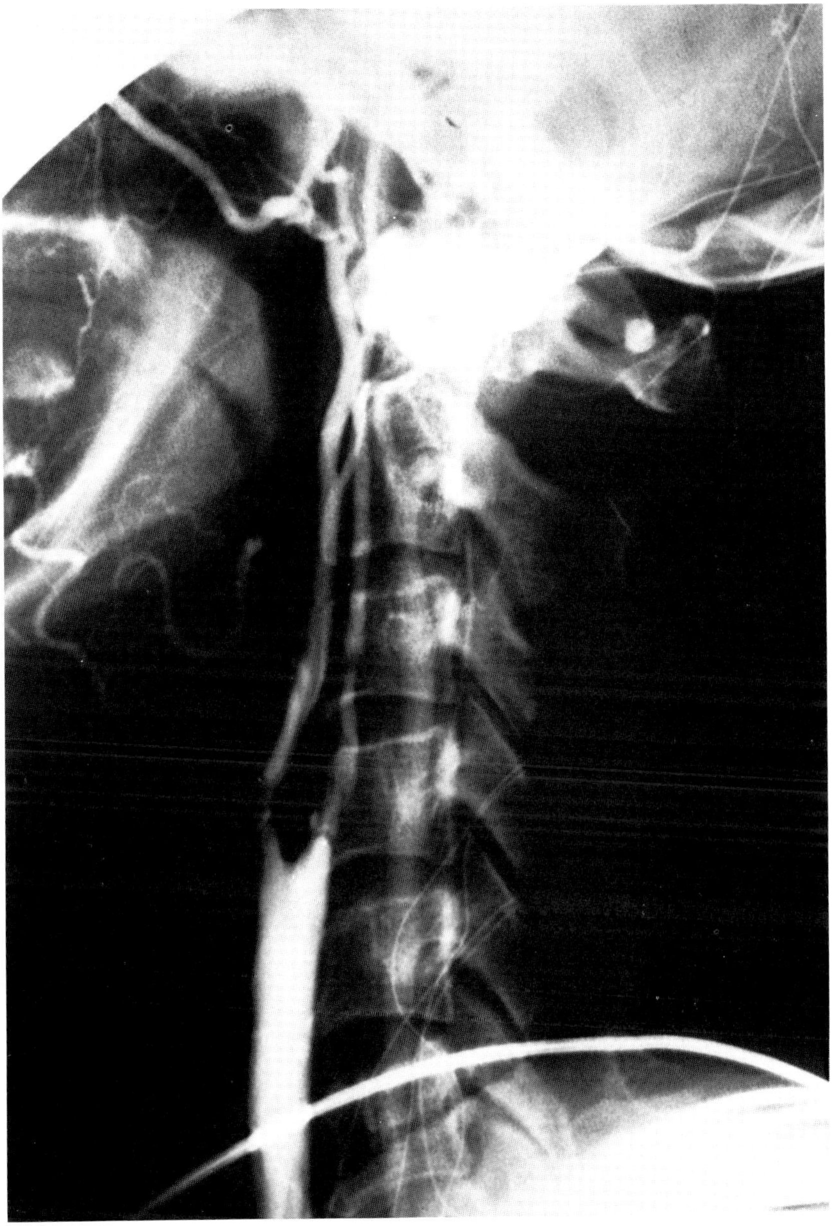

Figure 9 (c) Postangioplasty angiogram showed restoration of the internal carotid artery.

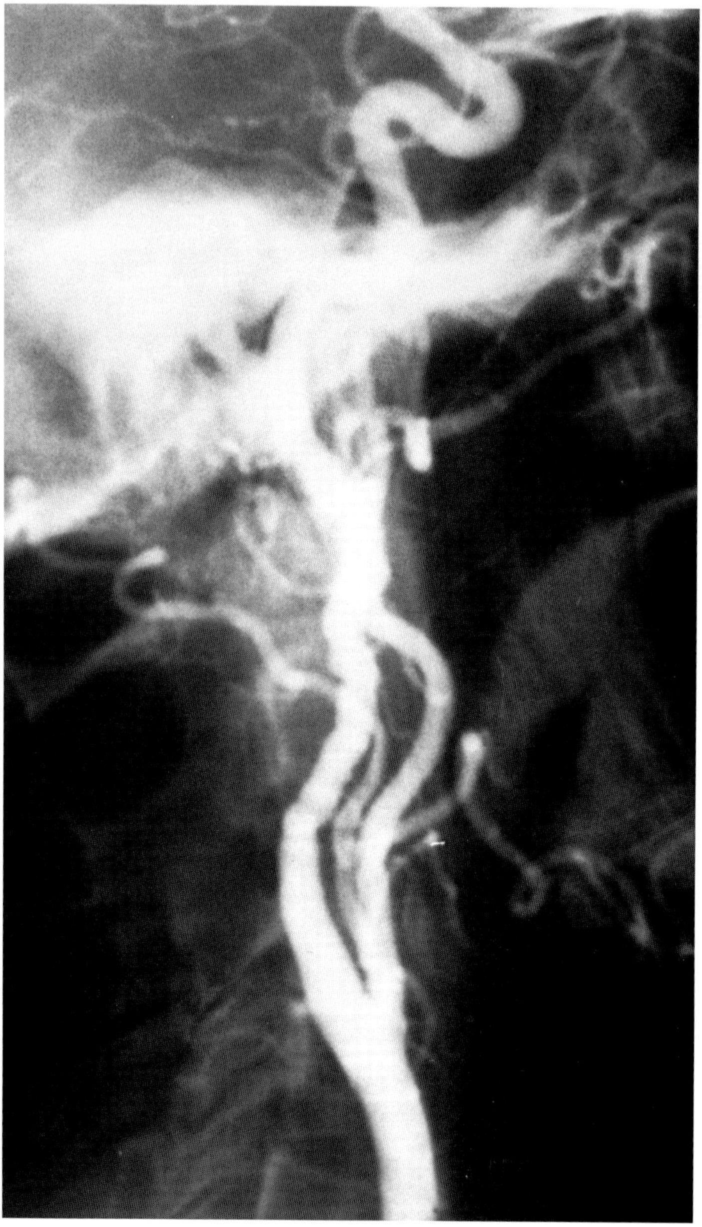

Figure 10 (a) Left common carotid angiography showed fibromuscular dysplasia of the left internal carotid artery.

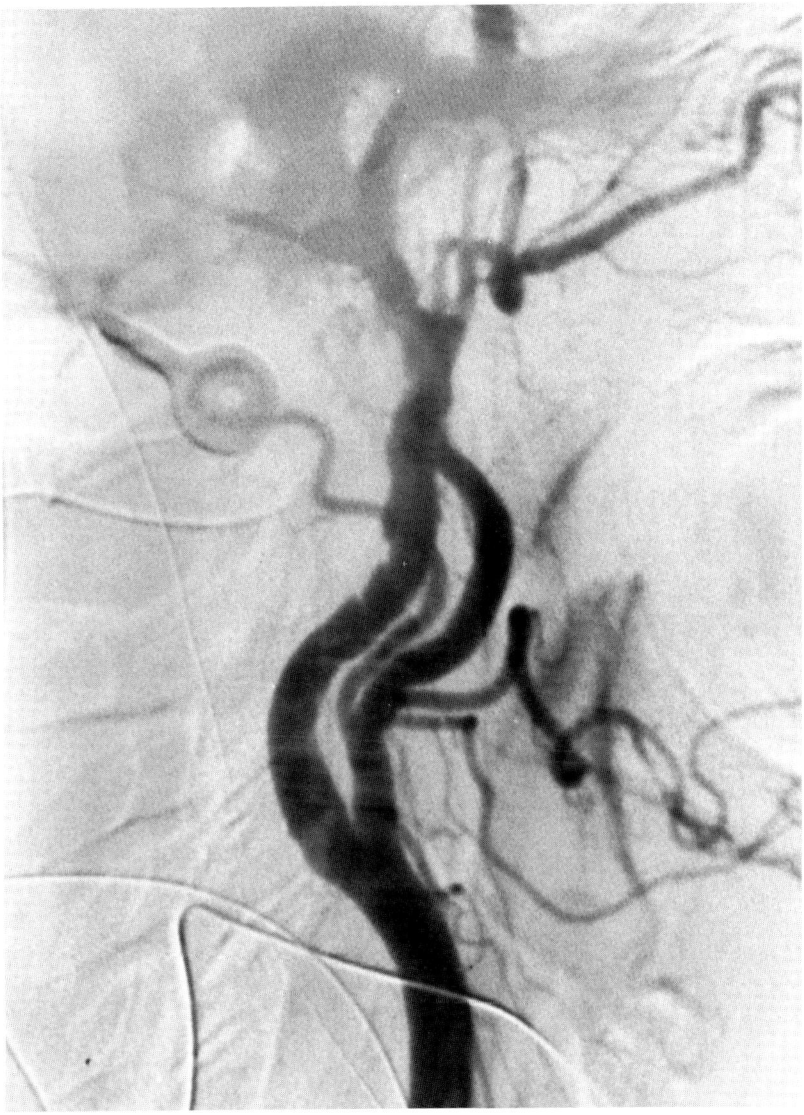

Figure 10 (b) Postangioplasty showed better caliber of dysplastic segment, but transverse clefts.

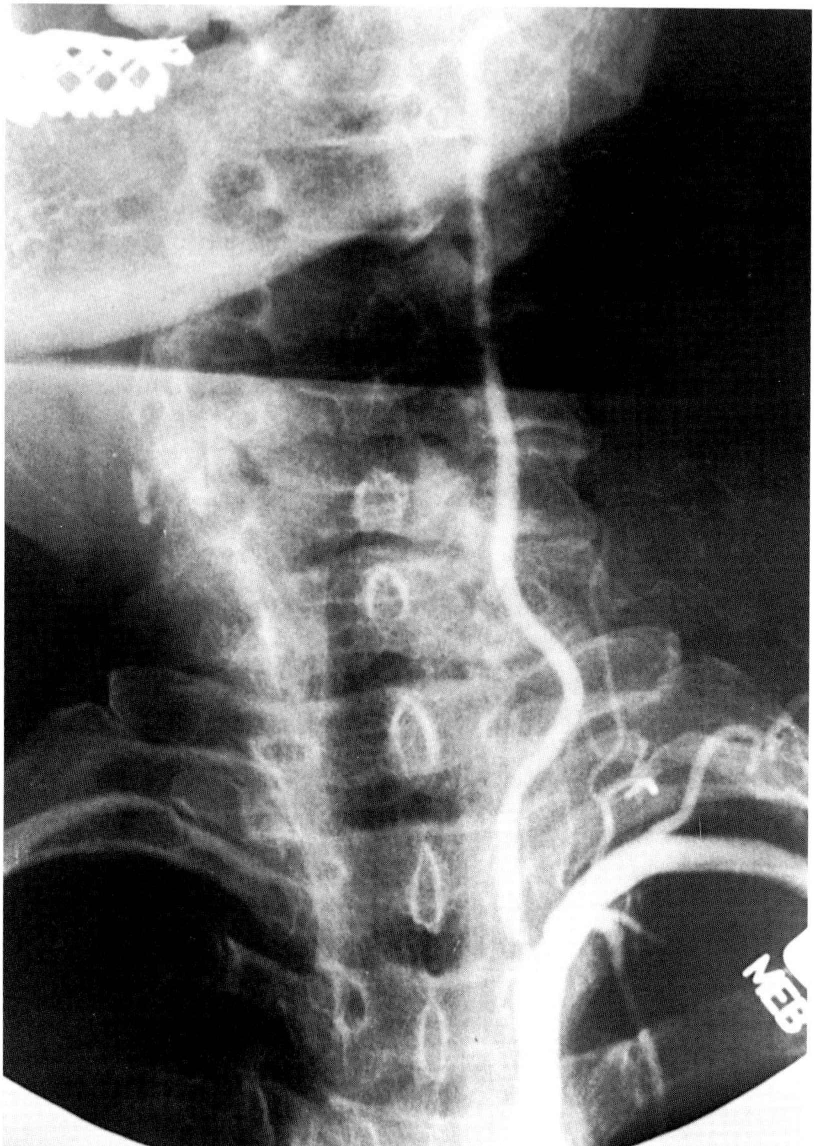

Figure 11 (a) Left subclavian angiogram showed severe stenosis of the left vertebral artery origin.

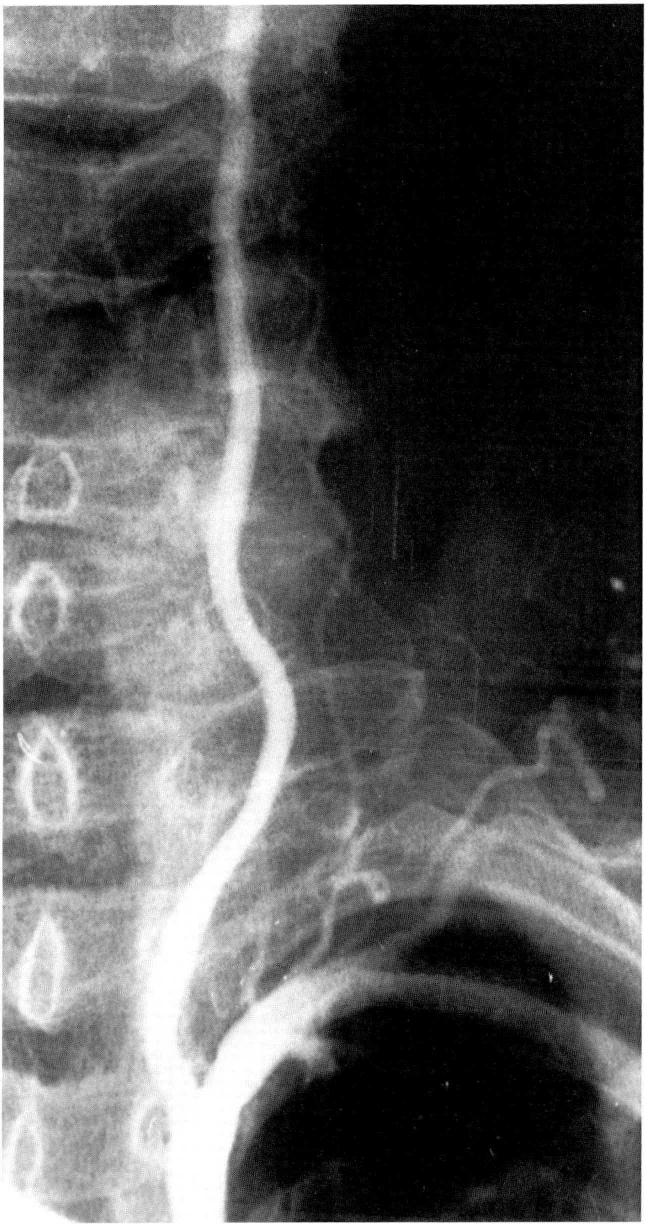

Figure 11 (b) After angioplasty the stenotic segment was restored to normal.

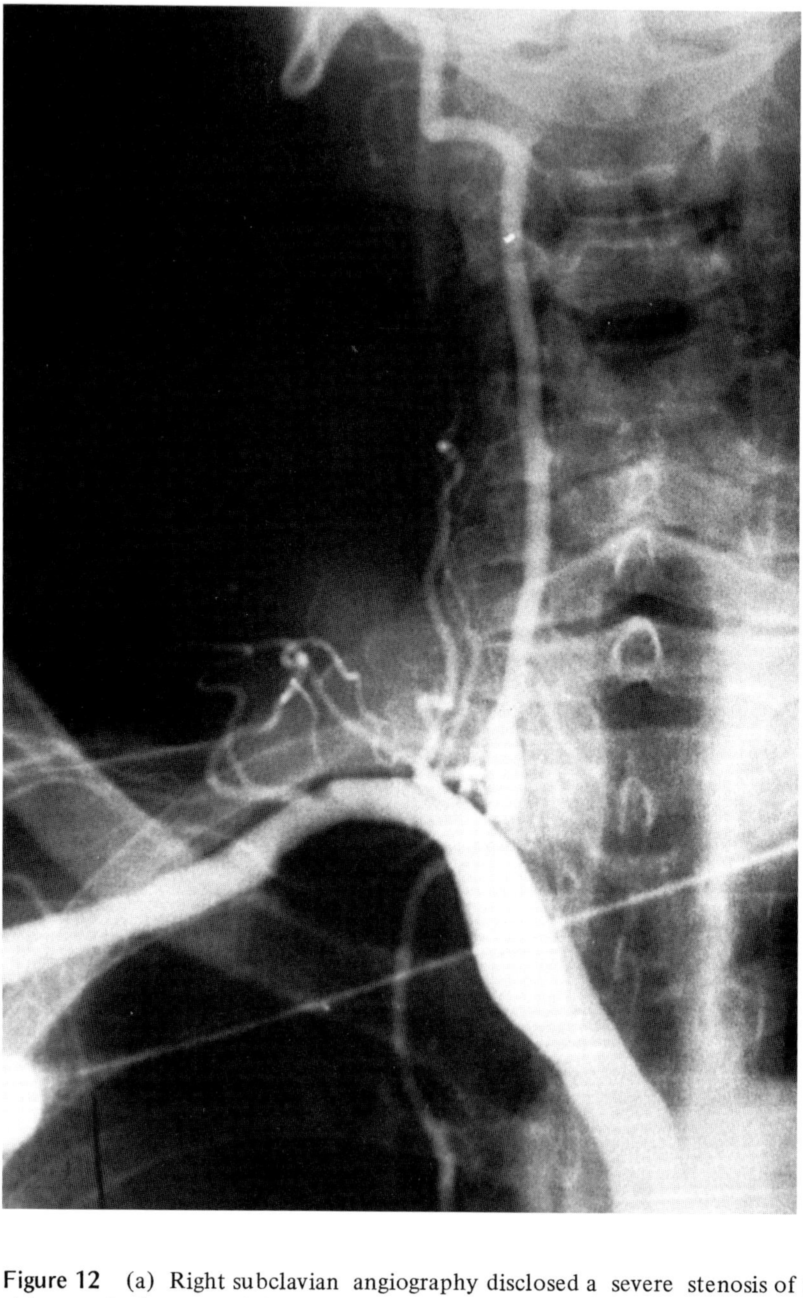

Figure 12 (a) Right subclavian angiography disclosed a severe stenosis of the right vertebral artery origin.

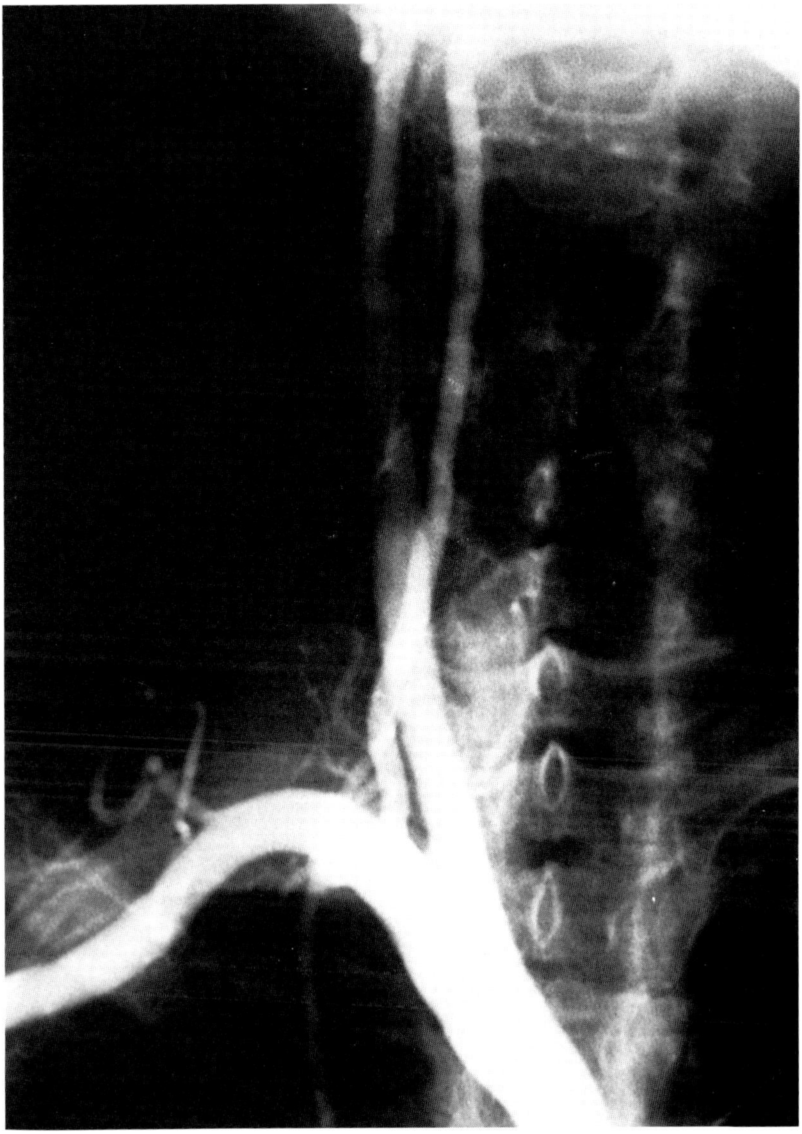

Figure 12 (b) Postangioplasty innominate angiography showed restoration of the right vertebral artery.

VI. VERTEBRAL AND BASILAR ARTERY STENOSIS

Vertebral artery stenosis mainly occurs at the origin from the subclavian artery and less frequently at the middle and distal segments. The etiology and progression of arteriosclerotic disease in this territory are uncertain. Baker et al. reported in 1965 that 8% of patients with vertebrobasilar insufficiency progress to stroke (56). However, later data have suggested that the risk of stroke for those patients with vertebrobasilar insufficiency may be as high as 7% per year and 20-62% over a period of 5 years (56-59). Intraoperative angioplasty and bypass of the vertebral artery origin has in the past been the surgical treatment of choice (56-58). However, surgery for vertebral artery stenosis is a rather complicated procedure. Surgical mortality has ranged from 1 to 3%, and morbidity may be as high as 13% (57-59).

Lesions of the vertebral artery are usually smooth without ulceration, unlike carotid bifurcation lesions. Motarjeme et al. in 1981 first reported successful PTA of vertebral artery stenosis in 11 patients (60). Schultz et al. (61) also reported successful dilatation of proximal vertebral artery stenosis through a right subclavian arteriostomy. Courtheoux et al. in 1985 reported successful dilation of vertebral artery stenosis in 23 of 24 patients (59). Thus far, initial reports on PTA of the vertebral artery appear very favorable (53,59-63). We have successfully performed PTA in 16 of 17 patients without complications (62,63) (Figs. 11 and 12).

Basilar artery stenosis is inaccessible by direct surgery. Sundt et al. reported the first balloon dilatation of basilar artery stenosis in 1980 (64). Two gravely ill patients with severe vertebrobasilar insufficiency were treated by PTA with good initial results. The long-term follow-up was not reported. Sundt et al. performed transluminal angioplasty by introducing a balloon catheter through a 19-gauge sheath. Surgical exposure of the extracranial vertebral artery at the base of the skull was achieved by resecting the arch of the atlas. The first dilatation used a 3-mm balloon with three inflations for 20 seconds. The second dilatation used a 3.7-mm balloon with two inflations (64).

We have performed angioplasty of the basilar artery in two cases (63). One patient with atherosclerotic stenosis was successfully dilated. However, the paient subsequently suffered a brainstem infarct. This was due to occlusion of small pontine arteries arising directly from the basilar artery. Basilar artery PTA carries the risk of branch occlusion of small brainstem perforating vessels. Thus, PTA for basilar stenosis is still a highly risky procedure.

VII. SUMMARY

Percutaneous transluminal angioplasty for brachiocephalic artery stenosis has been slow to evolve due to the inherent potential risk of dislodging emboli that may result in stroke. Our own experience and review of the recent literature indicate that PTA of brachiocephalic arteries is feasible. Angioplasty may be performed as an alternative procedure to treat hemodynamically significant atherosclerotic lesions of the subclavian, innominate, carotid, and vertebral arteries. It may also be performed in conjunction with other surgical procedures, such as coronary bypass, in order to treat patients who are at high risk for stroke.

Percutaneous transluminal angioplasty has been successfully performed on more than 200 patients with subclavian artery stenosis (5-29), 104 patients with carotid artery stenosis (29,33,42-55), 60 patients with vertebral artery stenosis (29,59-64), and 15 patients with innominate artery disease (29,34-36). Good patient selection is essential. A close working relationship between the neurologist, surgeon, and neuroradiologist is very important. As more experience is gained in this field, the indications for PTA of brachiocephalic arterial occlusion will likely increase. Thus far PTA has been performed with rather low morbidity and no procedure mortality. Long-term follow-up and comparison with surgical results are needed.

REFERENCES

1. Dotter CT, Judkins MP. Transluminal treatment of arteriosclerotic obstruction: description of a new technique and preliminary report of its application. *Circulation* 30:654-670, 1964.
2. Portsman W. Ein neuer korsett balloon katheter zur transluminalen rekanalisation nach doter unter besonderer berucksichtigung von obliterationen on den beckenarterien. *Radiol Diagn* 14:239-241, 1973.
3. Grüntzig A, Hopff H. Perkutane rekanalisation chronischer arterieller verschluse mit einem neuren dilatations-catheter. *Dtsch Med Wochenschr* 99: 2502-2505, 1974.
4. Morris GC, Lechter A, DeBakey ME. Surgical treatment of fibromuscular disease of the carotid arteries. *Arch Surg* 96:636-643, 1968.
5. Zeitler E, Holik B. Angiographische diagnostik. In: Raithel D (Ed.), *Zerebrale Insuffizienz durch extrakranielle gefahverschdusse*. Perimid, Erlangen, 1977, pp. 359-363.
6. Backman DM, Kim RM. Transluminal dilatation for subclavian steal syndrome. *Am J Radiol* 135:995-996, 1980.
7. Basche S, Ritter H, Gaerisch F, Grossman K, Heerklotz I, Schumann E. Percutaneous transluminal angioplasty of the subclavian artery. *Zentralbl Chir* 108(3):142-149, 1983.
8. Courtheoux, P, Theron J, Maiza D, Derlon JM, Pelouze GA, Henriet JP, Evrard C, Commeau P. Endoluminal angioplasty for atheromatous stenoses of supra-aortic trunks. The brachiocephalic arterial trunk, subclavian arteries. *J Radiol* 65(12):845-851, 1984.

9. Damouth HD Jr, Diamond AB, Rapporport AS, Renner JW. Angioplasty of sublcavian artery stenosis proximal to the vertebral origin. *Am J Neurolog Radiol* 4(6):1239-1242, 1983.
10. Galichia JP, Bajaj AK, Vine DL, Roberts RW. Subclavian artery stenosis treated by transluminal angioplasty: six cases. *Cardiovasc Intervent Radiol* 6(2):78-81, 1983.
11. Gordon RL, Haskell L, Hirsch M, Shifrin E, Weinman E, Romanoff H. Transluminal dilatation of the subclavian artery. *Cardiovasc Intervent Radiol* 8(1):14-19, 1985.
12. Grote R, Freyschmidt J, Walterbusch G. Percutaneous transluminal angioplasty in proximal subclavian stenoses. *ROFO* 138(6):660-664, 1983.
13. Hodgins GW, Dutton JW. Subclavian and carotid angioplasties for Takayasu's arteritis. *J Can Assoc Radiol* 33(3):205-207, 1982.
14. Kichikawa K, Nakagawa H, Yoshiya K, Ide K, Ohishi H, Uchida H, Iida N, Kyoi K, Utsumi S. Percutaneous transluminal angioplasty in a case of left subclavian and brachiocephalic artery stenosis due to aortitis syndrome. *Rinsho Hoshasen* 30(1):121-124, 1985.
15. Levien LJ, Fritz VU. Intra-operative transluminal angioplasty in the management of symptomatic aortic arch vessel stenosis. *S Afr J. Surg* 23(2): 49-52, 1985.
16. Lowman BG, Queral LA, Holbrook WA, Estes JT, Bayly B, Dagher FY. The correction of cerebrovascular insufficiency by transluminal dilatation: a preliminary report. *Am Surg* 49(11):621-624, 1983.
17. Mathias K, Staiger J, Thron A, Splliner G, Heiss HW, Konrad-Graf S. Perkutane katheterangioplastik der arteria subclavia. *Dtsch Med Wochenschr* 105:16-31, 1980.
18. Moore TS, Russell WF, Parent AD, Parker JL, Smith RR. Percutaneous transluminal angioplasty in subclavian steal syndrome: recurrent stenosis and retreatment in two patients. *Neurosurgery* 11(4):512-517, 1982.
19. Motarjeme A, Keifer JW, Zuska AJ. Percutaneous transluminal angioplasty of the brachiocephalic arteries. *AJR* 138(3):457-462, 1982.
20. Motarjeme A, Keifer JW, Zuska AJ, Nabawi P. Percutaneous transluminal angioplasty for treatment of subclavian steal. *Radiology* 155(3):611-613, 1985.
21. Olbert F, Mendel H, Muzika N, Schlegl A. Percutaneous transluminal vasodilatation. Long-term results and report on experience with a new system of catheters: transaxillary technic. *Wien Klin Wochenschr* 95(15): 528-536, 1983.
22. Pernes JM, Brenot P, Seuro M, Angl C, Ferrer J, Renaudin JM, Fabiani JN, D'Allaines C, Gaux JC. Percutaneous endoluminal angioplasty of the supra-aortic arterial trunks. Immediate and remote results. *Presse Med* 12(17): 1075-01078, 1984.
23. Rabkin IKH, Matevosov AL, Shekhter IUI. X-ray endovascular dilatation of the subclavian artery. *Grudn Khir* 2:76-78, 1984.
24. Schlosser V. Subclavian steal syndrome: correction by transthoracic or extra-anatomic repair. *Vasc Surg* 18:289-293, 1984.

25. Theron J, Courtheoux P, Henriet JP, Pelouze G, Derlon JM, Maiza D. Angioplasty of supra-aortic arteries. *J Neuroradiol* 11(3):187-200, 1984.
26. Theron J, Melancon D, Ethier R. Subclavian steal syndromes and their treatment by angioplasty. Hemodynamic classification of subclavian artery stenoses. *Neuroradiology* 27(3):265-270, 1985.
27. Tsai FY, Hieshima G, Mehringer CM, Gallacher DJ, Lewis G, Pribram HFW. Arterial digital subtraction angiography with particulate intravascular embolization and angioplasty. *Surg Neurol* 22:204-212, 1984.
28. Tsai FY, Yoon JW. Hieshima G, Tiu G, Shah D, Higashida R, Pribram HFW. Percutaneous transluminal angioplasty of subclavian steals. Presented at RSNR Nov. 18, 1985.
29. Zeitler E, Berger G, Schmitt-Ruth R. Percutaneous transluminal angioplasty of the supra-aortic arteries. In: Dotter CT, Gruntzig A, Schoop W, Zeitler E (Eds.), Springer-Verlag, Berlin, 1983, pp. 245-261.
30. Dietrich EB, Garrett HB, Ameriso J, Crawford ES, El-Bayer M, DeBakey ME. Occlusive disease of the common carotid and subclavian arteries treated by carotid subclavian bypass. *Am J Surg* 114:800-808, 1967.
31. Crawford ES, DeBakey ME, Morris GC Jr, Howell JF. Surgical treatment of occlusion of the innominate, common, carotid and subclavian arteries. *Surgery* 65:17-31, 1969.
32. Beebe HG, Start K, Johnson ML, Jolly PC, Hill LD. Choice of operation for subclavian-vertebral arterial disease. *Am J Surg 139:616-623, 1980.*
33. Lowman B, Queral L, Holbrook W, Estes J, Bayly B. The treatment of innominate artery stenosis by intraoperative transluminal angioplasty. *Surgery* 5:565-568, 1981.
34. Garrido E, Garofola J. Intraluminal dilatation of the innominate artery before extracranial-intracranial bypass: case report. *Neurosurgery* 12(5): 581-583, 1983.
35. Kobinia G, Bergmann H Jr. Angioplasty in stenosis of the innominate artery. *Cardiovasc Intervent Radiol* 6:82-85, 1983.
36. Tsai FY, Matovich V, Hieshima G, Shah DC, Mehringer CM, Tu G, Higashida R, Pribram HFW. Percutaneous transluminal angioplasty of the carotid artery. *Am J Neurolog Radiol* 7:349-358, 1986.
37. DeBakey ME, Crawford ES, Cooley DA, Morris GC Jr, Garrett E, Fields WS. Cerebral arterial insufficiency. One to 11 years result following arterial reconstructive operation. *Am J Surg* 161:921-945, 1965.
38. West H, Burton R, Roon AJ, Malone JM, Goldsteon J, Moore WS. Comparative risk of operation and expectant management for carotid artery disease. *Stroke* 10:117-121, 1979.
39. Brown OW, Kerstein MD. The surgical management of transient ischemic attacks. *Angiology* 34:12-21, 1984.
40. Riles TS, Imparato AM, Mintzer R, Baumann EG. Comparison of results of bilateral and unilateral carotid endarterectomy five years after surgery. *Surgery* 91:258-262, 1982.
41. Loftus CM, Quest DO. Current status of carotid endarterectomy for atheromatous disease. *Neurosurgery* 12:718-723, 1983.

42. Kerber CS, Cromwell LD, Lehden OL. Catheter dilatation of proximal carotid stenosis during distal bifurcation endarterectomy. *Am J Neurolog Radiol* 1:348-349, 1980
43. Mathias K, Mitlermeyer C, Ensinger H, Neff W. Percutane katherdilatation von karotisstenosen. *Fortschr Roetgenstr* 133:348-361, 1980.
44. Mullan S, Duda EE, Patro NAS. Some examples of balloon technology in neurosurgery. *J Neurosurg* 52:321-329, 1980.
45. Belan A, Vesela M, Vanek I, Weiss K, Peregram JH. Percutaneous transluminal angioplasty of fibromuscular dysplasia of the internal carotid artery. *Cardiovasc Intervent Radiol* 5:79-81, 1982.
46. Tievsky AL, Dray EM, Mardiat JG. Transluminal angioplasty in postsurgical stenosis of the extracranial carotid artery. *Am J Neurolog Radiol* 1:348-349, 1980.
47. Hasso AN, Bird CR, Zinek DE, Thompson JR. Fibromuscular dysplasia of the internal carotid artery. Percutaneous transluminal angioplasty. *Am J Neurolog Radiol* 2:175-180, 1981.
48. Hodgins GW, Dutton JW. Sublcavian and carotid angioplasties for Takayasu's arteritis. *J Can Assoc Radiol* 33:305-307, 1982.
49. Wiggli U, Gratzl O. Transluminal angioplasty of stenotic carotid arteries: case report and protocol. *Am J Neurolog Radiol* 4:793-795, 1983.
50. Vitek JJ. Percutaneous transluminal angioplasty of the external carotid artery. *Am J Neurolog Radiol* 4:796-799, 1983.
51. Pritz MB, Smolin MF. Treatment of tandem lesions of the extracranial carotid artery. *Neurosurgery* 15:233-236, 1984.
52. Freitag G, Freitag J, Koch RD, Wagemann W. Percutaneous angioplasty of carotid artery stenoses. *Neuroradiology* 28:126-127, 1986.
53. Kachel R, Ritter H, Grossmann K, Glasee FH. Ergebnisse der perkutanen transluminalen dilatation (PTD) von hirngefabstenosen. *Fortschr Roentgenstr* 144:338-342, 1986.
54. Namaguchi Y, Puyau FA, Provenza LJ, Richardson DE. Percutaneous transluminal angioplasty of the carotid artery. *Neuroradiology* 26:527-530, 1984.
55. Tsai FY, Matovich VB, Hieshima GB, Higashida R, Shah DC, Ashraf A, Pribram HFW. Practical aspects of percutaneous transluminal angioplasty of the carotid artery. *Acta Radiol* 369:127-139, 1986.
56. Baker RN, Carroll-Ramseyer J, Schauartz WS. Prognosis in patients with transient ischemic attacks. *Neurology* 18:1157-1165, 1968.
57. Cartlidge NEF, Whisnant JJP, Elveback lR. Carotid and vertebral basilar transient cerebral ischemic attacks. *Mayo Clin Proc* 52:117-120, 1977.
58. De los Reyes RA, Ausman JI, Diaz FG, Pak H, Pearce JE, Dujouny M. The surgical management of vertebrobasilar insufficiency. *Acta Neurochir* 68:203-216, 1983.
59. Courtheoux P, Tournade A, Theron J, Henriet JP, Maiza D, Derlon JM, Pelouze G, Evrard C. Transcutaneous angioplasty of vertebral artery atheromatous ostial stricture. *Neuroradiology* 27:259-264, 1985.

60. Motarjeme A, Keifer JW, Zuska AJ. Percutaneous transluminal angioplasty of the vertebral arteries. *Radiology* 139:715-717, 1981.
61. Schultz H, Yeung HP, Chin MC, Terbrugge K, Ginsberg R. Dilatation of vertebral artery stenosis. *N Engl J Med* 304:733, 1981.
62. Higashida RT, Hieshima GB, Tsai FY, Bentson JR, Halbach VV. Percutaneous transluminal angioplasty of the subclavian and vertebral arteries. *Am J Neurolog Radiol* 369: 124-126, 1986.
63. Higashida RT, Hieshima GB, Tsai FY, Halbach VV, Bentson JR, Norman D, Newton TH. Transluminal angioplasty of the vertebral and basilar artery. *Am J Neurolog Radiol* 8:745-750, 1987.
64. Sundt TM Jr, Smith HC, Campbell JK, Vlietstra RE, Cucchiara RF, Stanson AW. Transluminal angioplasty for basilar artery stenosis. *Mayo Clin Proc* 55:673-680, 1980.

13

Intracerebral Hemorrhage

John H. Neal and Steven L. Giannotta
University of Southern California School of Medicine, Los Angeles, California

I. INCIDENCE AND ETIOLOGY

Spontaneous intracerebral hemorrhage (ICH) accounts for approximately 10% of strokes in the United States and Western Europe (1-3). Over 20,000 such cases are diagnosed each year, yielding a net incidence of 9/100,000 in the U.S. population (4). The Japanese were initially thought to have a significantly higher incidence of ICH than Americans. However, recent reports suggest that the incidence of spontaneous intracerebral hematoma in Japan is similar to that in the United States (5).

Hypertension is the most common factor associated with ICH but varies in incidence from 40% to 90%, depending on the series consulted (6-9). Rupture of an intracranial aneurysm is the next most frequent factor, accounting for approximately 20% of ICH. Vascular malformations and coagulopathies account for another 5%. Hemorrhage into a preexisting tumor may account for up to 10% of ICH; metastatic tumors—e.g., melanoma, choriocarcinoma, renal cell carcinoma, and bronchogenic carcinoma—are most responsible (6,9,10). Occasionally, significant hemorrhages are seen in glioblastoma and oligodendroglioma as well as papillomas of choroid plexus.

Unusual causes of ICH include dural sinus or cortical vein thrombosis, mycotic aneurysms, and arteritis. Amyloid angiopathy has become a more frequently recognized factor in hemorrhages occurring in patients over 65 years of age. Hemorrhage into a preexisting infarction or following revascularization procedures such as endarterectomy are unusual and are typically associated with hypertension (11). Hemorrhagic encephalitis and various toxic or metabolic etiologies such as amephetamine abuse contribute a small percent to the overall incidence.

II. TOPOGRAPHY

An important factor in determining the etiology and subsequent management of ICH is the anatomical location. The topography of hypertensive ICH has been well categorized (12-14). Approximately 60% of such lesions occur in the basal ganglia or thalamus; putamenal hemorrhage occurs two to three times more frequently than thalamic hemorrhage. Hemorrhage in the lobar white matter near the cortical junction accounts for 10-20% of ICH. The remaining 25% of hypertensive ICH occurs infratentorially, with pontine hemorrhage slightly more frequent than cerebellar hemorrhage.

Intraventricular hemorrhage often accompanies hypertensive ICH and explains blood in the cerebrospinal fluid with parenchymal hematoma. Huge hemorrhages or cortical-white matter hemorrhages may rupture into the subarachnoid space or, rarely, subdural space.

Intracerebral hemorrhage resulting from aneurysmal rupture is rarely found in the absence of subarachnoid hemorrhage (15). Aneurysms tend to cluster near the anterior communicating and middle cerebral complexes; ICH from aneurysmal rupture usually occurs in the frontal and temporal lobes (16). Intracerebral hemorrhage from vascular malformations can occur in any location but is often situated superficially in the white matter or cortex. Hemorrhages from tumors occur in the common distribution of metastatic lesions. Thus, the frontal and parietal areas as well as the cerebellum are likely sites. Amyloid angiopathy results in hemorrhage that is predominantly subcortical and, while having little predilection for a given lobe, most often results in supratentorial hemorrhage (17).

III. DIAGNOSIS

A. Clinical Presentation

Neurological signs and symptoms from ICH depend largely on the location and size of the hemorrhage. Putamenal and thalamic hemorrhages frequently present with progressive hemiparesis or hemiplegia, usually in association with sensory loss. Visual field defects may be prominent; aphasia may occur if the dominant hemisphere is involved. Eye deviation opposite the side of the paralysis in putamenal hemorrhage and paresis of vertical gaze in thalamic hemorrhage are not uncommon. In cortical and subcortical hemorrhage, headache may be a prominent complaint. Seizures are not uncommon and are often focal.

Pontine hemorrhage, usually devastating, typically presents with rapidly progressive reduction in level of consciousness (18). Total paralysis may occur, with cessation of respiration within a few hours of symptoms. Cerebellar hemorrhage frequently occurs in the region of the dentate nucleus. This is accompanied by severe headaches, usually in the occipital region but occasionally in the frontal area as well. Severe ataxia, vomiting, and dysarthria are frequent; nuchal rigidity appears late. Ipsilateral 6th nerve or 7th nerve paresis is not uncommon with cerebellar hematoma.

The history is critical in determining etiologies of spontaneous ICH, especially in the absence of hypertension. Hematological disorders and the use of anticoagulants must be evaluated. A history of a pre-existing seizure disorder suggests underlying lesions such as a vascular malformation or neoplasm.

B. Imaging

Computerized tomography (CT) is the investigation of choice for the diagnosis of intracerebral hemorrhage (19). This imaging modality demonstrates the exact location of the hemorrhage, along with edema or hydrocephalus. The age of the clot can be determined by variation in lesion density. Contrast infusion with CT is helpful in patients without hypertension or in patients where the hematoma is located in an uncharacteristic area for hypertensive hemorrhage. Tumor, arteriovenous malformation, or aneurysm may be identified without using other imaging techniques. This may have a major impact on the treatment plan and will frequently clarify the need for angiography. Angiography should be performed in all instances where an aneurysm or vascular malformation is likely. Patients lacking a clear cause for ICH should also be investigated with angiography. The timing of angiography will depend on the clinical course of the patient.

IV. INITIAL MANAGEMENT

The approach to the patient with suspected ICH should be no different than for any acute neurological dysfunction. Adequate airway and respiratory support should be established as needed. Endotracheal intubation is performed for patients presenting in coma, for those who are unable to protect their airway, and for those who display an inadequate ventilatory effort. Blood pressure should be determined and venous access established for administration of appropriate fluids and pharmacological agents. Wide swings in blood pressure, especially hypertension, are common in the initial period following ICH. Intravenous sodium nitroprusside with concomitant intraarterial pressure monitoring is an effective method of controlling such elevations. Continuous cardiac monitoring for arrhythmias is essential. Hypotension from cardiac or other etiologies can be devastating due to the impact on cerebral perfusion pressure. Thus, fluid replacement and vascular access remain essential. During the initial evaluation, blood samples for basic laboratory studies including CBC, chemistries, coagulation studies, toxicology screen, and arterial blood gases are obtained. Computerized tomography scanning follows stabilization and examination of the patient.

V. TREATMENT

Traditionally, treatment of intracerebral hemorrhage has been divided into medical and surgical approaches (20,21). For optimal care, these two forms of therapy should not be considered competitive. A combined approach utilizing both surgical and medical modalities will most often yield satisfactory results.

Patients with suspected or documented intracerebral hemorrhage should be managed in a neurological or neurosurgical intensive care unit equipped with the latest monitoring equipment and staffed by personnel knowledgeable in neurological assessment. Such monitoring capabilities should include cardiac rhythm, arterial pressures, cardiac output indexes, intracranial pressure monitoring, blood gas analysis, and EEG. Since management is in part predicated on the etiology of the hemorrhage, and since discussion of management of all the causes of intracerebral hematomas is beyond the scope of this chapter, the focus here will be on the treatment of hypertensive intracerebral hemorrhage.

Any management scheme designed to treat the patient with an intracerebral hematoma must control local cerebral tissue pressure and intracranial pressure (ICP) (22). Patients who remain awake and alert following their ictus have either normal intracranial pressure or adequately compensated elevation of intracranial pressure. Unless deterioration occurs, management consists of supportive care with reduction of risk factors for recurrent hemorrhage. It is in those patients who deteriorate following their arrival at the medical center, or who present in coma, that management modalities for reduction of intracranial pressure should be considered.

A. Supportive Care

Intracranial Pressure Monitoring

Rational treatment of elevated ICP requires an objective index of intracranial pressure level (23). This is particularly true of patients who present in coma or who have begun to deteriorate following an intracerebral hemorrhage. Ventricular catheterization is a relatively safe and accurate method of moment-to-moment measurement of intracranial pressure. The procedure is usually performed at the bedside in the neurosurgical intensive care unit; local anesthesia and intravenous sedation are used as necessary. A frontal approach is usually employed. After the skin is shaved and prepped, the scalp is infiltrated with lidocaine. A 5-mm incision is made anterior to the coronal suture in the midpupillary line. A 3/16-inch hand drill is used to perforate the cranium. The dura is punctured, and a silicone elastic ventricular catheter is passed into the frontal horn of the lateral ventricle. The catheter is connected to a fluid-coupled transducer, which yields the characteristic ICP waveform on the monitor. The catheter is then sutured into place, and a full head dressing is applied. Prophylactic antibiotics are not used. Sterile technique and proper care of the system (including replacement of the catheter every 3-5 days as long as monitoring is indicated) ensures a highly acceptable infection rate. Rarely, a significant hemorrhage follows ventriculostomy. With identification of pre-existing coagulopathies and proper technique, such complications should be minimal.

Armed with continuous information on the state of the intracranial pressure, the clinician is able to more intelligently manage patients with intracranial mass lesions. However, cerebral perfusion pressure (CPP) measurements may be at least as important in the management of patients with elevated ICP. The CPP is calculated as the mean arterial pressure minus the intracranial pressure. Perfusion pressures below 60 torr are associated with ischemic neurological damage (24). Perfusion pressures below 70 torr may induce intracranial pressure waves (spontaneous severe elevations in ICP), further reducing the cerebral perfusion pressure. Extreme elevations in CPP may produce or exacerbate cerebral edema (24). Systemic hypertension, above levels required to maintain an adequate CPP, should be avoided.

Positioning

It has been routine neurosurgical practice to raise the head of the bed for patients with elevated intracranial pressure (25,26). Several studies have suggested that gravity increases venous return, thereby reducing intracranial pressures. Rosner and Coley evaluated this issue in a systematic way. They discovered that following head elevation, cerebral perfusion pressure may fall, resulting in severe elevations of intracranial pressure (27). Head elevation in this study was frequently associated with reductions in mean arterial pressure, thereby reducing CPP. Reduction in arterial pressure following head elevation is more common in patients with reduced intravascular volume or compromised cardiac status. The goal, with respect to head positioning, is to maintain CPP above 75 torr. In the presence of inadequate CPP, the head is positioned to maximize cardiac filling and minimize elevation of ICP. In patients with compromised cardiac status and reduced circulating plasma volume, a flow-directed, balloon-tipped catheter is positioned to allow close monitoring of cardiac indices and wedge pressure. This will provide the most rapid re-establishment of circulating volume while avoiding cardiac overload.

3. *Hyperventilation and Oxygenation*

Respiratory support is critically important in patients with intracranial mass lesions. Intracranial pressure can often be reduced acutely by hyperventilation. Cerebral blood flow decreases 1-2 ml/min/100 g for each milimeter decrease in P_{CO_2} (28,29). ICP responds to hyperventilation in 2-30 minutes, with a mean of 8 minutes (30). There is variable effect and duration of action of hyperventilation in patients with elevated ICP. Return of ICP to previous levels frequently occurs within an hour. Maximal vasoconstriction appears to occur at a P_{CO_2} of 20 mmHg. Below this level cerebral hypoxia can occur as a result of intense vasoconstriction (26). The goal, then, is to maintain P_{CO_2} in the range of 25-30 mmHg.

B. Medical Therapy

1. *Osmotherapy*

Osmotic agents are routinely used for ICH patients who deteriorate or have uncontrollable elevations in intracranial pressure (ICP). Mannitol has been the agent of choice for a number of theoretical and practical reasons. Mannitol acts by establishing an osmotic gradient between the vascular space and brain, resulting in the exit of interstitial fluid (31). Additionally, mannitol may reduce CSF production and improve brain microcirculation by reducing blood viscosity (32).

It is best to administer mannitol in intravenous bolus doses. Each time ICP becomes elevated above normal (15-20 torr) and cannot be reduced by other measures, 0.25 g/kg mannitol is administered. Doses as high as 1-1.50 g/kg are given when maximal reductions in ICP are desired. Supplemental adminstration of furosemide can potentiate and prolong the effect of mannitol on intracranial pressure (33). Frequent monitoring of serum electrolytes and fluid balance is mandatory in patients undergoing osmotherapy for control of ICP.

3. *Steroids*

The use of adrenocortical steroids in patients with intracranial mass lesions has been widespread, although controversial. Certainly their effectiveness is more dramatic in treating edema surrounding cerebral neoplasms than it is with other conditions (34). When used in a 9-day, double-blind, placebo-controlled trial in supratentorial ICH, there was no demonstrable reduction in mortality; there was, however, a significant increase in complications (infections, gastrointestinal hemorrhage, and diabetes) for those patients treated with dexamethasone (35). Steroids thus appear to have little, if any, place in the management of ICH.

3. Barbiturates

In situations of uncontrollable intracranial pressure despite all other available therapies, barbiturates may reduce ICP. It is not clear whether barbiturate therapy produces an improvement of neurological outcome. On an anecdotal basis, certain patients do respond favorably to barbiturates. Their use should be considered in situations where other methods of controlling ICP have failed.

4. Seizure Control

Sezures are more common with ICH in the subcortical area than in the basal ganglia or thalamus. However, anticonvulsant prophylaxis is recommended in all patients with supratentorial intracerebral hemorrhage. Seizure activity may have a negative effect on intracranial pressure as well as on perfusion and oxygenation of compromised brain (36,37). Diphenylhydantoin (loading dose 15 mg/kg; maintenance 5 mg/kg/day) can be used for routine seizure prophylaxis. Valium (5-10 mg IV) or lorazepam (1-2 mg IV) is used to control active seizures or status epilepticus.

VI. SURGICAL THERAPY

Surgical therapy of ICH is directed toward removing clots, identifying and treating the source of the hemorrhage, and relieving hydrocephalus if present. Surgical techniques, when used selectively in a meticulous and comprehensive management program, can be an effective method of reducing intracranial pressure and improving morbidity. However, current surgical techniques and guidelines for their use all require improvement. Indications for surgical removal of intracerebral hemorrhages are either neurological deterioration or uncontrollable elevations in intracranial pressure in otherwise salvageable patients. Prognosis for survival and ultimate recovery is largely dependent on the level of consciousness at the time of presentation, the size and location of the clot, and the age and clinical condition of the patient. Surgical therapy to remove the clot can be expected to improve outcome only in patients who are not immediately devastated by the acute hemorrhage. It is therefore the secondary effects of ICH that may be ameliorated by surgery. These secondary effects result in progressive elevation of intracranial pressure by a combination of mass effect of the hematoma and resultant edema. Hydrocephalus may also result from obstruction of a ventricular outlet pathway causing a further increase in intracranial pressure.

The timing of surgical intervention remains critical (23,38,39). A patient with an acceptable level of consciousness who is allowed to deteriorate to the point of transtentorial herniation is unlikely to benefit by any form of surgical or medical therapy. This again emphasizes the need for careful monitoring of intracranial pressure and cerebral perfusion pressure along with neurological signs. On the basis of such careful monitoring three groups of patients can be defined (40-42). The first group are patients who are alert on presentation, have small hematomas, and/or have low intracranial pressure. Barring systemic complications, these patients tend to make the best recoveries and may not require any specific intervention other than supportive care and avoidance of systemic complications. The second group of patients have severe neurological deficits or are deeply comatose on admission; they usually have large hematomas and severely increased ICP. These patients tend to die from herniation secondary to increased ICP in spite of surgical and/or medical therapy. Attempts to accurately categorize these patients are critical so that sophisticated, time-consuming, and expensive therapies are not utilized needlessly. A third group consists of patients who initially are alert or stuporous and then deteriorate neurologically, often with elevations in ICP. It is in this group that vigorous attempts to control intracranial pressure by medical and surgical means are instituted.

To control ICP, an intraventricular pressure monitor is placed and supportive ventilatory and pharmacological methods are utilized. Evacuation of small amounts of ventricular fluid is used to control hydrocephalus and to supplement osmotic and ventilatory therapy for reducing intracranial pressure. If these methods fail to improve the patient's neurological status, or fail to control the cerebral perfusion pressure or intracranial pressure, surgical evacuation of the clot is considered. Patients with large white-matter clots and cerebellar hematomas are most likely to fall into this category. These patients may benefit from meticulous surgical removal prior to coma-producing elevations in intracranial pressure. Thus, treatment should be individualized, with emphasis placed on preventing complications of ICH; surgical evacuation of the hematoma is reserved for patients who deteriorate in spite of medical therapy. Development of a stereotactically and endoscopically controlled evacuaton of ICH may further reduce morbidity and mortality (43-45).

VII. SELECTED ASPECTS OF MANAGEMENT

Patients with spontaneous ICH are frequently bedridden for prolonged periods of time. These patients may experience numerous complications. One potential life-threatening complication is deep venous thrombosis (DVT) and subsequent pulmonary embolism. This is particularly vexing in the ICH patient, since anticoaglation may exacerbate the underlying neurological condition (46,47). Under those circumstances, external pneumatic calf compression can reduce the incidence of DVT (48). In patients with known pulmonary emboli, ligation or the placement of a caval umbrella is probably the optimal treatment to prevent further embolization when anticoagulation is hazardous. If anticoagulation with heparin is necessary, there should be a 7-day interval between the removal of the clot and the institution of heparin therapy (49). Meticulous control of blood pressure is mandatory in this circumstance.

Patients with malignant brain tumors may be at risk for intracerebral hemorrhage if treated with anticoagulant medications. In such cases, antiplatelet agents may help avoid thrombotic complications. Anticoagulation with heparin and warfarin is reserved for those who are at high risk for pulmonary embolization. Given adequate control of the blood pressure, the risk of anticoagulation appears acceptable given the long-term benefits in avoiding embolization (50).

VIII. CONCLUSION

There is still much controversy regarding optimal management of spontaneous ICH. Many pathophysiological and methodological issues need further study. Treatment should be individualized, with emphasis placed on preventing complications of ICH while using surgical evacuation of the hematoma in patients who deteriorate despite optimal nonsurgical therapy. In patients with severe neurological deficit and large supratentorial hematomas, outcome tends to be poor regardless of therapy. Future progress requires further studies of intracranial physiology and dynamics, early surgery, and alternative surgical modalities such as stereotactic evacuation.

REFERENCES

1. Hansen BS, Marquardsen J. Incidence of stroke in Frederiksberg, Denmark. *Stroke* 8:663-665, 1977.
2. Herman B, Schulte BDM, van Luijk JH, Leyten ACM, Frenken CWGM. Epidemiology of stroke in Tilburg, The Netherlands. *Stroke* 11:162-165, 1980.
3. Kunitz SC, Gross CR, Heyman A, Kase C, Mohr JP, Price TR, Wolf PA. The pilot stroke data bank: definition, design, and data. *Stroke* 15:740–746, 1984.
4. Robins M, Braun HM. Incidence. In: Weinfeld FD (Ed.), *The National Survey of Stroke*, Chap. 4; Stroke 12(Suppl 1):I-45-I-57, 1981.
5. Kanaya H. Epidemiology of hypertensive ICH in Japan. In: Pia HW, Langnard C, Zierski J. (Eds.), *Spontaneous Intracerebral Hematomas: Advances in Diagnosis and Therapy.* Springer-Verlag, Berlin, 1980, pp. 98-99.
6. McCormick WF, Rosenfeld DB. Massive brain hemorrhage: a review of 144 cases and examination of their causes. *Stroke* 4:946-954, 1973.
7. Mutlu N, Berry RG, Alpers B. Massive cerebral hemorrhage. *Arch Neurol* 8: 644-661, 1963.

8. Ransohoff J, Derby B, Kricheff I. Spontaneous intracerebral hemorrhage. *Clin Neurosurg* 18:247-266, 1971.
9. Scott M. Spontaneous intracerebral hematoma caused by cerebral neoplasms. *J Neurosurg* 42:338-342, 1975.
10. Mandybur TI. Intracranial hemorrhage caused by metastatic tumors. *Neurology* 27:650-655, 1977.
11. Solomon RA, Loftus C, Quest DO, Cornell JW. Incidence and etiology of intracerebral hemorrhage following carotid endarterectomy. *J Neurosurg* 64:29-34, 1986.
12. Fisher CM. Clinical syndrome in cerebral thrombosis, hypertensive hemorrhage, and ruptured saccular aneurysm. *Clin Neurosurg* 22:117-147, 1974.
13. Fisher CM. The pathology and pathogenesis of intracerebral hemorrhage. In: Field WS (Ed.), *Pathogenesis and Treatment of Cerebrovascular Disease*, C. C. Thomas, Springfield, Illinois, 1961, pp. 295-317.
14. Freytag E. Fatal hypertensive intracerebral hematomas: a survey of the pathologic anatomy of 393 cases. *J Neurol Neurosurg Psychiatry* 31:616-620, 1968.
15. Housepian E, Pool JL. A systematic analysis of intracranial aneurysms from the autopsy file of The Presbyterian Hospital. *J Neuropathol Exp Neurol* 17:409-423, 1958.
16. Crompton MR. Intracerebral hematoma complicating ruptured cerebral berry aneurysms. *J Neurol Neurosurg Psychiatry* 25:378-386, 1962.
17. Kase C, Mohr JP. General features of intracerebral hemorrhage. In: Barnett HJM, Mohr JP, Stein BM, Yatso FM (Eds.). *Stroke*. Churchill Livingstone, New York, 1986, pp. 497-523.
18. Ojemann RG, Heros RC. Spontaneous brain hemorrhage. *Stroke* 14:468-474, 1983.
19. Wiggins WS, Moody DM, Toole JF, Laster DW, Ball MR. Clinical and computerized tomographic study of hypertensive intracerebral hemorrhage. *Arch Neurol* 35:832-833, 1978.
20. McKissock W, Richardson A, Taylor J. Primary intracerebral hemorrhage: A controlled study of surgical and conservative treatment in 180 unselected cases. *Lancet* 2:221-226, 1961.
21. Waga S, Yamamoto Y. Hypertensive putamenal hemorrhage: treatment and results. Is surgical treatment superior to conservative one? *Stroke* 14:480-485, 1983.
22. Sinar EJ, Mendelow AD, Graham DI, Teasdale GM. Experimental intracerebral hemorrhage: effect of a temporary mass lesion. *J Neurosurg* 66:568-576, 1987.
23. Papo I, Janny P, Caruselli G, Colnet G, Luongo A. Intracranial pressure time course in primary intracerebral hemorrhage. *Neurosurgery* 4:504-511, 1979.
24. Durward QJ, Del Maestro RF, Amacher AL, Farrar JK. The influence of systemic arterial pressure and intracranial pressure on the development of cerebral vasogenic edema. *J Neurosurg* 59:803-809, 1983.
25. Kenning JA, Toutant SM, Saunders RL. Upright patient positioning in the management of intracranial hypertension. *Surg Neurol* 15:148-152, 1981.

26. Ropper AH, O'Rourke D, Kennedy SK. Head position, intracranial pressure and compliance. *Neurology* 32:1288-1291, 1982.
27. Rosner MJ, Coley IB. Cerebral perfusion pressure, intracranial pressure, and head elevation. *J Neurosurg* 65:636-641, 1986.
28. Reivich M. Arterial P_{CO_2} and cerebral hemodynamics. *Am J Physiol* 206: 25-35, 1964.
29. Reivich M. Regulation of the cerebral circulation. *Clin Neurosurg* 16:378-418, 1968.
30. James HE, Langfitt TW, Kumar VS, Ghostline SY. Treatment of intracranial hypertension: analysis of 105 consecutive recordings of intracranial pressure. *Acta Neurochir* 36:189-200, 1977.
31. Brown FD, Johns L, Jafur JL, Crockard HA, Mullan S. Detailed monitoring of the effect of mannitol following experimental head injury. *J Neurosurg* 50:423-432, 1979.
32. Burke AM, Quest DO, Chien S, Cerri C. The effects of mannitol on blood viscosity. *J Neurosurg* 55:550-553, 1981.
33. Pollay M, Fullenwider C, Roberts A, Stevens A. Effect of mannitol and furosemide on blood-brain osmotic gradient and intracranial pressure. *J Neurosurg* 59:945-950, 1983.
34. Tellez H, Bauer RB. Dexamethasone as treatment in cerebrovascular disease. A controlled study in intracerebral hemorrhage. *Stroke* 4:541-546, 1973.
35. Poungvarin N, Bhoopat W, Viriyavejakul A, et al. Effects of dexamethasone in primary supratentorial intracerebral hemorrhage. *N Engl J Med* 316: 1229-1233, 1987.
36. Knoblich OE, Gaab M, Weber W. ICP and EEG in various forms of cerebral seizures. In: Shulman K, Marmarou A, Miller JD, Becker DD, Hockwald GM, Brock M (Eds.), *Intracranial Pressure*. Springer-Verlag, Berlin, 1980, pp. 183-187.
37. Matsuda M, Nakasu S, Handa J. Intracranial pressure responses to electroencephalographic changes in epileptic seizures and barbiturate coma therapy. In: Nagai H, Ishii S, Brock M (Eds.), *Intracranial Pressure*. Springer-Verlag, Berlin, 1983, pp. 793-795.
38. Kaneko M, Koba T, Yokoyama T. Early surgical treatment for hypertensive intracerebral hemorrhage. *J Neurosurg* 46:579-583, 1977.
39. Kaneko M, Tanaka K, Shimada T, Sato K, Vemura K. Long-term evaluation of ultra-early operation for hypertensive intracerebral hemorrhage in 100 cases. *J Neurosurg* 58:838, 1983.
40. Duff TA, Ayeni S, Levin A, Manucher J. Nonsurgical management of spontaneous intracerebral hematoma. *Neurosurgery* 9:387-393, 1981.
41. Suzuki A, Yasui N, Ito Z, Vemura K. Sequential changes of the epidural, the ventricular, and the surrounding tissue pressure in hypertensive intracerebral hemorrhage. In: Ishii S, Nagai H, Brock M (Eds.), *Intracranial Pressure*. Springer-Verlag, Berlin, 1982, pp. 721-725.
42. Tazawa T. Mizukami M, Kawase T, Usami T, Togashi O, Hyodo A, Eguchi T. Size of hematoma and time course of intracranial pressure in patients

with hypertensive intracerebral hemorrhage. In: Ishii S, Nagai H, Brock M (Eds.), *Intracranial Pressure*. Springer-Verlag, Berlin, 1983, pp. 716-720.

43. Auer LM. Endoscopic evacuation of intracerebral haemorrhage. *Acta Neurochir* 74:124-128, 1985.
44. Backlund EO, von Holst H. Controlled subtotal evacuation of intracerebral hematomas by stereotactic technique. *Surg Neurol* 9:99-101, 1978.
45. Higgins AC, Nashold BS. Stereotactic evacuation of large intracerebral hematoma. *Appl Neurophysiol* 43:3-5, 1980.
46. Powers SK, Edwards MSB. Prophylaxis of thromboembolism in the neurosurgical patient: a review. *Neurosurgery* 10(4):509-513, 1982.
47. Swann KW, Black PMcL. Deep vein thrombosis and pulmonary emboli in neurosurgical patients: a review. *J Neurosurg* 61:1055-1062, 1984.
48. Black PMcL, Baker MF, Snook CP. Experience with external pneumatic calf compression in neurology and neurosurgery. *Neurosurgery* 18(1):440, 1986.
49. Schaible KL, Smith LJ, Fessler G, Rachlin JR, Brown FD, Mullan S. Evaluation of the risks of anticoagulation therapy following experimental craniotomy in the rat. *J Neurosurg* 63:959-962, 1985.
50. Choucair AK, Silver P, Levin VA. Risk of intracranial hemorrhage in glioma patients receiving anticoagulant therapy for venous thromboembolism. *J Neurosurg* 66:357-358, 1987.

14

Medical Treatment of Aneurysmal Subarachnoid Hemorrhage

Harold P. Adams, Jr.
University of Iowa, Iowa City, Iowa

I. INTRODUCTION

Subarachnoid hemorrhage (SAH) accounts for approximately 8% of all acute cerebrovascular events. Ruptured saccular aneurysms are its most common cause. In the 1960s, the Cooperative Aneurysm Study found ruptured aneurysms in 3321 of the 6368 patients with SAH (1). With advances in neuroradiological diagnostic studies, aneurysms will be found in more than 80% of patients with SAH. This discussion will be limited to the treatment of patients with ruptured aneurysms.

Approximately 5% of American adults have intracranial saccular aneurysms (2). A minority of these lesions rupture. The incidence of SAH is 11/100,000 (3); more than 26,000 Americans annually have SAH. Unlike other forms of stroke, the frequency of SAH has not declined over the last 30 years (3). Subarachnoid hemorrhage is a disease of all ages; the average age is approximately 55 years. Approximately 20% of patients are older than 65. The incidence of SAH is greater in women than in men. Most patients are previously healthy, active adults. Traditional risk factors for vascular disease, such a diabetes mellitus or hypertension, are not applicable for SAH. Oral contraceptives (4), smoking (5), or acute alcohol intoxication (6) may promote aneurysmal rupture. Some families have more than one member with SAH.

Delays in diagnosis of SAH are common. In approximately 25% of cases, physicians do not initially recognize the nature or seriousness of the patient's complaints (7). Delayed diagnosis is more common among the least seriously ill patients; these patients are most likely to respond to acute treatment. Rerupture may occur during the period of delay. Prompt recognition of SAH is therefore necessary to improve outcome. Computerized tomography (CT) or cerebrospinal fluid (CSF) examinations will establish the diagnosis of SAH in most suspected cases. Besides confirming SAH, CT demonstrates acute complications such as hydrocephalus, intraventricular hemorrhage, or intracerebral hemorrhage (8). Arteriography is required to demonstrate the aneurysm, particularly if it is smaller than 1 cm in diameter.

Despite increased interest in SAH and better management of this condition, it remains a highly fatal disease. Fogelholm (9) reviewed the natural history of SAH in Finland. Within 24 hours of SAH, 25% of patients are dead. Another 10% die within 2 weeks. The overall mortality by 3 months after SAH is 40%. Whisnant et al. (10) reported the likelihood of survival based on a population study in Rochester, Minnesota. The probability of survival is influenced by the patient's clinical condition and the interval from SAH. If a patient is seen within 24 hours of SAH, the probability of 60-day survival is 55%. If the patient lives 2 weeks, the likelihood of survival increases to 88%. The 60-day survival rate is 70% among alert patients and drops to 15% among patients in poor condition. Many survivors are disabled by the SAH and its complications (Table 1). In 1981, the Cooperative Aneurysm Study reported results of therapy among patients seen within 3 day of SAH (11). Among 174 patients initially in good condition, 15.5% were disabled 3 months later. At 3 months after SAH, 24.6% of poor-condition patients were disabled. Weir and Aronyk (12) reported similar findings.

The leading causes of death and disability are (1) the neurological or medical effects of the initial SAH, (2) cerebral arterial vasospasm and ischemia, and (3) rebleeding. Medical complications include atelectasis, pneumonia, respiratory failure, gastrointestinal bleeding, cardiac arrhythmias, pulmonary edema, hyponatremia, hypokalemia, hypovolemia, and inappropriate secretion of antidiuretic hormone. Neurological consequences include convulsions, acute or chronic hydrocephalus, cerebral edema, increased intracranial pressure, and

Table 1 Complications of Aneurysmal Subarachnoid Hemorrhage

Neurological	Medical
Intraventricular hematoma	Atelectasis or hypoventilation
Intracerebral hematoma	Aspiration pneumonia
Subdural hematoma	Pulmonary edema
Cerebral edema	Cardiac arrhythmias
Acute or chronic hydrocephalus	Myocardial infarction
Convulsions	Deep vein thromobosis or pulmonary embolism
Rebleeding	Dehydration
Vasospasm, cerebral ischemia	Hyponatremia
	Hypertension/hypotension
	Gastrointestinal bleeding

major brain injuries. Some of these effects are sufficiently devastating that many patients die or become disabled despite any treatment. In particular, many of the deaths occurring during the first 24 hours cannot be avoided.

Vasospasm, with secondary cerebral infarction, is now considered to be the leading cause of death or long-term disability after SAH. Cerebral arterial vasospasm can be detected by arteriography in more than 70% of patients; approximately 30% of all patients develop symptoms of cerebral ischemia after SAH (13,14). Symptomatic vasospasm peaks at approximately 7-10 days after SAH, although arterial narrowing can persist for several weeks or longer. Vasospasm is most likely to occur in seriously ill patients; in patients with prominent meningeal signs (14); in patients with focal, thick collection of subarachnoid blood on CT (15); or in patients with early cortical enhancement on CT (16).

Recurrent hemorrhage is the other leading cause of death and disability. Rebleeding occurs within 2 weeks of SAH in 20% of cases (10). Recurrent bleeding peaks on the day of SAH, when it reaches 3% (17). Daily rebleeding rates for the next 10 days are approximately 2% (10). For the remainder of the first month, rebleeding happens at a rate of 0.5%/day (10). After 30 days following SAH, rebleeding occurs at a rate of 3%/year. Rebleeding adversely impacts on outcome of acute SAH. The prognosis of an initially alert patient who has rebleeding drops to that of an initially comatose patient (18). Approximately two-thirds of the patients who have acute rebleeding die.

Therapy of SAH is aimed at treatment of the acute effects of the initial bleed, prevention of rebleeding, and prevention of vasospasm and its ischemic consequences. A team of physicians, including neurologists and neurosurgeons assisted by consultants such as neuroradiologists, intensive care specialists, and neuroanesthesiologists, are required for the successful treatment of these critically ill patients.

II. INITIAL CARE

Subarachnoid hemorrhage is a medical emergency. Patients require immediate evaluation and treatment. Patients with suspected SAH who are at remote, small community hospitals should be evacuated by air or land ambulance to a major medical center as soon as possible. Primary care physicians generally refer these patients unless the immediate outlook is hopeless. Treatment begins as soon as emergency personnel reach the patient or when the patient enters the emergency room (Table 2). Upon arrival at the hospital, approximately 60% of the patients are alert, 20% are drowsy, 10% are stuporous, and 10% are comatose. A few patients are delirious or agitated.

Airway obstruction, aspiration, and respiratory failure need to be anticipated and managed promptly. Intubation of comatose patients is performed even if there is no sign of airway obstruction. Besides securing the airway, hyperventilation of patients with increased intracranial pressure is facilitated if an endotracheal tube is in place. Supplemental oxygen is given. Vital signs and neurological parameters are measured frequently, at least every 15 minutes. In particular, changes in consciousness are looked for. Early medical complications are cardiac arrhythmias, pulmonary edema, severe vomiting, and gastrointestinal bleeding. Acute neurological complications are convulsions, cerebral edema, acute hydro-

Table 2 Emergency Treatment of a Patient with Aneurysmal Subarachnoid Hemorrhage

Constant medical and nursing attention
Cardiac monitoring and airway support
Frequent measurements of vital signs and neurological parameters
Diagnostic studies
Intravenous access with normal saline
Pain: meperidine or codeine
Agitation: diazepam or phenobarbital
Nausea and/or vomiting: trimethobenzamide
Convulsions: phenytoin or phenobarbitol
Cerebral edema: furosemide, dexamethasone, mannitol, hyperventilation
Surgical evacuation of hematoma
Hypertension: sodium nitroprusside
Cardiac arrhythmias: ? propranolol

cephalus, and increased intracranial pressure. Rebleeding peaks during the first 24 hours; it can occur in the emergency room (17). Rebleeding should be suspected if the patient suddenly complains of increasingly severe headache followed by altered consciousness. Patients may have a "seizure"; rather than a convulsion, this seizure often is transient extensor posturing, which results from massive increases in intracranial pressure. Systemic hypertension frequently accompanies the episode of recurring hemorrhage. Agitation, restlessness, and pain tend to induce recurrent bleeding.

Emergency laboratory work includes arterial blood gases, complete blood count, platelet count, prothrombin time, partial thromboplastin time, blood glucose, serum electrolytes, and blood urea nitrogen. Blood for typing and cross match for transfusion is obtained in case an emergency operation is necessary. A complete electrocardiogram and chest roentgenogram are also obtained.

A careful general medical examination is warranted. The neurological examination should be performed carefully because some signs can be very subtle. Meningeal signs are usually present but may not be marked for several hours. Changes in state of alertness, grogginess, lethargy, or drowsiness are present in approximately one-third of patients. A minority have focal neurological deficits (19). Monoparesis or hemiparesis are most frequently found. A unilateral oculomotor nerve palsy suggests an aneurysm arising at the origin of the posterior communicating artery from the internal carotid artery. Retinal hemorrhages are found in 20% of patients after SAH. Retinal hemorrhages are highly suggestive of SAH as a cause of nontraumatic coma (20).

In most cases, SAH can be confirmed by CT. The CT is abnormal in more than 95% of patients studied on the day of SAH (11). If CT is delayed by several days, its yield drops quickly. Besides demonstrating subarachnoid blood, CT also visualizes intracerebral or intraventricular blood. Hydrocephalus or mass effect can also be seen. Computerized tomography is also useful in predicting survival. Diffuse or thick, localized collections of subarachnoid blood, intraventricular blood, or intracerebral blood found on early CT are poor prognostic signs (21).

Almost every patient with disturbed consciousness has an abnormal CT. The CT scan is most likely to be normal among alert patients (11). If CT reveals intracranial blood, CSF examination is usually not necessary. If the CT is not diagnostic, lumbar puncture is required to make the diagnosis of SAH. Lumbar puncture is generally safe in an alert patient who has a normal CT. Physicians sometimes err by avoiding lumbar puncture in this situation. Once SAH is established, arteriography is needed to demonstrate the aneurysm. The results of CT (a localized collection of blood) provide a clue for the site of the aneurysm, and in 5-20% of patients the aneurysm will be visualized. This situation is especially true in cases with giant aneurysms.

Medical care in the emergency room and during radiological investigations is tailored to each patient. An intravenous access line is placed, using normal saline; the line is primarily for administration of emergency drugs. Because some patients have excessive release of antidiuretic hormone after SAH, hyponatremia can result. The usual management of hyponatremia is strict fluid restriction, but this has not provided a favorable outcome after SAH. Nibbelink et al. (22) noted no reduction in mortality or rebleeding with a daily restriction of 1500 ml/day. Water and sodium losses are major after SAH (23,24), making strict fluid restriction dangerous (25). Hypoosmolar fluids such as 5% dextrose in water should be avoided. Daily intake of fluids should be approximately 2000-2500 ml.

Alert patients complain of severe headache; they should receive parenteral analgesics, such as codeine or meperidine. Agitated patients are given diazepam or phenobarbital. Patients who are nauseated or are vomiting can receive trimethobenzamide. Phenothiazines are avoided because they can lower the seizure threshold, reduce blood pressure, or induce dystonic reactions. Convulsions occur in 26% of patients after SAH (26). The prophylactic use of anticonvulsants is debatable (26), but the use of phenytoin or phenobarbital is reasonable. Phenobarbital is used for both its sedative and anticonvulsant effects. Most patients are hypertensive immediately after SAH, which may promote rebleeding. The blood pressure often will normalize when pain, nausea, and agitation are relieved or when intracranial hypertension is reduced. If the blood pressure remains markedly elevated despite treatment, antihypertensive agents should be given. Sodium nitroprusside in a continuous infusion is effective and the dosage is titrated to the patient's response. Diazoxide is avoided because of the possibility of an "overshoot" and because of its long duration of action.

Emergency treatment of intracranial hypertension is required in critically ill, comatose patients. The risks of uncal herniation and of cerebral ischemia are high. Hyperventilation is supplemented by 40 mg of dexamethasone and 50 mg of furosemide. Dexamethasone is given in a dosage of 10 mg every 6 hours. Intravenous mannitol is given in a dose of 0.25 g/kg over 20 minutes (27). Mannitol will reach effective blood levels within 20 minutes; intracranial pressure should remain controlled for 4-6 hours. Mannitol can be repeated in 4-6 hours (28). The total daily dose of this drug should not exceed 2 g/kg. Management of fluids becomes critical if several doses of mannitol are given. Hypernatremia, hyperosmolarity, and dehydration are complications of repeated doses of this drug.

Surgical intervention to evacuate a hematoma is potentially a life-saving measure. However, the results of surgery are disappointing mainly because an intracranial hematoma adds to the gravity of the patient's condition. Ljunggren et al. (29) reported a postoperative mortality of 42% and a good outcome in 16%.

Table 3 Medical Treatment of a Patient with a Recent Aneurysmal Subarachnoid Hemorrhage

Absolute bed rest	Antiembolic hose
Quiet environment, restricted visitors	Frequent turns, gentle range-of-motion exercises
Cardiac monitoring for at least 24 hr	Antacids
Vital signs and neurological checks every hour for 24 hours, then reduced in frequency	Analgesics
	Sedatives
	Antiemetics
Intake and output measured every 6 hours	Anticonvulsants
	Antihypertensives
Intravenous access using normal saline	Aminocaproic acid
High-fiber soft diet supplemented by stool softeners	
Intake to be at least 2000 ml/day	

III. MEDICAL TREATMENT

Not all patients with SAH will be ideal candidates for early operation; therefore early medical treatment will remain very important (Table 3). The primary goals of early medical care are prevention of recurrent hemorrhage and prevention of cerebral vasospasm and its ischemic consequences. Early medical therapy is deemed successful if a patient is in good condition at the time of surgery approximately 10-14 days after SAH.

The foundation of supportive medical therapy is absolute bed rest for the first 2 weeks after SAH in an attempt to prevent rebleeding. A quiet environment, conducive to rest and free of distractions, is sought. Patients are in single-bed rooms, lights are dimmed, and visitors are restricted. Patients are not allowed to watch television or receive telephone calls. To avoid atelectasis, patients are encouraged to take frequent deep breaths. More seriously ill patients require suctioning and gentle pulmonary toilet. Vigorous physical and respiratory therapy are avoided. Patients are turned frequently and the extremities are actively or passively moved. Antiembolic stockings reduce the risk of deep vein thrombosis. External pneumatic calf compression further reduces the risks of deep vein thrombosis, postphlebotic syndrome, and pulmonary embolism (30). Daily care such as shaving or brushing teeth is performed by the nursing staff. Nurses or relatives feed the patient.

Alert patients are given a soft, high-fiber diet, supplemented by stool-softening drugs. They do not receive tobacco, alcohol, or caffeine-containing beverages. All patients receive a slow intravenous infusion with normal saline. Daily intake of fluids should be 2-2.5 liters. Intake is increased if output is more than

1.5 liters or if insensible loss is major. Total blood volume and red blood cell mass are reduced following SAH (23), and plasma volume and sodium stores are low (25). Hyponatremia occurs secondary to inappropriate secretion of antidiuretic hormone and as the result of sodium loss. Fluid restriction to correct hyponatremia is potentially dangerous because it leads to further decline in blood volume, increased viscosity, and hemoconcentration (25). Fluid restriction may be particularly dangerous at the time of vasospasm. A depleted intravascular volume may be an important difference between asymptomatic and symptomatic vasospasm (24).

Sedation is achieved with phenobarbital in a daily dosage of 120-180 mg or diazepam in a daily dosage of 20-40 mg. Analgesia is achieved with acetomenophen, codeine, or meperidine. Morphine is not prescribed because of its respiratory depressant action. Aspirin is avoided because of its antiplatelet effects. Antacids and occasionally cimetidine are administered. Using this regimen, the Cooperative Aneurysm Study found that the mortality of SAH was 54.6% in good condition patients (31). Rebleeding occurred in 50.0%. Poor condition patients had a mortality of 81.6%. These results are very disappointing.

One of the acute medical complications is cardiac arrhythmias. Patients dying of SAH have focal areas of subendocardial and myocardial necrosis (32). Elevations of creatine kinase and changes in the electrocardiogram can be found (33). The MB component of creatine kinase is elevated, reflecting cardiac ischemia (33). Electrocardiographic changes include inversion of T waves, prolongation of the Q-T interval, pathological Q waves, and depression or elevation of the S-T segment (34,35). The pathological Q waves and changes in the S-T segment predict poor outcome. The cardiac effects result from direct toxicity or systemic hypertensive responses induced by elevated catecholamines. Release of norepinephrine is stimulated by the posterior hypothalamus and requires an intact hypothalamo-spino-adrenal axis (34). Propranolol and phentolamine may prevent the cardiac complications of SAH and reduce mortality (36,37). Further investigation of these therapies is warranted.

Elevated blood pressure is a common physical finding after SAH. The mortality is higher among patients with systemic hypertension (38). Elevated blood pressure is a nonspecific phenomenon. It may result from (1) elevated blood catecholamines; (2) consequences of pain, anxiety, or agitation (see Ref. 3); and or (3) intracranial hypertension. Drug-induced hypotension may lessen transmural pressure and reduce the risk of early rebleeding. However, hypotension may provoke cerebral ischemia in a patient who has cerebral arterial vasospasm. Antihypertensive drugs have been used in patients with SAH for more than 30 years; their use remains the subject of controversy. Slosberg (39) reported favorable results, but the Cooperative Aneurysm Study did not find significant reduction in mortality or rebleeding when drug-induced hypotension was compared to bed rest (38). With drug-induced hypotension, rebleeding occurred within 2 weeks in 17.4% of patients and 26.3% by one month. In another randomized study, antihypertensive therapy was compared to antifibrinolytic drugs (40). Mortality and rebleeding were much higher among patients receiving antihypertensive drugs. The protective effects of antifibrinolytic drugs was negated by the addition of drug-induced hypotension. These findings were confirmed by the Cooperative Aneurysm Study (17). Drug-induced hypotension did not prevent rebleeding and predisposed to development of cerebral ischemia. Mortality among patients treated with drug-induced hypotension was more than 20%.

Antihypertensive drugs may still play a role in treatment. Previous trials used methyldopa, reserpine, thiazide diuretics, or apresoline to achieve blood pressure control (38). In patients with marked hypertension, a rapidly acting drug such as sodium nitroprusside can be intravenously administered. An advantage of this drug is its short duration of action. Control of agitation, pain, or intracranial pressure may lead to a lowering of blood pressure in an acutely ill patient. Antihypertensive drugs might not be required under these circumstances. If antihypertensive drugs are administered, some precautions are in order. Lowering blood pressure in a patient with intracranial hypertension may promote cerebral ischemia. Cerebral ischemia may result from reduction in blood pressure in a patient who has vasospasm. Antihypertensives should be discontinued if focal neurological signs consistent with cerebral ischemia develop. Care to avoid dehydration, hemoconcentration, or hypotension is in order to reduce the possible ischemic consequences of vasospasm. Chapter 8 discusses this topic in more detail.

IV. ANTIFIBRINOLYTIC DRUGS

Recurrent hemorrhage is a major cause of death and disability; medical measures to prevent such a complication during the first 2 weeks after SAH are critical. Prolonged bed rest and drug-induced hypotension have not been effective. Antifibrinolytic drugs may be useful in preventing rebleeding Despite almost 20 years of experience, antifibrinolytic therapy after SAH remains controversial (41). Much of the controversy has been generated by methodological problems of previous studies (42).

Upon aneurysmal rupture, a clot forms around the aneurysm. Antifibrinolytic drugs may help stabilize the perianeurysmal clot and prevent early rebleeding (43). The rent in the aneurysmal wall is occluded by the clot. The clot may help stabilize the aneurysm and inhibit rebleeding. At the time of SAH, fibrinolytic forces are activated. Plasminogen activators increase in arterial and meningeal tissues (44). Fibrin degradation products and available plasminogen activity are elevated (45-50). Antifibrinolytic drugs may help stabilize the perianeurysmal clot and prevent early rebleeding (43).

Aminocaproic acid and tranexamic acid are the two most commonly used drugs. Both drugs have free amino and carboxylic groups, which are required for their antifibrinolytic activity (51). On the basis of per-milligram activity, tranexamic acid has six times the antifibrinolytic activity of aminocaproic acid. Both drugs are competitive inhibitors of plasminogen activators (52). They are also noncompetitive inhibitors of plasmin. The fibrin clot is stabilized, and serum and CSF plasminogen activity drops with administration of the drugs (49,50). Fibrin split products fall in the CSF (47); plasma fibrinogen, prothrombin time, partial thromboplastin time, platelet count, and other coagulation factors are not altered. Qualitative inhibition of platelet function and prolongation of the template bleeding time occur with large doses of aminocaproic acid (53). Aminocaproic acid inhibits ADP or collagen-induced platelet aggregation in a dose-dependent manner.

These drugs are rapidly absorbed by the gastrointestinal tract; maximal concentrations occur within 2 hours of a single oral dose. For a sustained effect, oral doses of aminocaproic acid must be given every 2 hours (54). When given in an intravenous bolus, the antifibrinolytic effects of the drugs are almost instantaneous. Effective blood levels of aminocaproic acid are 130 μg/ml. If the drugs are given as a continuous intravenous infusion without a loading dose, a serum steady state is achieved in 24-36 hours. Aminocaproic acid is not protein-bound; it is free in the plasma (55). Both drugs are rapidly excreted by the kidney; a single intravenous dose is cleared entirely within 12 hours (51). A single intravenous dose does not have any long-lasting effect. Clearance is slower with an intravenous infusion than it is when the drug is given orally or in a single intravenous dose (43). Therefore, a loading intravenous bolus followed by a continuous infusion is the best method for treating a patient with recent SAH.

Antifibrinolytic drugs cross the blood-brain barrier, and levels are detected in CSF within 30 minutes of intravenous administration (56). With a continuous infusion, presumed therapeutic effects in the CSF are achieved in 24-36 hours (47). Intrathecal administration has been attempted. By this route, CSF concentrations fall below detectable levels after 24-36 hours (57). Intrathecal administration of antifibrinolytic drugs is not recommended.

In 1981, Ramirez-Lassepas (41) reviewed the clinical studies of antifibrinolytic therapy for SAH that had been published up to that time. These studies will not be reviewed here. Since 1981, several reports have appeared. The Cooperative Aneurysm Study reported the results of antifibrinolytic therapy in 1114 patients (58). The 2-week mortality was 10.7%, and the rebleeding rate was 10%. Another series compared 100 patients treated with antifibrinolytic drugs with 100 controls (59). Rebleeding was lowered by antifibrinolytic drugs, but mortality was not influenced. Chowdhary and Sayed (60) compared the results of treatment with aminocaproic acid to results with tanexamic acid. Outcome was similar with both drugs. Fodstad et al. (61) reported the outcome of 30 patients receiving tranexamic acid in comparison with 29 controls; mortality and rebleeding occurred at similar rates. Rebleeding was delayed among the patients receiving tranexamic acid. A favorable response to treatment with tranexamic acid and kallikrein was noted in another report (62). Flamm (63) reported six instances of rebleeding among 92 patients treated with aminocaproic acid. In 1982, Fodstad (64) reported the results of treatment of 53 patients with tranexamic acid in comparison to 52 control patients. With treatment, mortality was 25% and the rebleeding rate was 13%. Among control patients, mortality was 19% and rebleeding occurred in 31%.

In 1984, the Cooperative Aneurysm Study reported the outcome in 467 patients treated with antifibrinolytic drugs and 205 patients not given these drugs (17). All patients were treated within 3 days of SAH. This was not a randomized study, but prognostic factors and adjunctive medical management were comparable in both groups. Rebleeding was significantly reduced by antifibrinolytic therapy. Rebleeding was 11.7% among patients given the drugs and 19.4% among the controls. Rates of recurrent hemorrhage were similar in the two treatment groups during the first 36 hours after SAH. Thereafter, rebleeding was much lower among patients receiving antifibrinolytic drugs. The 36-hour lag in the therapeutic effect of antifibrinolytic drugs may reflect the delay in reaching therapeutic blood and CSF levels. Despite the reduction in recurrent hemorrhage, mortality was not reduced by antifibrinolytic drugs. Rebleeding was the leading cause of death among patients who did not receive antifibrinolytic drugs. Focal ischmemic deficits were the primary cause of mortality among patients given antifibrinolytic treatment.

Vermeulen et al. (64) performed a randomized double-blind study of tranexamic acid in 479 patients treated within 72 hours of SAH. 285 patients had aneurysms found by arteriography. Tranexamic acid was given in a daily dose of 6 g for the first week; then a dose of 4 g/day was administered. Tranexamic acid significantly reduced the rate of rebleeding. The impact of antifibrinolytic drugs was not noted until 2-3 days after onset of treatment. Mortality and disability after SAH were not eased by the use of antifibrinolytic drugs. The causes of death among patients receiving tranexamic acid were rebleeding 23% and infarction 45%. Of mortality among patients given placebo, 51% was due to rebleeding and 27% to infarction. Vermeulen and colleagues concluded that antifibrinolytic therapy was not justified in the management of patients with recent SAH because mortality was not lowered.

A major concern is the potential for complications of antifibrinolytic drugs. Large doses of drugs that may promote coagulation may predispose to deep vein thrombosis, pulmonary embolism, or myocardial infarction (66,67). However, these complications are unusual. The Cooperative Aneurysm Study reported that pulmonary embolism occurred in 0.7% of 1114 patients (58). Rates of deep vein thrombosis or pulmonary embolism were no higher among treated patients than among controls (17,65). Disorders of platelet function and prolongation of the bleeding time accompany large doses of aminocaproic acid (53). However, bleeding disorders are not significantly increased by the administration of antifibrinolytic drugs (17). Other medical complications are infrequent. Diarrhea is a common side effect of the oral administration of tranexamic acid (58). These drugs are not hepatotoxic or nephrotoxic.

Prolonged administration of aminocaproic acid can induce an acute myopathy (68-72). Patients present with a sudden onset of muscle pain, tenderness, and weakness. Myoglobinuria is found; acute tubular necrosis can result. Serum levels of muscle enzymes are elevated. A myopathic pattern is found on electromyography. The etiology of aminocaproic acid myopathy is not known. It may be the result of direct toxicity, an autoimmune reaction, or microthrombotic events. This complication only follows the long-term administration (greater than 3 weeks) of aminocaproic acid in a total dose exceeding 500 g and can be avoided by limiting the duration of antifibrinolytic therapy.

Seizures (73,74) or an encephalopathy (75) can develop in patients receiving antifibrinolytic drugs. These are rare events and are not indications for avoiding antifibrinolytic therapy. Other causes should be sought for seizures or altered mental status before attributing these symptoms to antifibrinolytic therapy in a patient with SAH.

Hydrocephalus is a complication of SAH. Any factor that prolongs the presence of blood clots in the subarachnoid space and around the arachnoid villi will predispose to the development of hydrocephalus. Using echoencephalography, Knibestol et al. (76) noted severe and protracted ventricular dilatation in patients given antifibrinolytic drugs. Park (77) reported symptomatic hydrocephalus in 31% of 48 patients treated with aminocaproic acid and in 10% of control patients. The recent report of the Cooperative Aneurysm Study confirms that hydrocephalus is a complication of antifibrinolytic therapy (17). Hydrocephalus was found in 13.5% of patients given antifibrinolytic drugs, and it developed in 6.8% of patients not receiving these drugs. Antifibrinolytic drugs approximately double the risk of hydrocephalus after SAH. Hydrocephalus is a cause of neurological deterioration after SAH; it should be considered in any patient who develops a decline in neurological status. Hydrocephalus is a treatable condition and is usually not as devastating as recurrent bleeding. The increased risk of hydrocephalus is apparently not sufficiently great to prohibit the use of antifibrinolytic drugs.

Cerebral infarction secondary to cerebral arterial vasospasm is a leading cause of disability or death after SAH. In 1973, Kagstrom and Palma (78) predicted that antifibrinolytic drugs would increase the frequency of ischemic complications after SAH. Anything that prolongs the subarachnoid clot could predispose to the development of vasospasm. Instances of spontaneous thrombosis of aneurysms or cerebral arteries have been reported (79,80). In 1974,

Sonntag and Stein (81) reported three patients who developed an "arteriopathy" while taking aminocaproic acid. These patients had arterial narrowing demonstrated by arteriography. They probably had vasospasm rather than an arteritis. No other instances of "vasculitis" secondary to antifibrinolytic drugs have been reported. In the last few years, several reports have reported that cerebral ischemia is a possible complication of antifibrinolytic therapy (58,59, 61,64). Approximately 20% of 1114 patients treated by the Cooperative Aneurysm Study developed ischemia during the first 14 days after SAH (58). Mortality and morbidity due to cerebral ischemia are the primary reasons that antifibrinolytic drugs have not been more effective in improving outcome after SAH. The two large studies confirm this opinion.

The Cooperative Aneurysm Study found that focal ischemic deficits had occurred within 14 days of SAH in 32.4% of patients taking these agents (17). Ischemic complications appeared at the same rate in both groups of patients until the fifth day after SAH. Thereafter the frequency escalated rapidly in the treated patients. The Dutch-British randomized trial provided similar results (65). Cerebral infarction was the leading cause of death in patients treated with tranexamic acid; the rate was significantly increased. Ischemic complication developed at the same rate in both treated and control groups during the first 4 days. Then the rate rose steeply among patients treated with tranexamic acid.

The etiology of the ischemic complications of antifibrinolytic drugs is not known. Maintaining subarachnoid clots may increase the extent and severity of vasospasm (17). The drugs may promote intravascular sludging, microthrombosis, or fibrin-platelet embolism. A combination of factors is likely. If antifibrinolytic drugs are prescribed, the physician should remain alert to the possibility of cerebral ischemic complications. The drugs should be discontinued if focal ischemic symptoms appear. The risk of cerebral ischemia may be lessened if dehydration and hypotension are avoided. Drugs such as calcium channel blockers that may prevent vasospasm may be useful adjuncts to antifibrinolytic therapy.

V. CEREBRAL VASOSPASM AND CEREBRAL INFARCTION

In the past, the role of vasospasm in the outcome after SAH was the subject of lively debate (82). It is now accepted that vasospasm produces cerebral infarction after SAH, and the combination is the leading cause of death and disability after SAH (13,14,83). Prevention or amelioration of vasospasm and cerebral ischemia is a critical component in the management of recent SAH. In the 1950s, the term "vasospasm" was applied to the arterial narrowing found on arteriograms performed 7-10 days after SAH. Vasospasm probably is a misnomer for this particular vascular process. Vasospasm was thought to be a sustained, spastic contraction of intracranial arteries, yet it is a much more ominous vasculopathy. Marked pathological changes occur in the walls of arteries, arterioles, capillaries, and veins (84). The adventitia is invaded by lymphocytes, monocytes, and plasma cells (84). The media becomes swollen and necrotic; later there is fibrosis with deposition of type V collagen (85). The endothelial lining desquamates. The intima proliferates, and changes occur in the internal elastic lamina (84,85). Many severe changes similar to the healing phase of acute atheroma appear (84). The lumen of the artery can be held in a contracted phase for weeks after SAH (85).

The etiology and mechanism of vasospasm are not known. Several hypotheses have been proposed; these are the subject of two recent reviews (13,83). Any etiology must explain the approximately 1 week lag between SAH and the peak of vasospasm and the 1 to 2-week duration of the phenomenon. The local nature of the vasculopathy with its close relationship to the site of the aneurysm should also be explained. The vasospasm-inducing factor must be present in blood and normally should be inactive. Some mechanism, poorly understood at present, activates a spasmogenic factor after SAH (86). Vasoactive substances such as serotonin have been proposed as the cause, but specific antagonists are not effective (87). Vasospasm likely is a multifactorial process that increases arterial permeability and disturbs the blood-brain barrier (83).

Calcium may play an important role in vasospasm and cerebral ischemia. Transmembrane influxes of calcium lead to smooth muscle contraction (88,89). Reduction in intracellular calcium can produce vasodilation, and reduced calcium flux can prevent vasospasm. During ischemia, calcium homeostasis is disturbed, mitochondrial function is abnormal, and cell membranes are damaged. Slowing calcium flux may prevent ischemia from becoming infarction (88). Drugs that block calcium channels may ease vasospasm or prevent secondary infarction.

Vasospasm influences outcome after SAH, regardless of medical or surgical treatment (90,91). The mortality is approximately 9% among patients without vasospasm but becomes 26% if vasospasm is severe and generalized (92). Weir et al. (93) noted that 50% of their patients died when vasospasm was present before surgery. In another series, symptomatic vasospasm developed in 41 of 112 patients (94). Four patients died, and 15 had ischemic sequelae. Vasospasm peaks 4-12 days after SAH; it is rare during the first 48 hours or after 2 weeks (13,14,83,95). It is more likely to develop in poor condition patients, women, patients with markedly abnormal electrocardiogram, and patients with marked nuchal rigidity. The risk of vasospasm is apparently not influenced by age, hypertension, diabetes mellitus, or atherosclerosis. Patients with thick clots in the subarachnoid space found on operation will have a high probability of developing vasospasm (96). This complication is more likely to occur in patients with marked collections of subarachnoid blood found on CT. Focal, thick collections are the most dangerous (15,16). Contrast enhancement of cortex of the brain on early CT also predicts vasospasm (97). Acute hydrocephalus on CT may also predict vasospasm (98,99). Black (98) reported that vascular spasm developed in 84% of patients who had hydrocephalus and in 18% of patients without hydrocephalus.

Symptoms of ischemia develop in 20-30% of all patients with recent SAH. Clinical manifestations appear indolently and often wax and wane. New or persistent headache is often an initial complaint (100). Confusion, somnolence, and depressed consciousness follow. Later, focal deficits appear often induced by hypotension, surgery, or dehydration (83). Most patients eventually develop focal dysfunction (99). Hemiparesis, paraparesis, hemisensory loss, anosognosia, aphasia, or mutism occur (99). Symptoms reflect ischemia in the areas perfused by the anterior or middle cerebral arteries (13). Multiple deficits and confusion may reflect generalized or watershed ischemia (99). The differential diagnosis of neurological decline several days after SAH includes hypoxia, hyponatremia, hydrocephalus, convulsions, rebleeding, postoperative complications, or medical complications. Blood and CSF examinations plus CT eliminate most of the other causes of the neurological deficits. CT and arteriography confirm infarction and vasospasm. Cerebral blood flow studies or transcranial pulsed Doppler evaluations may be helpful (83).

Several medical or surgical treatments have been proposed to prevent vasospasm (Table 4). Vasodilators and antagonists or biogenic amines have been tried but are not useful (87). Lavage of the subarachnoid space with removal of clots is said by some to prevent vasospasm (101,102). Early intracranial surgery, however, may induce vasospasm. Hence the value of early operation in prevention of vasospasm has not been established.

Calcium channel blocking drugs are used to forestall vasospasm (103). Drugs that have prominent cardiac depressant or hypotensive effects will not be useful. Verapamil or nifedipine are not effective. Drugs that have selective protective cerebral actions, such as nimodipine or nicardipine, appear to hold the most promise (88,104,105). In a controlled trial, Allen et al. (103) treated 116 patients with recent SAH; 60 received a placebo, and 56 were given oral nimodi-

Table 4 Medical Treatment to Prevent Cerebral Ischemia After Subarachnoid Hemorrhage

Prevention of vasospasm	Symptomatic vasospasm
1. Adequate hydration	1. Stop antifibrinolytic drugs and antihypertensives
2. Avoid hyponatremia	2. Hypervolemic hemodilution: dextran, albumin, plasmanate, colloids
3. Nimodipine or nicardipine	3. Drug-induced hypertension: dopamine
4. ? Surgery	

pine. Rates of symptomatic vasospasm were comparable in the two groups. Severe neurological sequelae and death were more common among the control patients. They concluded that nimodipine was effective.

Auer (106) treated 65 patients with early intracranial surgery supplemented by nimodipine. At the time of operation, the subarachnoid space was lavaged using a solution containing nimodipine. Postoperatively, the patients received intravenous nimodipine, later replaced by oral doses. Good or excellent outcomes were found in 49 patients (75%). Among 49 better condition patients, 45 (92%) had good or excellent results. Ljunggren et al. (107) reported similar results. Severe arterial narrowing was demonstrated by arteriography in only three of 38 patients treated with the nimodipine regimen. If these figures are matched by other investigators, a major breakthrough will have been achieved. Nicardipine has the same attributes as nimodipine but is also water-soluble. It can be administered intravenously, a major advantage in the care of critically ill patients.

Calcium channel blocking drugs appear to offer great promise in avoiding vasospasm. They have not been successful in reversing the arterial narrowing once it has developed (82). Questions remain about dosage, route of administration, duration of therapy, and which drug is preferable. Further studies on the usefulness of calcium ion entry blockers in patients with recent SAH have been reported (107a,107b). One study used nicardipine, the other evaluated nimodipine. Adams et al. reported a dose escalation study of nicardipine in 60 patients treated within one week of SAH (107a). At the highest dosage, they noted a lower than expected frequency of ischemic deficits and vasospasm. The large doses of nicardipine were well tolerated. Nicardipine is now being evaluated in a randomized trial to prove efficacy. Seiler et al. (107b) studied 70 patients who were given nimodipine and were followed by transcranial Doppler ultrasound measurements of blood flow velocity. They noted reduced severity of vasospasm, especially in high-risk patients. Calcium channel blockers may be most effective in patients with internal carotid or middle cerebral artery aneurysms (108).

Even if vasospasm is not prevented or reversed, treatment may ameliorate ischemic consequences. If medical therapy forestalls infarction, vasospasm becomes a less important phenomenon. During the last several years, a variety of treatments have been proposed to treat vasospasm. In reality, these therapies are directed toward ameliorating ischemia. Regimens include isoproterenol and lidocaine (109, reserpine and kanamycin (110), sodium nitroprusside (111), and isoproterenol and aminophylline (112). Initial reports were encouraging with all these therapies. However, widespread favorable clinical results have not been substantiated, and animal studies have been negative (113). Most of these regimens included at least one vasopressor; the benefits may reflect improved perfusion because autoregulation is impaired after SAH. Cerebral blood flow becomes pressure-dependent and can be improved by elevating cerebral perfusion pressure. Reducing intracranial pressure or raising mean blood pressure improve cerebral perfusion pressure. If antihypertensive drugs are used to reduce the risk of rebleeding, they should be discontinued if the patient develops signs of cerebral ischemia. Drug-induced hypertension will usually reverse developing ischemic signs. Elevating mean blood pressure by 20-40 mmHg can be accompanied by prompt neurological improvement. Dopamine is the most commonly used vasopressor; a 200-mg ampule is mixed with 250-500 ml of normal saline. It is given in a constant infusion, and the dosage is titrated to the blood pressure response. Elevating blood pressure is difficult if calcium channel blocking drugs are continued. Vigorous elevation of the blood pressure may induce rebleeding; it should be used with caution if the aneurysm has not been obliterated by surgery. Myocardial ischemia or cardiac arrhythmias can also complicate this therapy.

Cerebral circulation can also be improved by reducing viscosity. Volume expansion increases flow through microcirculatory pathways in ischemic brain by reducing cellular aggregation and arteriovenous shunting (112). Hence, the first step is to avoid dehydration. Hyponatremia should be corrected. Several measures such as venesection with removal of a unit of blood improve the rheological characteristics of blood and increase cerebral blood flow. Lowering of the hematocrit to 35-40% will improve viscosity without reducing the oxygen-carrying capacity of blood. Hemodilution with colloid solutions, albumin, plasmanate, or low molecular weight dextran will also decrease viscosity (83). Giannotta et al. (114) noted partial or complete recovery in 15 of 17 patients with vasospasm. They used low molecular weight dextran. Other researchers have noted similar favorable results using other agents (115). Marked expansion of intravascular volume can be successfully and safely achieved (116). However, volume expansion can be complicated by cardiac failure and pulmonary edema (115). Low molecular weight dextran does prolong bleeding and occasionally causes anaphylaxis. Therefore, many physicians avoid this agent after SAH.

Volume expansion has been successfully combined with drug-induced hypertension. Kassell et al. (115) treated 58 patients with volume expansion, antidiuretic drugs, drugs that block vagal depressor responses, and vasopressors. Ischemic deficits were reversed in 47 patients, of whom 43 had permanent recovery. Fifteen patients remained unchanged or deteriorated. Ten probably had cerebral infarction before treatment began. Three patients had progressive vasospasm despite treatment. Rebleeding occurred in three of 16 individuals who received this treatment before the aneurysm had been surgically treated. This combined therapy is relatively safe and effective. Because the use of antidiuretic drugs can make management of hyponatremia more difficult, they probably should not be used in this circumstance (13).

Other therapies have included mannitol, heparin, dipyridamole, barbiturates, prostacyclin, and nizofenone. Mannitol increases cerebral perfusion pressure by reducing intracranial pressure. Because it also influences red blood cell deformability, microcirculation can be improved. Heparin could prevent intravascular clotting and microembolism in narrowed arteries. The use of an anticoagulant in a patient with recent SAH may be dangerous. While most of the ischemic consequences of vasospasm are secondary to hypoperfusion, fibrin-platelet embolism may play a critical role. Spontaneous platelet aggregation with release of thromboxane may also play a critical role in the evolution of the arterial narrowing. Antiplatelet aggregating drugs such as aspirin, ticlopidine, or dipyridamole are being investigated. A blinded, controlled study found no significant improvement with dipyridamole (117). Prostacyclin may also be an effective local vasodilator. Prostacyclin has been reported to prevent the consequences of vasospasm (118). Further investigation is needed. Kassell et al. (119) tried high-dose barbiturates in critically ill patients who had failed other treatments; the results were disappointing. While barbiturate-induced coma might provide some protection in less critically ill patients, the usefulness of this therapy appears small. Ohta et al. (120) reported that nizofenone may protect against ischemia in patients with vasospasm. Nizofenone is reported to be a free radical scavenger, an antiedema agent, and a drug useful to reduce cerebral metabolism. The investigators noted good functional recovery in 73% of 78 treated patients and in 56% of 90 control patients. Further evaluation of this form of treatment is needed.

At present, the optimal treatment of vasospasm appears to be parenteral administration of a calcium channel blocking drug supplemented by adequate hydration as prophylaxis. If symptoms of ischemia appear, hypervolemic hemodilution is instituted. If the neurological state does not improve, vasopressors are given and calcium channel blocking drugs are discontinued.

VI. OTHER CAUSES OF NEUROLOGICAL DETERIORATION

A large number of medical or neurological complications can provoke deterioration after SAH. Medical complications include pneumonia, pulmonary edema, pulmonary embolism, atelectasis, hypoventilation, cardiac arrhythmias, severe hypotension, thrombophlebitis, myocardial infarction, or gastrointestinal bleeding. Neurological side effects include cerebral edema, intracerebral or subdural hematoma, convulsions, or hydrocephalus. Neurological deterioration can result from complications of arteriography, medical therapy, or surgical therapy (121,122).

Acute deterioration is due not only to rebleeding but to other causes as well (123,124). Seizures, ischemia, or medical complications can cause sudden declines in neurological status. Patients can have more than one cause of altered consciousness; many are reversible (125). Hypoxia, acidosis, or hyponatremia may be missed. Hydrocephalus causes progressive obtundation without focal signs of dysfunction (126). These neurological and medical complications must be anticipated, recognized, and promptly treated (127). Successful management of these less frequent complications will assist in improving the outcome of SAH.

VII. DECISION FOR SURGERY

Some physicians still question the necessity and utility of intracranial surgery in patients with ruptured aneurysms (39). Surgery, even if delayed, effectively reduces the long-term risk of rebleeding. Rebleeding occurs at an annual rate of 3% for at least 10 years after SAH; two-thirds of the time it is fatal (128). In most instances, surgery prevents this complication. A common question is: When is the optimal time for surgery?

In the 1950s and 1960s, surgeons reported prohibitively high rates of complications after early surgery. They found inflamed meninges and edematous brains; dissections were difficult. Premature aneurysmal rerupture occurred during operation. The Cooperative Aneurysm Study did not find reduced morbidity and mortality with intracranial surgery compared to medical measures. Early intracranial operations were generally abandoned at that time. Delayed operation was safer (129). During the last 20 years, however, operative techniques and neuroanesthesia have improved. In particular, operating microscopes are now widely used. As a result of these improvements and because a large number of patients died before surgery, neurosurgeons are again advocating early operations (130-133).

The reasons for delaying surgery are (1) intracranial dissections are easier, (2) prematuare intraoperative aneurysmal rerupture is less likely to occur, (3) the brain is less edematous and fragile, (4) postoperative vasospasm is milder, and (5) postoperative complications are fewer (134). Reasons for early surgery are (1) operative obliteration of the aneurysm is the best method to avoid rebleeding, (2) lavage of the subarachnoid space and removal of clots may prevent vasospasm, (3) a clipped aneurysm expedites treatment of vasospasm-induced ischemia, (4) side effects of medical therapy are avoided, and (5) the length of hospitalization may be shortened (134).

The International Cooperative Study on the Timing of Aneurysm Surgery has evaluated the optimal time for operative intervention. This collaborative study was performed at 68 major medical centers around the world; it was headed by Dr. Neal F. Kassell of the University of Virginia. The study enrolled 3521 patients seen within 3 days of SAH. At the time of admission, the neurosurgeon selected the time for surgery. Results were analyzed by the selected, not actual, time of surgery. Patients were grouped into intervals of 0-3, 4-6, 7-10, 11-14, or 15+ days after SAH.

Intracranial surgery was done in 83% of the patients. The interval influenced the frequency of surgery. Operations were done in 92% of those who had planned early surgery. More than one-third of the patients who had delayed scheduled operations never had surgery. Many of these patients died or had complications that prohibited operation. Among those patients who reached surgery, postoperative results were superior among those who had delayed surgery. Among those patients who were alert upon admission, postoperative results were comparable for either delayed or very early (within 48 hours) operation. Patients with surgery in the interval of 7-10 days had poorer outcomes than those treated at other intervals. If only postoperative results are analyzed, the conclusion would be that delayed surgery was superior to early surgery.

However, overall management results, including the patients who did not have surgery, are different. The overall management outcomes were almost identical among those patients who had early or delayed operations. Early operation was not associated with increased rates of complications; while it significantly lowered the risk of rebleeding, this effect was negated by death or disability due to vasospasm. The results did not prove that early operation was superior or worse than early medical therapy and delayed surgery. Early operations are a useful management choice in good condition patients with recent SAH. However, patients should be selected for early surgery on a case-by-case basis.

VIII. CONCLUSIONS

Several advances are occurring in the medical and surgical treatment of SAH and should improve prognosis. Patients are often critically ill during the first days after SAH. Acute neurological complications cause morbidity and mortality in the first hours after SAH, so that efforts to prevent rebleeding and vasospasm ischemia take precedence.

Early management includes control of cerebral edema and increased intracranial pressure. Marked arterial hypertension is treated medically. Agitation, nausea, and pain are controlled. Patients are given anticonvulsants. If early intracranial operation is planned, antifibrinolytic drugs are not administered. However, many patients are not eligible for early operation. If surgery is delayed, antifibrinolytic drugs may be given for 10-14 days. Adequate hydration, avoiding hyponatremia and hypotension, and administration of calcium channel blocking drugs may prevent the ischemic complications of vasospasm. Hypervolemic hemodilution and drug-induced hypertension are used for symptomatic vasospasm. As further data accrue, there is reason to expect important advances in the symptomatic care of this critically ill group of patients.

REFERENCES

1. Locksley HB, Sahs AL, Knowler L. Report of the cooperative study of intracranial aneurysms and subarachnoid hemorrhage. General survey of cases in the central registry and characteristics of the sample population. *J Neurosurg* 24:922-932, 1966.
2. McCormick WF. Pathology and pathogenesis of intracranial saccular aneurysms. *Semin Neurol* 4:291-303, 1984.
3. Phillips LH II, Whisnant JP, O'Fallon WM, et al. The unchanging pattern of subarachnoid hemorrhage in a community. *Neurology (NY)* 30:1034-1040, 1980.
4. Royal College of General Practitioners. Further analyses of mortality in oral contraceptive users. *Lancet* 1:541-546, 1986.
5. Bell BA, Symon L. Smoking and subarachnoid hemorrhage. *Br Med J* 1: 577-578, 1979.
6. Hillbom M, Kaste M. Alcohol intoxication. A risk factor for primary subarachnoid hemorrhage. *Neurology (NY)* 32:706-711, 1982.
7. Adams HP Jr, Jergenson DD, Kassell NF, et al. Pitfalls in the recognition of subarachnoid hemorrhage. *JAMA* 244:794-796, 1980.
8. Adams HP Jr, Kassell NF, Torner JC, et al. CT and clinical correlations in recent aneurysmal subarachnoid hemorrhage. A preliminary report of the Cooperative Aneurysm Study. *Neurology (Cleve)* 33:981-988, 1983.
9. Fogelholm R. Subarachnoid hemorrhage in middle-Finland. Incidence, early prognosis and indications for neurosurgical treatment. *Stroke* 12: 296-301, 1981.
10. Whisnant JP, Phillips LH II, Sundt TM Jr. Aneurysmal subarachnoid hemorrhage. Timing of surgery and mortality. *Mayo Clin Proc* 57:471-475, 1982.
11. Adams HP Jr, Kassell NF, Torner JC, et al. Early management of aneurysmal subarachnoid hemorrhage. A report of the Cooperative Aneurysm Study. *J Neurosurg* 54:141-145, 1981.
12. Weir B, Aronyk K. Management, mortality and timing of surgery for supratentorial aneurysms. *J Neurosurg* 54:146-150, 1981.
13. Heros RC, Zervas NT, Varsos V. Cerebral vasospasm after subarachnoid hemorrhage. An update. *Ann Neurol* 14:599-608, 1983.
14. Chyatte D, Sundt TM Jr. Cerebral vasospasm after subarachnoid hemorrhage. *Mayo Clin Proc* 59:498-505, 1984.
15. Kistler JP, Crowell RM, David KR, et al. The relation of cerebral vasospasm to the extent and location of subarachnoid blood visualized by CT scan. A prospective study. *Neurology (Cleve)* 33:424-436, 1983.
16. Mizukami M, Takemae T, Tazawa T, et al. Value of computed tomography in the prediction of cerebral vasospasm after aneurysm rupture. *Neurosurgery* 7:583-586, 1980.
17. Kassell NF, Torner JC, Adams HP Jr. Antifibrinolytic therapy in the acute period following aneurysmal subarachnoid hemorrhage. Preliminary observations from the Cooperative Aneurysm Study. *J Neurosurg* 61:225-230, 1984.

18. Aoyagi N, Hayakawa I. Analysis of 223 ruptured intracranial aneurysms with special reference to rerupture. *Surg Neurol* 21:445-452, 1984.
19. Adams HP Jr. Clinical manifestations and diagnosis of subarachnoid hemorrhage. *Semin Neurol* 4:304-314, 1984.
20. Keane JR. Retinal hemorrhage. Its significance in 100 patients with acute encephalopathy of unknown cause. *Arch Neurol* 36:691-694, 1979.
21. Adams HP Jr, Kassell NF, Torner JC. Usefulness of computed tomography in predicting outcome after aneurysmal subarachnoid hemorrhage. A preliminary report of the Cooperative Aneurysm Study. *Neurology* 35:1263-1267, 1985.
22. Nibbelink DW, Torner JC, Burmeister LF. Fluid restriction in combination with antifibrinolytic therapy. In: Sahs AL, Nibbelink DW, Torner JC (Eds.), *Aneurysmal Subarachnoid Hemorrhage*. Urban & Schwarzenberg, Baltimore, 1981, pp. 307-330.
23. Maroon JC, Nelson PB. Hypovolemia in patients with subarachnoid hemorrhage. Therapeutic implications. *Neurosurgery* 4:223-226, 1979.
24. Solomon RA, Post KD, McMurtry JG III. Depression of circulating blood volume in patients after subarachnoid hemorrhage. Implications for the management of symptomatic vasospasm. *Neurosurgery* 15:354-361, 1984.
25. Wijdicks EFM, Vermeulen M, Hijdra A, et al. Hyponatremia and cerebral infarction in patients with ruptured intracranial aneurysms. Is fluid restriction harmful. *Ann Neurol* 17:136-140, 1985.
26. Hart RG, Byer JA, Slaughter JR, et al. Occurrence and implications of seizures in subarachnoid hemorrhage due to ruptured intracranial aneurysms. *Neurosurgery* 8:417-421, 1981.
27. Marshall LF, Smith RW, Rauscher LA, Shapiro HM. Mannitol dose requirements in brain-injured patients. *J Neurosurg* 48:169-172, 1978.
28. Winn HR, Almaani WS, Berga SL, et al. The long term outcome in patients with multiple aneurysms. Incidence of late hemorrhage and implications for treatment of incidental aneurysms. *J Neurosurg* 59:642-651, 1983.
29. Ljunggren B, Brandt L, Sundbarg G, et al. Early management of aneurysmal subarachnoid hemorrhage. *Neurosurgery* 11:412-418, 1982.
30. Black P McL, Crowell RM, Abbott WM. External pneumatic calf compression reduces deep venous thrombosis in patients with ruptured intracranial aneurysms. *Neurosurgery* 18:25-28, 1986.
31. Nibbelink DW, Torner JC, Henderson WG. Cooperative study of intracranial aneurysms and subarachnoid hemorrhage. Report on a randomized treatment study. IV—A regulated bedrest. *Stroke* 8:202-218, 1977.
32. Koskelo P, Punsar S, Sipila W. Subendocardial hemorrhage and ECG changes in intracranial bleeding. *Br Med J* 1:1479-1480, 1964.
33. Fabinyi G, Hunt D, McKinley L. Myocardial creatine kinase isoenzyme in serum after subarachnoid hemorrhage. *J Neurol Neurosurg Psychiatry* 40:818-820, 1977.
34. Marion DW, Segal R, Thompson ME. Subarachnoid hemorrhage and the heart. *Neurosurgery* 18:101-106, 1986.

35. Stober T, Kunze K. Electrocardiographic alterations in subarachnoid hemorrhage. Correlation between spasm of the arteries of the left side of the brain and T inversion and QT prolongation. *J Neurol* 227:99-113, 1982.
36. Neil-Dwyer G, Walter P, Cruickshank J, et al. Effect of propranolol and phentolamine on myocardial necrosis after subarachnoid hemorrhage. *Br Med J* 2:990-992, 1978.
37. Elliott HL, Campbell BC, Morgan I. Beta blockade in subarachnoid hemorrhage. *Br Med J* 2:1370-1371, 1978.
38. Nibbelink DW, Torner, JC, Henderson WG. Randomized treatment study. Drug-induced hypotension. In: Sahs AL, Nibbelink DW, Torner JC (Eds.), *Aneurysmal Subarachnoid Hemorrhage*. Urban & Schwarzenberg, Baltimore, 1981, pp. 77-106.
39. Slosberg PS. Zero percent mortality due to recurrent hemorrhage in follow-up of medically treated ruptured single intracranial aneurysms. A 23-year study. *Trans Am Neurol Assoc* 104:180–183, 1980.
40. Nibbelink DW. Considerations in the treatment of stroke. Cooperative aneurysm study. Antihypertensive and antifibrinolytic therapy following subarachnoid hemorrhage from ruptured intracranial aneurysm. In: Whisnant JP, Sandok BA (Eds.), *Cerebral Vascular Diseases*. Grune & Stratton, New York, 1975, pp. 155-165.
41. Ramirez-Lassepas M. Antifibrinolytic therapy in subarachnoid hemorrhage caused by ruptured intracranial aneurysm. *Neurology (NY)* 31:316-322, 1981.
42. Vermeulen M, Muizelaar JP. Do antifibrinolytic agents prevent rebleeding after rupture of a cerebral aneurysm? A review. *Clin Neurol Neurosurg* 82:25-30, 1980.
43. Norlen G, Thulin CA. The use of antifibrinolytic substances in ruptured intracranial aneurysms. *Neurochirurgica (Stuttg.)* 12:100-102, 1969.
44. Fodstad H, Kok P, Algers G. Fibrinolytic activity of cerebral tissue after experimental subarachnoid hemorrhage. Inhibitory effect of tranexamic acid (AMCA). *Acta Neurol Scand* 64:29-46, 1981.
45. Tovi D, Nilsson IM. Increased fibrinolytic activity and fibrin degradation products after experimental intracerebral hemorrhage. *Acta Neurol Scand* 48:403-415, 1972.
46. Alvarez Garijo JA, Vilches JJ, Aznar JA. Preoperative treatment of ruptured intracranial aneurysms with tranexamic acid and monitoring of fibrinolytic activity. *J Neurosurg* 52:453-455, 1980.
47. Fodstad H, Pilbrant A, Schannong M, et al. Determination of tranexamic acid (AMCA) and fibrin/fibrinogen degradation products in cerebrospinal fluid after aneurysmal subarachnoid hemorrhage. *Acta Neurochir* 58:1-13, 1981.
48. Sawaya R, Sonnino V, McLauren RL, et al. Monitoring of antifibrinolytic therapy following subarachnoid hemorrhage. *J Neurosurg* 58:699-707, 1983.
49. Burchiel KJ, Schmer G. A method for monitoring antifibrinolytic therapy in patients with ruptured intracranial aneurysms. *J Neurosurg* 54:12-15, 1981.

50. Burchiel KJ, Hoffman JM, Bakay RAF. Quantitative determination of plasma fibrinolytic activity in patients with ruptured intracranial aneurysms who are receiving aminocaproic acid. Relationship of possible complications of therapy to the degree of fibrinolytic inhibition. *Neurosurgery* 14:57-63, 1984.
51. Markwardt F. Synthetic inhibitors of fibrinolysis. *Hand Exp Pharmacol* 46:511-577, 1978.
52. Prentice CRM. Indications for antifibrinolytic therapy. *Thromb Diath Haemorrh (Stuttg)* 34:634-643, 1975.
53. Glick R, Green D, Tsao C-H, et al. High dose ϵ-aminocaproic acid prolongs the bleeding time and increases rebleeding and intraoperative hemorrhage in patients with subarachnoid hemorrhage. *Neurosurgery* 9:398-401, 1981.
54. Nibbelink DW. Antifibrinolytic activity during administration of epsilon aminocaproic acid. *Stroke* 2:555-558, 1971.
55. Fish SS, Pancorbo S, Berkseth R. Pharmacokinetics of epsilon-aminocaproic acid during peritoneal dialysis. *J Neurosurg* 54:736-739, 1981.
56. Tovi D, Thulin CA. Ability of tranexamic acid to cross the blood-brain barrier and its use in patients with ruptured intracranial aneurysms. *Acta Neurol Scand* 48:257, 1972.
57. Heidrich R, Markwardt F, Endler S, et al. Antifibrinolytic therapy of subarachnoid hemorrhage by intrathecal administration of *p*-aminomethylbenzoic acid. *J Neurol* 219:83-85, 1978.
58. Adams HP Jr, Nibbelink DW, Torner JC, et al. Antifibrinolytic therapy in patients with aneurysmal subarachnoid hemorrhage. *Arch Neurol* 38:25-29, 1981.
59. Ameen AA, Illingworth R. Antifibrinolytic treatment in the preoperative management of subarachnoid hemorrhage caused by ruptured intracranial aneurysms. *J Neurol Neurosurg Psychiatry* 44:220-226, 1981.
60. Chowdhary UM, Sayed K. Comparative clinical trial of epsilon aminocaproic acid and tranexamic acid in the prevention of early recurrence of subarachnoid hemorrhage. *J Neurol Neurosurg Psychiatry* 44:810-813, 1981.
61. Fodstad H, Forssell A, Liliequist B, et al. Antifibrinolysis with tranexamic acid in aneurysmal subarachnoid hemorrhage. A consecutive controlled clinical trial. *Neurosurgery* 8:158-165, 1981.
62. Guidetti B, Spallone A. The role of antifibrinolytic therapy in the preoperative management of recently ruptured intracranial aneurysms. *Surg Neurol* 15:239-248, 1981.
63. Flamm ES. Antifibrinolysis and the preoperative management of subarachnoid hemorrhage. In: Hopkins LN, Long DM (Eds.), *Clinical Management of Intracranial Aneurysms*. Raven Press, New York, 1982, pp. 49-58.
64. Fodstad H. Antifibrinolytic treatment in subarachnoid hemorrhage. Present state. *Acta Neurochir* 63:233-244, 1982.
65. Vermeulen M, Lindsay KW, Murray GD, et al. Antifibrinolytic treatment in subarachnoid hemorrhage. *N Engl J Med* 311:432-437, 1984.
66. Farina ML, Levat A, Paino R. Myocardial infarction during antifibrinolytic treatment of subarachnoid haemorrhage. *Thromb Haemost (Stuttg)* 42: 1347-1348, 1979.

67. Levat A, Minella C, Farino ML, et al. Potential hazards of antifibrinolytic treatment in subarachnoid hemorrhage. *Thromb Haemost* (*Stuttg*) 44:170, 1980.
68. MacKay AR, U HS, Weinstein PR. Myopathy associated with epsilon-aminocaproic (EACA) therapy. *J Neurosurg* 49:597-601, 1978.
69. Britt CW, Jr, Light RR, Peters BH, et al. Rhabdomyolysis during treatment with epsilon-aminocaproic acid. *Arch Neurol* 37:187-188, 1980.
70. Brodkin HM. Myoglobinuria following epsilon-aminocaproic acid (EACA) therapy. *J Neurosurg* 53:690-692, 1982.
71. Brown JA, Wollmann RL, Mullan S. Myopathy induced by epsilon-aminocaproic acid. *J Neurosurg* 57:130-134, 1982.
72. Vanneste JAL, Van Winngaarden GK. Epsilon aminocaproic acid myopathy. *Eur Neurol* 21:242-248, 1982.
73. Feffer SE, Parray HR, Westring DW. Seizure after infusion of aminocaproic acid. *JAMA* 240-2468, 1978.
74. Yamaura A, Nakamura T, Makino H, et al. Cerebral complication of antifibrinolytic therapy in the treatment of ruptured intracranial aneurysm. *Eur Neurol* 19:77-84, 1980.
75. Wysenbeek AJ, Sella A, Vardi M, et al. Acute delirious state after ϵ-aminocaproic acid. *Lancet* 1:221, 1978.
76. Knibestol M, Karadayi A, Tovi O. Echoencephalographic study of ventricular dilatation after subarachnoid hemorrhage, with special reference to the effect of antifibrinolytic treatment. *Acta Neurol Scand* 54:57-70, 1976.
77. Park BE. Spontaneous subarachnoid hemorrhage complicated by communicating hydrocephalus. Epsilon aminocaproic acid as a possible predisposing factor. *Surg Neurol* 11:73-80, 1979.
78. Kagstrom E, Palma L. Influence of antifibrinolytic treatment on the morbidity in patients with subarachnoid hemorrhage. *Acta Neurol Scand* 48: 257-258, 1972.
79. Fodstad H, Liliequist B. Spontaneous thrombosis of ruptured intracranial aneurysms during treatment with tranexamic acid (AMCA). Report of three cases. *Acta Neurochir* 49:129-144, 1979.
80. Hoffman EP, Koo AH. Cerebral thrombosis associated with amicar therapy. *Radiology* 131:687-689, 1979.
81. Sonntag VKH, Stein BM. Arteriopathic complications during treatment of subarachnoid hemorrhage with epsilon-aminocaproic acid. *J Neurosurg* 40: 480-485, 1974.
82. Millikan CH. Cerebral vasospasm and ruptured intracranial aneurysm. *Arch Neurol* 32:433-449, 1975.
83. Kassell NF, Sasaki T, Colohan ART, et al. Cerebral vasospasm following aneurysmal subarachnoid hemorrhage. *Stroke* 16:562-572, 1985.
84. Hughes JT, Schianchi PM. Cerebral arterial spasm. A histological study of necrospy of the blood vessels in cases of subarachnoid hemorrhage. *J Neurosurg* 48:515-525, 1978.
85. Smith RR, Clower BR, Grotendorst GM, et al. Arterial wall changes in early human vasospasm. *Neurosurgery* 16:171-176, 1985.

86. Cook DA. The pharmacology of cerebral vasospasm. *Pharmacology* 29:1-16, 1984.
87. Wilkins RH. Attempted prevention or treatment of intracranial arterial spasm. A survey. In: Wilkins RH (Ed.), *Cerebral Arterial Spasm*. Williams & Wilkins, Baltimore, 1980, pp. 542-555.
88. Weir B. Calcium antagonists, cerebral ischemia and vasospasm. *Can J Neurol Sci* 11:239-246, 1984.
89. Gelmers HJ. The role of calcium and the significance of calcium antagonists in some neurological and neurosurgical diseases. *Clin Neurol Neurosurg* 85:213-224, 1983.
90. Artiola I, Fortuny L, Adams CBT. Predicting outcome in patients with intracranial aneurysms with the help of microsurgery. *J Neurol Neurosurg Psychiatry* 44:615-620, 1981.
91. Richardson JTE. Arterial spasm and recovery from subarachnoid haemorrhage. *J Neurol Neurosurg Psychiatry* 39:1134-1136, 1976.
92. Torner JC, Kassell NF, Wallace RB, et al. Preoperative prognostic factors for rebleeding and survival in aneurysm patients receiving antifibrinolytic therapy. Report of the Cooperative Aneurysm Study. *Neurosurgery* 9:506-513, 1981.
93. Weir B, Rothberg C, Grace M, et al. Relative prognostic significance of vasospasm following subarachnoid hemorrhage. *Can J Neurol Sci* 2:109-114, 1975.
94. Ropper AH, Zervas NT. Outcome 1 year after SAH from cerebral aneurysm. Management morbidity, mortality and functional status in 112 consecutive good-risk patients. *J Neurosurg* 60:909-914, 1984.
95. Kwak R, Niizuma H, Ohi T, et al. Angiographic study of cerebral vasospasm following rupture of intracranial aneurysms I. Time of the appearances. *Surg Neurol* 11:257-262, 1979.
96. Tomasello F, Albanese V, Picozz P, et al. Relation of cerebral vasospasm to operative findings of subarachnoid blood around ruptured aneurysms. *Acta Neurochir* 60:55-62, 1982.
97. Tazawa T, Mizukami M, Kawase T, et al. Relationship between contrast enhancement on computed tomography and cerebral vasospasm in patients with subarachnoid hemorrhage. *Neurosurgery* 12:643-648, 1983.
98. Black P McL. Hydrocephalus and vasospasm after subarachnoid hemorrhage from ruptured intracranial aneurysms. *Neurosurgery* 18:12-16, 1986.
99. Hijdra A, Van Gijn J, Stefanko S, et al. Delayed cerebral ischemia after aneurysmal subarachnoid hemorrhage. Clinicoanatomic correlations. *Neurology* 36:329-333, 1986.
100. Fisher CM, Roberson GH, Ojemann RG. Cerebral vasospasm with ruptured saccular aneurysm. The clinical manifestations. *Neurosurgery* 1:245-248, 1977.
101. Mizukami M, Kawase T, Usami T, et al. Prevention of vasospasm by early operation with removal of subarachnoid blood. *Neurosurgery* 10:301-307, 1982.

102. Taneda M. Effect of early operation for ruptured aneurysms on prevention of delayed ischemic symptoms. *J Neurosurg* 57:622-628, 1982.
103. Allen GS, Ahn HS, Preziosi TJ, et al. Cerebral arterial spasm. A controlled trial of nimodipine in patients with subarachnoid hemorrhage. *N Engl J Med* 308:619-624, 1983.
104. Meldrum BS. Calcium entry blockers and cerebral function. An introduction. In: Godfraind T, Herman AG, Wellens D (Eds.), *Calcium Entry Blockers in Cardiovascular and Cerebral Dysfunctions.* M. Nijhoff, Boston, 1984, pp. 207-219.
105. Wellens D. Twenty-seven calcium entry blockers in development. A new chapter in pharmacology. In: Godfraind T , Herman AG, Wellens D (Eds.), *Calcium Entry Blockers in Cardiovascular and Cerebral Dysfunctions,* M. Nijhoff, Boston, 1984, pp. 25-42.
106. Auer LM. Acute operation and preventive nimodipine improves outcome in patients with ruptured cerebral aneurysms. *Neurosurgery* 15:57-66, 1984.
107. Ljunggren B, Brandt L, Saveland H, et al. Outcome in 60 consecutive patients treated with early aneurysm operation and intravenous nimodipine. *J Neurosurg* 61:864-873, 1984.
107a. Adams H, Flamm E, Beck D, Godersky J, Pinto R. A study of nicardipine in prevention of infarction after subarachnoid hemorrhage. *Stroke* 18:281, 1987.
107b. Seiler RW, Grolimund P, Zurbrugg HR. Evaluation of the calcium antagonist nimodipine for the prevention of vasospasm after aneurysmal subarachnoid hemorrhage. *Stroke* 18:281, 1987.
108. Saveland H, Ljunggren B, Brandt L, et al. Delayed ischemic deterioration in patients with early aneurysm operation and intravenous nimodipine. *Neurosurgery* 18:146-150, 1986.
109. Sundt TM. Management of ischemic complications after subarachnoid hemorrhage. *J Neurosurg* 43:418-425, 1975.
110. Heros RC, Zervas NT, Negoro M. Cerebral vasospasm. *Surg Neurol* 5:354-362, 1976.
111. Allen GS. Cerebral arterial spasm. Part 8. The treatment of delayed arterial spasm in human beings. *Surg Neurol* 6:71-80, 1976.
112. Flamm ES, Ransohoff J. Treatment of cerebral vasospasm by control of cyclic adenosine monophosphate. *Surg Neurol* 6:223-226, 1976.
113. Noseworthy TW, Weir B, Boisvert D, et al. Effect of reserpine-kanamycin treatment on chronic vasospasm after platelet enriched subarachnoid hemorrhage in primates. *Neurosurgery* 14:193-197, 1984.
114. Giannotta SL, McGillicuddy JE, Kindt GW. Diagnosis and treatment of postoperative cerebral vasospasm. *Surg Neurol* 8:286-290, 1977.
115. Kassell NF, Peerless SJ, Durward QJ, et al. Treatment of ischemic deficits from vasospasm with intravascular volume expansion and induced arterial hypertension. *Neurosurgery* 11:337-343, 1982.
116. Pritz MB, Giannotta SL, Kindt GW, et al. Treatment of patients with neurological deficits associated with cerebral vasospasm by intravascular volume expansion. *Neurosurgery* 3:364-368, 1978.

117. Shaw MDW, Foy PM, Conway M, et al. Dipyridamole and postoperative ischemic deficits in aneurysmal subarachnoid hemorrhage. *J Neurosurg* 63:699-703, 1985.
118. Fukomori T, Tani E, Maeda Y, et al. Effects of prostacyclin and indomethacin on experimental delayed cerebral vasospasm. *J Neurosurg.* 59: 829-834, 1983.
119. Kassell NF, Peerless SJ, Drake CG, et al. Treatment of ischemic deficits from cerebral vasospasm with high dose barbiturate therapy. *Neurosurgery* 7:593-397, 1980.
120. Ohta T, Kikuchi H, Hashi K, et al. Nizofenone administration in the acute stage following subarachnoid hemorrhage. Results of a multi-center controlled double-blind clinical study. *J Neurosurg* 64:420-426, 1986.
121. Peerless SJ. Pre- and postoperative management of cerebral aneurysms. *Clin Neurosurg* 26:209-231, 1979.
122. Crowell RM, Zervas NT. Management of intracranial aneurysm. *Med Clin N Am* 63:695-713, 1979.
123. VanCrevel H. Pitfalls in the diagnosis of rebleeding from intracranial aneurysms. *Clin Neurol Neurosurg* 82:1-9, 1980.
124. Vermeulen M, VanGijn J, Hijdra A, et al. Causes of acute deterioration in patients with a ruptured intracranial aneurysm. *J Neurosurg* 60:935-939, 1984.
125. Majim Al-Din AS, Jamieson DG. Reversible causes of altered consciousness after spontaneous subarachnoid haemorrhage. *Br Med J* 284:180–181, 1982.
126. Van Gijn J, Hijdra A, Wijdicks EFM, et al. Acute hydrocephalus after aneurysmal subarachnoid hemorrhage. *J Neurosurg* 63:355-362, 1982.
127. Weir B. Medical aspects of the preoperative management of aneurysms. A review. *Can J Neurol Sci* 6:441-450, 1979.
128. Graf CJ, Nibbelink DW. Cooperative study on intracranial aneurysms and subarachnoid hemorrhage. Report on a randomized treatment study. III. Intracranial surgery. *Stroke* 5:557-601, 1974.
129. Drage CG. Management of cerebral aneurysm. *Stroke* 12:273-283, 1981.
130. Hunt WE, Miller CA. The results of early operation for aneurysm. *Clin Neurosurg* 24:208-215, 1976.
131. Sand K, Saito I. Timing and indication of surgery for ruptured intracranial aneurysms with regard to cerebral vasospasm. *Acta Neurochir* 41:49-60, 1978.
132. Hori S, Suzuki J. Early intracranial operations for ruptured aneurysms. *Acta Neurochir* 46:93-104, 1979.
133. Kassell NF, Boarini DJ, Adams HP Jr, et al. Overall management of ruptured aneurysm. Comparison of early and late operation. *Neurosurgery* 9:120-128, 1981.
134. Sahs AL, Kassell NF. Aneurysmal subarachnoid hemorrhage. An appraisal. *Mayo Clin Proc* 57:529-530, 1982.

15

Medical Therapy of Cerebral Ischemia

Mark Fisher
University of Southern California School of Medicine, Los Angeles, California

I. INTRODUCTION

Secondary prevention of cerebral infarction has traditionally been the major focus of attention for patients experiencing symptoms of cerebral ischemia. Risk factor reduction, the use of platelet antiaggregant agents, and surgical revascularization of extracranial carotid arteries are the major features of stroke prevention programs. Treatment of stroke risk factors, particularly aggressive therapy for hypertension, has undoubtedly contributed to the decline in the incidence of stroke over the past 40 years. The use of aspirin is beneficial, albeit modestly. The proper role of surgical therapy will be defined by prospective trials currently underway; their results should be known by the early 1990s. In contrast, medical therapy for acute cerebral ischemia is very much in its infancy. This area of investigation contains the possibilities for a substantial transformation in modern neuromedicine.

II. DIAGNOSTIC EVALUATION IN CEREBRAL ISCHEMIA

There is far from general agreement as to what constitutes the appropriate diagnostic evaluation of the patient with acute cerebral ischemia. This includes the use of lumbar puncture, noninvasive evaluation of cranial circulation, the use of arteriography, and the choice of method for brain imaging. Lumbar puncture (LP) remains a useful, if erratically utilized, diagnostic modality. It is certainly reasonable to perform lumbar puncture on all patients presenting with symptoms of cerebral ischemia. However, many physicians seem to believe that this is an improper carryover from a bygone era, before computerized tomography (CT) provided images of the brain. It is true that hemorrhagic infarction is best dèmonstrated by CT. It is also true that LP has a low diagnostic yield, if the latter is defined as the percentage of patients in whom substantive information is provided that is not readily available from other modalities. Nevertheless, LP remains the only method for diagnosing "cryptic" meningoencephalitis, including neurosyphilis, which can present with symptoms of cerebral ischemia. It may be that LP can also provide supplementary information on which of the large cardiogenic infarcts are likely to undergo "hemorrhagic transformation," i.e., which will convert from a bland to a hemorrhagic infarct on CT. While these issues have not been explored in a systematic fashion, anecdotal evidence suggests their potential importance. Lumbar puncture should be performed, at the very least, on any patient with either unusual presentations of cerebral ischemia (e.g., prolonged course of stroke progression) or signs suggesting etiologies other than atherothromboembolic disease (e.g., light-near dissociation), in the absence of mass effect on CT.

When lumbar puncture is performed, there are several considerations that are unique for stroke patients. Since LP should be performed only in the absence of significant mass effect, the development of cerebral edema must be considered. Vasogenic cerebral edema usually becomes prominent beginning 24-48 hours postinfarct; lumbar puncture should thus usually be performed very early following any large infarct or delayed until signs of edema have resolved. A second consideration concerns LP and anticoagulation. There is a small risk of spinal subdural or epidural hematoma in patients undergoing LP followed by heparin infusion (1). If anticoagulation is anticipated, the following guidelines are suggested:

1. Lumbar puncture should be performed by an experienced physician, in order to minimize the possibility of a traumatic tap
2. A 22-gauge spinal needle, if available, may also help reduce the risk of a traumatic tap
3. There should be a delay of at least 1 hour between performance of LP and initiation of heparinization
4. Loading doses of heparin are rarely necessary unless the patient has active progression of symptoms of an ischemic infarct.

Arteriography for stroke patients is often a controversial issue. The two central considerations are whether arteriograms are "appropiate" and, if so, what is the best time to perform the study. The issue of appropriateness of arteriography usually focuses on the "risk/benefit ratio," i.e., whether the information gained by performing the study is likely to yield information that is important enough to overshadow the small but real risk of the procedure. The risk/benefit ratio can sometimes be lessened by using arteriograms performed with digital technology. These arterial catheterization-requiring "digital arteriograms," which are sometimes confused with venous injection "digital subtraction angiography" (DSA), provide adequate visualization of the carotid bifurcation and rather mediocre images of the intracranial vasculature. Digital arteriograms are best suited for the neurologically stable patient being considered for carotid endarterectomy. They are generally inadequate for the search for an embolic fragment or a branch occlusion of an intracranial artery.

The risks of stroke from conventional arteriography are largely dependent on the technical abilities of the neuroradiologist, and range up to 5% (2). An additional issue is whether arteriography in the acute state is associated with more risk than a study performed when the patient is stable. There has been no documentation of a "time-dependent" risk of arteriography following stroke, despite the clear theoretical risks of neurotoxicity, platelet activation, and reduced erythrocyte deformability associated with contrast media and arteriography.

The benefits obtained from arteriography are most difficult to quantitate, particularly in the face of newer imaging modalities such as magnetic resonance imaging. Arteriography is unquestionably necessary if a surgical procedure is seriously contemplated. A more difficult question is the necessity of arteriography in association with acute medical therapy. Arteriographic information will certainly be helpful for analysis of results of acute stroke therapy protocols and will likely be essential in the understanding of the utility of fibrinolytic therapy in cerebral infarction. The logistic demands of emergency carotid arteriography arc of sufficient magnitude that the procedure is, and will likely remain, optional much of the time, at least in association with nonfibrinolytic stroke therapy.

The rolc of noninvasive examinations of the cranial vasculature remains unclear. Despite widespread claims for their utility, these procedures can yield data that are inaccurate and misleading. It is inappropriate to assume that the typical noninvasive laboratory of community hospitals or even academic centers are in any way comparable to state-of-the-art laboratories reporting their experience in the literature. Carotid ultrasound examinations are, at best, not helpful in the absence of dedicated carotid ultrasound technicians and appropriate technology (usually a duplex scanner). This is due to such technical features as adequacy of arterial imaging in the presence of excessive adipose tissue, distinguishing external from internal carotid arteries, and position of the bifurcation in relation to the mandible. Most noninvasive laboratories have never performed systematic comparisons between arteriograms and ultrasonic procedures; the sensitivity and specificity of tests in these laboratories are unknown. These tests are probably best used when clinical, laboratory, and imaging procedures suggest that symptomatic extracranial arterial disease is unlikely, e.g., presumed cardiogenic or lacunar stroke. In this setting, the thoughtful clinician can wisely use data that are often rather crude. Arteriography remains the imaging choice for suspected symptomatic carotid artery disease.

Transcranial doppler represents a new diagnostic modality with potentially significant impact on the evaluation of the acute stroke patient. The possibility of a noninvasive and logistically convenient method for measuring middle cerebral artery blood flow seems irresistible. However, the same caveat applied to duplex scanning of the bifurcation is in order here: Systematic comparisons of arteriograms and dopplers are needed in order to define the usefulness of this procedure.

Electrophysiologic studies of the acute stroke patient are of very limited value. For the patient with signs suggesting seizure activity, electroencephalography (EEG) will be helpful. However, EEG should not be performed routinely in patients with stroke. In addition, evoked potentials have no role in the routine management of the acute stroke patient. There is no evidence that evoked potentials provide information that is not easily elicited by a careful clinical evaluation of the stroke patient (3). Perhaps the only group of patients in whom evoked potentials may be helpful are those individuals with a possibly functional neurological deficit. Somatosensory evoked potentials may be useful in patients with suspected functional sensory symptoms. Again, however, standardization of the procedure using age-matched controls is crucial.

Echocardiography is an important component of the diagnostic workup of the acute stroke patient. Two-dimensional echocardiography is recommended for all patients under the age of 50 presenting with cerebral ischemia in whom mitral valve prolapse may be an important risk factor. Echocardiography is recommended for those stroke patients over 50 with signs or symptoms of coronary artery disease. This will help identify those patients with intracardiac thrombi associated with akinetic regions. The routine use of so-called "contrast echocardiography" to identify a patient foramen ovale represents a provocative consideration that awaits confirmatory studies (4).

Computerized tomography (CT) remains the imaging modality of first choice in acute stroke. The primary issue that such imaging must address is the possible presence of hemorrhage or an unsuspected process, e.g., a space-occupying lesion. CT scans are ideal for such questions. While magnetic resonance imaging is more sensitive in demonstrating infarction, its ability to distinguish hemorrhage from infarction appears to be less than CT (5). An unresolved issue is the use of contrast with CT in the acute stroke patient. The question of neurological deterioration with intravenous contrast injection remains unexplored. Contrast agents, in the concentration and dose used with CT, have the capacity to alter microcirculatory flow on the basis of reduction of erythrocyte deformability (6). It is uncertain whether these experimental findings have practical, clinical significance. Given this uncertainty, it is probably wise to reserve contrast infusion in acute stroke to those situations where diagnostic uncertainty increases the likelihood that useful additional information will be obtained from the procedure.

III. THERAPY OF CEREBRAL ISCHEMIA

Routine use of most acute therapies outlined in earlier chapters awaits performance of carefully designed clinical trials demonstrating their efficacy. For the present, acute stroke management focuses largely on supportive care. Clinical measures to avoid include: hypotonic intravenous fluids, which may accentuate cerebral edema; iatrogenic hypotension, which may transform a minor ischemic neurological deficit into a major deficit; and the use of sedatives, including haloperiodol and benzodiazepines, which may retard recovery of neuronal function (7,8). Oral feedings should begin promptly following demonstration of absence of dysphagia and aspiration. This can be assessed by watching the patient swallow one-third teaspoon of liquid, followed by larger volumes of liquid, soft foods, and solid foods. Patients capable of eating should be on a high-fiber diet (9). Range-of-motion exercises, performed with a physical therapist at the bedside, should begin promptly. These rather general measures of supportive care are probably best performed on the neurology ward. The necessity of a dedicated "stroke unit" is uncertain.

Drs. Brott and MacCarthy have outlined the use of antihypertensive agents in Chapter 8. The use of anticoagulation is described in Chapter 4. As Dr. Easton indicates, heparinization of patients with acute, partial, nonprogressive infarction is recommended with some reluctance. An alternative is to start such patients on aspirin.

The deteriorating stroke patient represents an often difficult clinical problem. In this setting, the most prudent course is to define the cause of deterioration as being "medical" (sepsis or electrolyte imbalance) or "neurological." The two most common neurologic etiologies are "stroke progression" and brain edema. The former is usually defined as stepwise progression of a focal neurological deficit during the first 48 hours poststroke, and can usually be distinguished from the sudden extension of a deficit suggesting a second, discrete infarction. As summarized in Chapter 4, heparinization remains the preferred therapy and appears to be effective in halting progression in approximately 50%

of patients (10). Poststroke edema typically presents with drowsiness, beginning between the second and fifth day poststroke. Computerized tomography scans will demonstrate mass effect, and pupillary asymmetry is common (11). Optimal treatment is mannitol at doses of 0.25 to 0.5 g/kg, at 4-6-hour intervals, and with careful attention to possible electrolyte abnormalities and serum osmolality(12). Hyperventilation, often used to treat raised intracranial pressure, is generally to be avoided in acute ischemic stroke. The effects of hyperventilation on perfusion of the infarct and peri-infarct region are unpredictable (13).

The current assessment of stroke monotherapies will undoubtedly evolve into analysis of a variety of combination therapies. The most likely candidates for combined stroke therapy are "reperfusion" plus "neuronal protection." This will probably take the form of combining fibrinolytic or hemorrheologic therapy with, for example, a calcium channel antagonist. The most exciting strategies for acute stroke therapy have only just begun to emerge from the laboratory. These approaches provide further focus on neuronal protection, with particular emphasis on blockade of excitatory amino acid receptors (14) and prevention of generation of oxygen free radicals (15). What will likely emerge is a complex strategy of reperfusion, reduction of thrombogenicity, and neuronal protection. We are fast approaching an era in which the patient with acute cerebral infarction is treated as aggressively as the patient with myocardial infarction. The current, correct emphasis on randomized, prospective, blinded trials should ensure that any such intervention will be beneficial for the patient.

ACKNOWLEDGMENT

Supported in part by Teacher-Investigator Development Award K07 NS 884 and NINCDS R01 NS 20989.

REFERENCES

1. Ruff R, Dougherty J. Complications of lumbar puncture followed by anticoagulation. *Stroke* 12:879-881, 1981.
2. Faught E, Troder S, Hanna G. Cerebral complications of angiography for transient ischemia and stroke: Prediction of risk. *Neurology* 29:4-15, 1979.
3. Karnaze D, Fisher M, Ahmadi J, Gott P. Short-latency somatosensory evoked potentials correlate with the severity of the neurological deficit and sensory abnormalities following cerebral ischemia. *Electroencephalog Clin Neurophysiol* 67:147-150, 1987.
4. Lechat P, Mas J, Lascault G, et al. Prevalence of patient foramen ovale in patients with stroke. *N Engl J Med* 381:1148-1152, 1988.
5. Brant-Zawadzki M. Ischemia. In: Stark D, Bradley W (Eds.), *Magnetic Resonance Imaging*. Mosby, St. Louis, 1988, pp. 299-315.

6. Fisher M, Meiselman H. Clinical implication of platelet activation and rheologic alterations associated with arteriography. *Stroke* 15:184, 1984.
7. Porch B, Wyckes J, Feeney D, Haloperidol, thiazides, and some antihypertensives slow recovery from aphasia. *Soc Neurosci Abstr* 11:52, 1985.
8. Schallert T, Hernandez T, Barth T. Recovery of function after brain damage: severe and chronic disruption by diazepam. *Brain Res* 379:104-111, 1986.
9. Reding M, McDowell F. Stroke rehabilitation. *Neurol Clin* 5:601-630, 1987.
10. Haley E, Kassell N, Torner J. Failure of heparin to prevent progression in progressing ischemic infarction. *Stroke* 19:10-14, 1988.
11. Ropper A, Shafran B. Brain edema after stroke. *Arch Neurol* 41:26-29, 1984.
12. Marshall L, Smith R, Rauscher L, Shapiro H. Mannitol dose requirements in brain-injured patients. *J Neurosurg* 48:169-172, 1978.
13. Raichle M, Plum F. Hyperventilation and cerebral blood flow. *Stroke* 3: 566-575, 1972.
14. Ozyurt E, Graham D, Woodruff G, McCulloch J. Protective effect of the glutamate antagonist MK 801 in focal cerebral ischemia in the cat. *J Cereb Blood Flow Metab* 8:138-143, 1988.
15. Cherchiari E, Hoel T, Safar P, Sclabassi R. Protective effects of combined superoxide dismutase and deferoxamine on recovery of cerebral blood flow and function after cardiac arrest in dogs. *Stroke* 18:869-878, 1987.

T

U,V

W,X

About the Editor

MARK FISHER is Associate Professor of Neurology at the University of Southern California School of Medicine, Los Angeles, where he directs stroke research and serves as a lecturer, consulting neurologist, and attending physician. His primary area of interest is cerebral vascular disease. A recognized authority in this field, Dr. Fisher has numerous publications to his credit and is the recipient of the Teacher-Investigator Development Award from the National Institutes of Health (NIH). He has lectured widely and has received research funding from the American Heart Association and the NIH. He is a member of many professional societies, including the American Academy of Neurology and International Society of Thrombosis and Haemostasis.